W9-AVH-716

The Resourceful
Mother's
Secrets to
Healthy Kids

The Resourceful Mother's *Secrets to* Healthy Kids

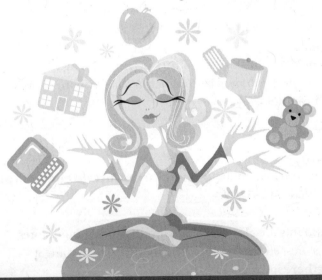

Understand Food, Understand Your Child

Meredith Deasley, BA, RNCP, RHN

Medical Disclaimer

The health information in this book is based on the training, experience and research of the author. Because each person and situation is unique, the reader should check with a qualified health professional before beginning a health program. Therefore, the author/publisher specifically disclaims any liability, loss, or risk, personal or otherwise, which is incurred as a consequence, directly or indirectly, of the use and application of the contents of this book.

Cover and book designed with ease by Heidy Lawrance and Cynthia Cake of *www.wemakebooks.ca* in Willowdale, Ontario.

Edited with flair by Janet Cocklin of *Always Get It Write.*

Photograph of Taylor and Paige Deasley on Dedication Page taken by *Here's My Baby!* See *www.heresmybaby.ca* for more information and to view their wonderful work.

Photograph of Meredith Deasley on Back Cover taken by *Catherine J. Capek Photography*. See *www.catherinejcapekphotography.com* for more information and to view her beautiful work.

How to Order:

Copies may be ordered online at **www.theresourcefulmother.com** or by calling **905–713–3299**.

Quantity discounts are also available for nutritionists, bookstores, health food stores, etc. For more information, please inquire at **meredith@theresourcefulmother.com**.

Visit us online at **www.theresourcefulmother.com**.

Mixed Sources
Cert no. SW-COC-000952
FSC © 1996 FSC

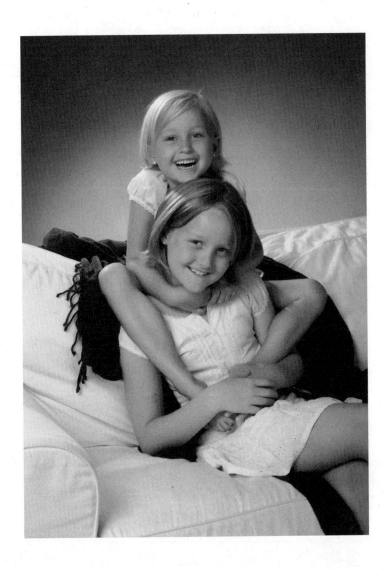

DEDICATION

I lovingly dedicate this book to my daughters, Taylor and Paige.
I thank you for opening up my soul and helping me find and fulfill my true
purpose. You have been, and continue to be, my greatest life teachers.

Most importantly, I thank you for every moment I have the
privilege of spending with you—you fill me with pure joy.

TABLE OF CONTENTS

Chapter 3
The Dirty Laundry List: Symptoms, Conditions and Disease

Chapter 4

Chapter 5

Chapter 6

Eat This! How to Feed Your Child 165

Chapter 7

**Let's Talk About it! Recommendations for Effectively
Communicating About Feeding Your Child Differently** 203

Chapter 8

Outside the Safety Zone:

Chapter 9

Help is Out There!

Chapter 10
The Food–Love Connection—When Food is A Form of Nurturing .

Appendix
Scrumptious Recipes . . . .

ACKNOWLEDGEMENTS

I would like to thank my brother, Jay Dodd, for being my enlightened witness in this world and for guiding me from the next. You are the person that propelled me into "officially" starting my business.

My husband, Craig, for always challenging me to reach greater heights. I wouldn't have wanted to grow alongside anyone other than you over the past 20 years. Thank you for holding the space for me, so that I could even entertain writing a book. I love you.

My mother, Maggie Gold, for your love and belief in me, your friendship, and your vast knowledge of health. You are the most knowledgeable nutritionist for adults that I know. Thank you for all the time spent discussing this book with me!

My father and step mom, Lionel and Lise Dodd, for your love, continual support and encouragement in getting this information out there and for sharing your numerous, excellent ideas for the book.

My sister, Danielle Dodd, for your can-do, cheerful attitude and assistance with my recipe section.

Jade Altavilla, for your infinite wisdom. Thank you for your vast knowledge of polarity therapy, other healing modalities and understanding of the human condition. You are the person that retrieved my soul. Without you, I could not have transferred my life learnings onto paper or into this world with the same effectiveness.

The management and teachers at CSNN, particularly Lorene Sauro, for your incredible expertise and the time you spent with me outside of class helping me understand the causes of food sensitivities and allergies. Your knowledge is absolutely invaluable. Thank you also for helping others become more aware of the value that nutritionists impart to the world.

The complementary/alternative practitioners who helped me relieve the symptoms in my girls before I determined the root causes and then continued to support us throughout the years. You, incredible people, know who you are. Dr. Murray Stewart, you were the first to help us, thank you for your infinite knowledge of chiropractic care and your strong desire to make a difference in the lives of others.

My good friend and nutritionist, Ingrid Davis, for getting me started conducting many of the seminars that I offer to this day. Thank you for the example you set, for your faith in me, in the human spirit and in God. You were also a wonderful help critiquing this book.

All the nutritionists who work tirelessly spreading the word about the power of food. My body, mind and spirit are motivated each and every time I am in your presence. Thank you, in particular, Susan Baker, for your belief in our work and for keeping us all together, growing in knowledge.

My amazing friends who never stopped believing in me. You listened and supported me as I worked on this project for over 6 years! I list your names alphabetically:

Niki Brinton, Camille Schappy, Jessica Cimmarusti, Sarah Clarke, Bea Cowan, Karyn Deasley, Carol Fazari, Jill Hewlett, Kari Horn, Debbie Kallitsis, Jodi Labelle, Denise Martin, Rebecca Martin, Kelly Mayo, Nadia Naylor, Krystal Pollock, Tammie Sarra and Elsa Shoniker. Jacquie Foran, Kim Hewitt and Susan Surtees, you were also extremely helpful in critiquing this material. Thank you from the bottom of my heart.

The experts in their fields that spent time and energy critiquing or proofreading my book: Shelley Black, Giovanna Capozza, Brenda Glashan, Mark Levine, Nicole Meltzer, Dr. Kristine Newman, Shauna Park, Frances Toews, and Lisa Walters. Thank you!

Christine Muskat, for looking after Taylor one afternoon a week so that I could write and for caring for both of my girls when I attended nutrition school. It is a rare ability to be able to sit and play like you do, Christine.

The babysitters at The Aurora Leisure Complex, particularly Liz, for tirelessly listening to me and offering ideas as I attempted to solve the mystery of what was making Taylor so sick.

Jimmy Duan, for your appreciation of who I have become and for spending a big part of one of your summers, typing research from numerous sources, allowing me to meet my goal for the completion of this book.

Debbie Kennedy, Sarah Ebbs, Jennifer Lumsden, and Brigitta Emes at Prenatal Plus Parenting Centre for opening my mind to all of the possibilities in delivering, raising and healing children and for continuing to impact other families in our community in the same way. Thank you for your support over all of these years!

Janet Cocklin of "Always Get It Write" for editing my work in the most efficient and best possible way. You were the first writing expert to read my whole book and the first member of "my book team".

Simone Gabbay for all of your support and recommendations, particularly Heidy Lawrance Associates, without whom I could not have published this book in the wonderful, easy manner in which I did.

James Gross, founder of Random Ink, for creating the finest title for this book. Thank you, James!

Heather Ebbs, for your professional and efficient work in creating the index.

Cheryl Stewart, my doula and Hilary Monk, my midwife, for helping me bring my daughters into this world. You had no idea how much their safe delivery would impact others.

All the authors whose work helped me grow into the person I am today. I could not have done it without you. You are my main advisors and what is so sad, is that there are too many of you to mention. I am now honoured to be in your ranks.

All the authors who helped me grow my knowledge of food and health. The most important one being Zoltan Rona MD, author of *Childhood Illness and the Allergy Connection*. Please see my bibliography for the names of the other authors who impacted me.

All the parents who believe in me and tell me that the lives of their children are more beautiful every day as a result of the wisdom my girls shared with me.

FOREWORD

Dr. Zoltan P. Rona practices Complementary Medicine in Toronto and is the medical editor of *The Encyclopedia of Natural Healing*. He has also published several Canadian best selling books including *Return to The Joy of Health* and *Childhood Illness and the Allergy Connection*. His new book, *Vitamin D, The Sunshine Vitamin* is available January 2010. His website is: *www.mydoctor.ca/drzoltanrona*

Very few of us were lucky enough to receive a course on how to keep our children both physically and mentally healthy. Even fewer of us were taught that what we feed or do not feed our children from Day One could have such an enormous influence on every aspect of our children's future lives. Longevity, vitality, freedom from recurrent illness, school performance, friendships, adult relationships as well as career success can all be heavily influenced by one's biochemistry in early life. The balance between environmental toxins and nutrient deficiencies has traditionally been ignored by most mainstream health care experts.

We have all been indoctrinated to rely on conventional medical advice for feeding our children, preventing illness as well as treating a long list of common childhood illnesses. Most of us seek Complementary Medicine only when we have exhausted other medical options or have experienced the damage caused to our children by prescription and over the counter drugs.

The deterioration of our children's health starts early enough with synthetic, sugar flavoured, packaged infant formulas. Later, our children are injected with countless vaccines that contain poisons such as mercury, aluminum, formaldehyde, squalene, foreign DNA and antibiotics. When our children suffer from disease, they are prescribed one of a long list of drugs. Despite all this, our children are not getting any healthier. Conventional advice on how to produce healthy kids has failed us as parents. Witness the alarmingly escalating childhood illnesses like asthma, autism spectrum disorders, ADD/ADHD, learning disabilities, suicide and childhood obesity.

Children of all ages are now commonly medicated with drugs that were previously only used by adults. Children who cannot sleep are often prescribed tranquilizers. Far too many make frequent trips to the child psychiatrist's office.

Many children with common health challenges could well be the victims of undiagnosed food allergies and do not necessarily suffer from a Prozac deficiency. Even some conventional pediatricians will now admit that recurrent middle ear infections could be linked to unsuspected allergies to milk and dairy products and that food dyes and additives could trigger ADHD.

The good news is that our children's biochemistry can be optimized without resorting to drugs. For some children, this could simply mean some basic changes in their dietary habits. For others, more physical activity is part of the answer. Most will require some sort of detoxification and nutritional supplementation. The overwhelming majority, however, will not require drugs, psychiatrists or social workers.

In the chapters that follow, Meredith Deasley will teach you the basics of how to keep your children as healthy as possible with down to earth, practical advice. Unlike most conventional medical texts, this book was written by one who actually experienced dealing with her children's health issues on a first hand basis. You will learn about the role of food allergies in causing chronic health problems. You will also learn techniques for recognizing, detecting and reversing food allergy related illness.

There is much information here on how you can help your child eliminate common harmful toxins that could be responsible for numerous psychological, psychiatric and physical problems. There is a wonderful section on medical alternatives as well as on the emotional connections to food selection and consumption. You will become an expert on how to shop for the right kinds of foods and beverages. There will be answers to commonly asked questions such as: Where do I shop? What kind of water do I drink at home? What about restaurant eating? What do I do about my children attending birthday parties at homes where junk foods are considered to be perfectly all right to feed kids?

There is still a great deal of resistance to implementing dietary and other changes in our schools, particularly with our conventional medical system that resists any change, as well as all the negatives associated with peer pressures. Parents who opt for healthier, non-toxic lifestyles are often confronted with many fear-based questions from friends and family like, "Aren't you worried that your kids will get the flu without the flu shot?" In making changes for the better, parents will have to deal with objections and criticism from numerous sources within the community. The pages that follow will discuss how you can successfully deal with these unpleasant issues as well. Take the time to read this book. After all, your children are well worth the trouble and will be better able to look after you in your older years.

Dr. Zoltan P. Rona, MD, MSc

INTRODUCTION

I believe that one of my main purposes in life, other than raising two wonderful, happy children, is to learn about health and then share that knowledge with you. In this book, I will explain to you the changes to our food since our parents raised us, how these changes to our food affect us, and how to feed and care for our children in today's world. The ultimate goal is for our children to be the healthiest and happiest possible so that they can live the lives they were born to live.

Many parents are not aware of the need to do things differently than our parents, when it comes to feeding our children. They notice the addition of the health aisles in the regular grocery stores, see health food stores expanding and the selection of organic foods growing, and know someone has found a new way to make money. Others are hearing or sensing that we need to change the way we eat and my even be open to change but do not understand why we need to do things differently. Some know why we need to change the way we eat but do not know how to get started. There is no question that the information that is circulating about health–in the newspapers, on the radio and amongst "experts"–is downright confusing. It's reported that children's allergies, asthma and other conditions are on the rise but often we do not hear that new medical research shows them to be food–related.

I remember doing one of my first seminars on the impact of food on our children and a parent saying afterward, "It's all just common sense, isn't it?" and I realized she was right. I hope to make common sense to you. I write to you primarily as a mother; I was a mother first, long before I received my designation in nutrition. My aim is to write to the parents who just want to know what to do to help their children. They don't want more choices, just the straight goods. In every part of this book, I have tried to write simply so that the confusion surrounding children's nutrition and well–being is dispelled.

This book is written for all the parents who struggle through each day, trying to do the hardest job in life, for the least amount of recognition …raising children in today's world. Many of you have been labeled neurotic or hypochondriacs or at the very least, you've followed a very lonely path all because your child is reacting to food, chemicals or other aspects of their environment. You may or may not be aware that food is the major culprit, but you certainly will be by the time you have finished reading this book.

In a way, I envy parents who lived at the turn of the century. Those families lived simply, on farms, putting themselves and their children to work each day in order to survive. There are times I wish I was a parent in the days when Dr. Spock's book was the bible of parenting and everyone agreed with and followed his methods of parenting, even though his information was later disproved. Today, parents have so many decisions to make, so many different ways of going about raising our children. Do we have a midwife–assisted or doctor–assisted birth at the hospital or give birth in a tub or deliver at home? Do we circumcise our son? Do we partake in stem cell storage? Do we vaccinate? Is my child stimulated too much or not enough? What type of schooling should my child have–Montessori, Waldorf, Private, Public or home study? What do I need to do to make my child healthy? Choice is absolutely wonderful and so is knowledge. The parents of today have both. Sometimes, I wish we didn't have either. There is no doubt that being a parent of today is a tough job. However, with every challenge comes our greatest lessons.

The children of today have a greater purpose

The children of today are different from those of the past. They are more sensitive, physically and emotionally. As a result, they are often harder to raise. Yes, we have all the gadgets and toys to keep our children happy–the self-pushing and timing swings, the exersaucers, the vibrating chairs–but you know what? The children and parents of today often need these inventions. For the most part, our kids are the fussiest, neediest and sickest of any generation. Children with medical conditions and disease are everywhere you look.

Somewhere along the way, man got carried away with industrialization, with making money, with only looking at the present and not at future repercussions. As a result, our air, water and food are the most contaminated they have ever been. Our sensitive children are reacting very badly as evidenced by the symptoms, conditions and diseases that they are contracting. Isn't it interesting that the children that live in the underdeveloped countries have no such issues with food?

The "Children of the Now", as they are referred to, need to be understood and loved the same as children of generations prior. However, they have a greater purpose. **These children are helping us clean up our planet, both environmentally and socially.** You see, when these sensitive children are not heard or understood, they become sick. Do not fear them. Learn from them; they are the world's biggest wakeup call. Their bodies will communicate with you; they will tell you all of the answers, if only you will listen.

Children's bodies communicate with us

Children are multi and extra sensory beings. They *see* more than us, particularly the little things, like the worm struggling to get home after the rainstorm or the coin lost in the dirt on which you stepped. They *hear* the sound of a train horn bellowing miles away. They *feel* more than us; they yelp at the temperature of the water, telling you it's too hot, when you thought the bath water was just right. They *taste* the cilantro in the guacamole and ask you why it tastes funny. They are wise and intuitive beyond belief. You think they are this way, noticing these subtleties, with a twinkle in their eyes because the world is new to them. Maybe that's part of it. But do you notice the adults with a twinkle in their eyes or those that laugh more than others? They are small in number, but they do exist. Those are the adults that have not lost their connection to the way life is supposed to be.

What fogs our vision, blocks our taste buds, ruins our sight, dulls our minds and breaks our connection to the way it's supposed to be? Food and emotions. Food that is not natural, alive or good quality, blocks our channels. You don't believe me? Look at the child that cannot close his mouth because it's too hard to breathe. Try eliminating the mucus–forming foods, particularly dairy and wheat, and watch your child transform. Look at the girl who has attention deficit disorder and such bad nightmares that she goes into school each day exhausted. How much better able to concentrate and understand life would she be, if you eliminated chemicals from her diet? Look at the 6–year–old child under such stress that they experience irritable bowel syndrome. I could share countless examples with you but I know you are understanding.

Dare to be different

Once you realize that the wonder and fascination in life does not need to end in early childhood, maybe you'll want to give your children the opportunity to experience this joy for the rest of their lives.

It is no longer possible for our children to have the quality of life they deserve unless we start going about things differently when it comes to feeding them. Over the decade that I've been raising children differently, I've been faced with many disbelievers but continued to do my own thing. My children's health is by no means perfect but it *is* different. They catch fewer colds, recover from them faster, have never been diagnosed with an infection or needed antibiotics, only have the occasional nightmare, are slim and muscular and have incredible academic prowess…..Oh now, here she goes, you're thinking. All right, I won't carry on any longer other than saying that because of the way my children eat, my life as a parent is easier, the lives of my children are easier and everyone that comes into contact with them is happier for it. Am I getting carried away? Don't take my word for it. Try the techniques discussed in this book. You'll see the difference. Raising children should not make you want to run for the hills every single day–the odd day, sure!

It is my most fervent wish that you will read this book, cover to cover, dare to be different and then look at me with that zest for life. I'll see the twinkle in your eye and know what you've been doing. I'll ask that you save the actual lives of other children by spreading the word, or simply setting an example of health. One day you might be asked, "Your son seems so much happier; what did you do differently?"

You might say, "I just learned how to feed him to help him reach his full potential." If you can answer in that way, it is obvious that you are doing the very best you possibly can for your child.

Our responsibility to our children

We have a responsibility as parents that the majority of us do not discuss. Many of us were raised by very strict parents and therefore, employ a more relaxed parenting style in raising our own children. As understandable as this is, when it comes to your child's nutrition, I implore you to be stricter.

In our household, our girls have a lot of freedom. They usually choose, with some parental guidance, what they wear, what activities they join, who their friends are, how their rooms look and how they spend their own money. When it comes to nutrition, they get to choose between the foods I offer, at which events they are going to eat unhealthy foods and how much they eat. But they eat nutritious foods every single day of their lives. Nutrition is simply too important to let children make all the decisions. I have told my girls that they mean too much to me for me to feed them badly.

I know children who eat candy every day, never touch a fruit or vegetable and whose beverage of choice is diet coke, consumed multiple times a day. These children are not being given the basics of life. When your child regularly wants to forgo eating vegetables and you let them because it's another battle you do not have the strength to fight, you are telling your child, whether you realize it or not, that their health doesn't matter.

The choices you make concerning what you feed your children will affect every single area of their lives. It will affect how they feel, how much energy, strength and brain power they have, how they look and whether they will age with vitality or not.

If the job of parenting was unanimously revered as the most important job one could have and we were paid lots of money to do it well, how differently would we view our jobs as parents? How differently would we view our children? For some of us, no differently. For many of us, very differently. I invite you to view your job as revered, as the most important job in the world. You know why? Because it is.

It is our responsibility as parents not only to provide the basics of life to our children but also to help these souls develop into the happiest, healthiest and finest human beings possible. How can we do this without accepting responsibility and giving our children the proper foundation?

Helping your child become healthier begins with you

No other relationship sets the tone for the life experience of each individual more powerfully than the relationship between parent and child. Therefore, the real healing of children begins with their parents. I believe in you. I encourage you to believe in yourself and your child. I've seen the incredible healing power of the human body. I've seen the amazing changes families have made to create a healthy, balanced life. It's yours for the taking. Have courage, have patience, and have faith. There is no greater accomplishment than raising a happy and healthy human being.

This book

In this book, you will learn about the symptoms, conditions, and diseases caused by food and help you determine which foods are the healthy ones and which ones are the culprits for your child and why (Chapters 1– 4). You will read about how to prevent, detect, minimize or eliminate reactions to food (Chapter 5). You will receive numerous ideas for feeding children healthily, with particular emphasis on the alternatives to the common allergens. Vitamins and minerals, that prevent, minimize and eliminate reactions to food, as well as improve overall health, are described in detail with helpful suggestions for getting them into your child's food or drinks (Chapter 6). When a child eats differently than the majority, a parent needs to know how to discuss these differences with their child and others, so that everyone understands the benefits of eating healthier alternatives to "regular" food (Chapter 7). Whether your child is reacting to foods or is simply eating the healthiest possible diet, you need to know how to handle eating out, holidays and special occasions, as well as traveling, so that your child doesn't miss out on any fun (Chapter 8)! Learn about a whole realm of alternative practitioners who can help minimize your child's reactions to foods and help build their immune system (Chapter 9). Lastly, our relationship to food mirrors our relationship to life. This material provides effective methods for helping your child be nourished by food (Chapter 10). There are also loads of recipes for tasty meals and snacks, devoid of common allergens (Appendix). Food sensitivities and allergies are a hidden epidemic. **By reading the material within these pages, you will have the tools to improve your child's health for life.**

OUR STORY

For as long as I can remember, I believed that having children would be the most important thing I would ever do. Now, I fully understand why. My 10-year-old and 8-year-old are teaching me all there is to know about life. My biggest task is to remain open and clear, so I can receive all of their teachings.

Before my children arrived, I had little interest in health. The concept that food could nourish me never entered my mind! After a stressful childhood, I entered the (just as) stressful corporate world, where I remained for ten years. I worked extremely hard as Lombard Canada's youngest manager, Canada Life's senior marketing analyst and then, as a Commercial Insurance Broker at HKMB Brokerage. I attended numerous parties and drank copious amounts of alcohol. Yes, I ate processed foods and lots of sugar. I put my trust in my medical doctor. She was the only person I consulted on a regular basis when it came to my health. I was open-minded about alternative therapies, but knew very little about them.

For eleven years, my husband, Craig, and I lived and loved life to the fullest knowing that our world would change once a little one arrived. People say that you are never fully ready for a child, but I can honestly say we were. We each had over 30 years of knowledge about the world to share with our child. We faced many challenges and had numerous accomplishments, individually and as a couple. I was determined to raise a happy child and do the "right thing" at all costs.

When I was pregnant with our first child, I was on top of the world… strong and proud. For the first time in my life, I gloried in walking around the house naked. I read many books on pregnancy, labour, and child rearing, attended pre-natal classes, visited the chiropractor and cranial osteopath (having heard that every pregnant woman should see these experts), practiced yoga and exercised three to four times a week. I so eagerly anticipated the arrival of this soul that had chosen me to be its mother.

After 42 *hours* of labour, our little girl, Taylor, was born and placed in an incubator at our local hospital. She was pretty badly cut from the two sets of forceps that were used to pull her out. It looked like she might have vision problems from the cut on her cornea that one of the forceps made. As I lay on the operating table with fire engine red blood all over myself, the floor, and the walls, I remember briefly wondering where it had all gone wrong. A little while later, I was allowed to spend time with my baby. All I'd said to her so far was, "Welcome to the world, little one," as my mother had said to me upon my birth. Luckily, Craig remembered our discussions about staying with our baby at all times, so he and his brother, Grant, took turns holding Taylor's hand and talking to her.

I had a lot of questions about what went on in that hospital, during and after Taylor's birth–things that shouldn't happen when staff deliver and care for as many babies as they do, day after day, year after year. Having said that, I was euphoric for days as a result of the miracle that had taken place within those walls. The sense of completeness I felt after giving birth was overwhelming and I fell in love with the world again.

Unfortunately, my labour with Taylor was only one of many challenges we faced together as a family. That first day, Taylor developed a rash all over her body from the detergent used on the hospital linens. Shortly after we put her in her own clothes, washed in Ivory Snow, her rash disappeared. That evening, a nurse's aid informed us that because Taylor's glucose level was low, she was going to feed Taylor a bottle of formula, even though I was breastfeeding. Taylor, luckily, took only 1 ounce of the formula before making it clear that she wanted no more. For the rest of Taylor's first full night on this earth, she had projectile vomiting and very painful gas. After caring for her for hours, it dawned on me that the formula must have been the cause. She had been peaceful prior to that feeding and I had heard that many infants react to cow's-milk-based formulas. I asked a nurse for confirmation of this the next morning. She looked at me as though I was crazy.

A week later, Craig and I took Taylor for her first regular doctor's check-up, other than the two trips we had made to Sick Kids Hospital to have the experts look at her eye to see if the forceps caused long-term damage (Taylor needs glasses as a result). Taylor's doctor told us that she was severely dehydrated and immediately sent us to the hospital. To make a long story short, she was not receiving enough breast milk despite having a "perfect latch". I later learned that I had what are called "tubular breasts" and that I would never have sufficient milk production to be able to breastfeed exclusively. I knew from our experience during Taylor's first night that I couldn't supplement my breast milk with a formula based on cow's milk, so we started feeding Taylor a soymilk formula. Here I was–a woman who wanted the best for her child and was pretty well obsessed with it–having a labour that put her baby in distress, learning that she'd allowed her baby to become dehydrated, and now, the final straw, having to feed Taylor formula, as opposed to breastfeeding exclusively! I was quickly losing my euphoria....

Less than a week after returning home from a horrendous five-day stay in the hospital, where we were able to get Taylor's weight back up, I ate a grilled-cheese sandwich. Within minutes of breast- and bottle-feeding, Taylor's projectile vomiting spanned three feet. Then, I knew for certain that dairy was out of the question for me, as long as I was breastfeeding Taylor. I quickly learned that Taylor wasn't just reacting to what she ate, but also to what I ate and passed on to her through my breast milk.

Unfortunately, cutting dairy and all gas producing foods out of my diet did not eliminate Taylor's tremendous amounts of gas pains, spitting up, and projectile vomiting. By the time she was three months old, I decided that my breastfeeding was doing her more harm than good. I was completely sold on the fact that breastfeeding was best; no one ever needed to convince me of that. At that point, however, I made one of my most difficult decisions yet and stopped breastfeeding my baby.

Two weeks later, Taylor started what I termed her "gas attacks," during which she would scream and cry at the top of her lungs, as if she'd been stung by a bee. The first time this happened, we were in a public place and I was only comforted by the fact that my husband was there with me, to shoulder the blame that we saw in strangers' eyes. These "attacks" were always in the evenings and they lasted for hours at a time. One night, she had colic for eight hours straight. Each time Taylor had a bout, I would be at my wit's end trying to determine the cause. Various friends and family members witnessed these attacks. The older generation kept reminding me that "babies cry." I knew in my heart that when a baby cries, there is a reason. I was bound and determined to get to the bottom of it. I was right, but it took me a long time to realize it.

HEALTH FACT

When a baby cries, there is a reason.

I have always been an avid reader, so I immediately turned to books and magazines to learn about this condition called "colic". All I was able to find out was that "colic" meant "unexplained crying" or "extreme gas". I took Taylor to her doctor and asked for her advice about Taylor's very bad case of colic. She simply said, "It's a normal thing for babies to go through," and "she will outgrow these reactions," without any concern or inclination to offer help in the meantime. I asked her about a link between colic and food allergies. She knew of no such link, but I believed that there was something in Taylor's formula to which she was allergic because her attacks started so soon after I began solely feeding her formula.

There was no way I was just going to sit back and watch my child suffer. Through further reading, I learned that chiropractors are often able to assist with colic by restoring balance to the body. I knew that my chiropractor specialized in treating children. Amazingly, he didn't charge for his work with children because he believed in what he did so much, that he didn't want any parent to be deterred from bringing their child to him due to lack of money.

Our chiropractor literally saved us. Following each appointment, Taylor was a different person. She had no or very little gas, fussiness, or other symptoms for four weeks following each treatment. Like clockwork, each month, the lengthy sessions of gas and crying would start up again and I would know it was time to book another appointment. Once, she did not improve the day after her "adjustment". I called our chiropractor and said, "You must have missed a spot." Sure enough, following our appointment that day, Taylor was fine.

By the way, many people say that "colic" happens at dinnertime each day because the atmosphere in the home changes at that hour. There's more stimulation as the husband comes home from work, then invariably turns on the TV or talks to his wife and generally "disrupts" the household. I don't believe that. I believe the real story is that after a day of being fed, the child acquires a build-up of substances that their body cannot assimilate properly and it is released through crying or fussiness.

Although chiropractic adjustments provided relief, I nevertheless wanted to find the root cause of Taylor's challenges. My continued research led me to learn that sugar is a common allergen. I decided to try Taylor on a soy-based formula that had no sugar. Wouldn't you know it, she wouldn't drink it! Needless to say, I put her back on her original formula.

When Taylor was about six months old, I decided to take her to the moms-and-tots swim class. Each time she swam, she developed a full-fledged cold. After three of these sessions, I mentioned the pattern to my mother-in-law, who later learned from a pediatrician on a radio show that Taylor could be allergic to chlorine. This fascinated me–she could be allergic to more than just food and a cold could be a symptom of an allergy. I began keeping an eye out for a company that could test Taylor's allergies safely. Thankfully, I knew she was too young for the invasive scratch test that is done at doctors' offices.

When Taylor was eleven months old, I found an advertisement for a company that did Interro Sensitivity Testing (does not differentiate between allergies and sensitivities) on babies and children. I went for this testing in my twenties, trying to determine the cause of my pimples and bloating. At the time, I found the test to be reasonably accurate. I decided to have Taylor tested in the same way.

Taylor's test results identified numerous problem foods, which even included certain fruits and vegetables! She reacted to all the common allergens–dairy, wheat, sugar, chemicals, eggs, chocolate, coffee, and citrus fruits, to name a few. I learned that one of Taylor's sensitivities was to corn. The second ingredient listed on her soymilk formula was corn syrup, not to mention the fact that her formula had sugar in it! You can imagine how I felt leaving this meeting, with such a long list of foods that Taylor could not eat–foods that form the basis of our North American diet. I was completely devastated and overcome by fear. The main and most basic function of a mother is to feed her child and now, I had no idea how. If it hadn't been for Taylor playing peek-a-boo with her blanket and me in the backseat of our car all the way home, I know I would have cried.

I waited one more month, until Taylor was a year old, and then took her off her formula. Her gas attacks disappeared. I then eliminated every food from her diet to which she could be reacting. Talk about a limited diet.

Knowing that cow's milk was not an option for Taylor, I decided to try almond milk for her, which someone had recommended. She became horribly constipated (apparently, carrageenan, a common ingredient in almond milk, is known to be a stomach irritant and can cause various digestive problems, including constipation in rare cases) but I didn't know this at the time. Thinking back, I don't know how many days went by that Taylor went without a bowel movement or only had a pellet-sized one. We never once remember having any diaper "explosions" which some children tend to have. Taylor had been constipated all along, from her formula and her solids, which we had started introducing when she was four months old. However, because she'd always been such a happy baby, other than when she was experiencing colic, we were never concerned about her lack of bowel movements.

Almond milk is not something you tell a lot of people your child is drinking nor is the fact that you take your child to the chiropractor and he "saves" you and your child. People just don't talk freely about their child's bowel movement frequency or consistency; it doesn't go over well. Then, there was the fact that I was desperately trying not to feed my child any of the foods listed in her sensitivity or allergy testing. Not to mention that I was also keeping her away from chlorine, grass and cat and dog hair, which I'd also had tested and found to be a problem. I was really feeling like I needed help at that point.

What happened to my daughter to make her so sensitive? What nutrients was Taylor missing by eating so few foods? How long would her diet have to be so sparse? Were there any alternatives to the foods she was reacting to? What could I do to reverse these sensitivities or allergies? Was there anything I could do for her physically when she was clearly in pain from constipation? You see, the only reason I even knew she was constipated from the almond milk, when I'd never recognized her to be constipated before, was that she was in pain. She hid behind furniture, wanting privacy while trying with all her might to have a bowel movement, for hours on end.

Finally, after a couple of weeks of this, we gave Taylor a laxative and it cleared her (It did not continue to help her though!). I learned that constipation is a symptom of a food sensitivity or allergic reaction. Up to that point, I only knew diarrhea to be a symptom, in terms of bowel movements. We didn't feed her almond milk again until years later.

We switched Taylor onto rice milk, which she could tolerate. Most rice milk is made from brown rice, not refined white rice, which lacks fibre and is, therefore, constipating. All of these "odd" milks were enriched with added vitamins and minerals.

By this point, I was having a hard time determining which solids to feed Taylor. Then someone gave her a piece of corn, without knowing about her sensitivities or allergies, and she seemed fine after eating it! I had a glimmer of hope–hope that the test had been wrong and Taylor did not have problems with so many foods. After all, I didn't want her to be a food-reactive child. I also didn't want her to be deprived, which I felt she was. For the next six months, I fed Taylor lots of things on her list of problem foods, except dairy, in very small amounts at first and then larger amounts, as time went on.

When Taylor was eighteen months, severe constipation and pain set in. I now know that her body went into overload. She might have been able to handle the odd food to which she was sensitive, but there was no way her body could handle these foods all day, every day. I had to eliminate any foods that were a problem right away. I had recently read an article in which the validity of Interro testing had been questioned, so I really didn't know where to begin eliminating food groups from Taylor's now vast diet. I also still didn't know the alternatives. In addition, I needed to learn what ingredients were in the food Taylor was eating and identify the food group it belonged to (for instance, whether couscous was made from wheat–which it is).

I went to the grocery store with the largest selection in our area and spent two hours scouring the shelves for foods Taylor could eat. At that time, pretty much everything had one of the common allergens in it, usually more than one. I was completely desolate. I started going to the health food store and studying the products that lined its shelves. I asked the employees a lot of questions and read every health magazine I could get my hands on. Even when I found foods that Taylor could eat, most of them tasted absolutely horrible. I am surprised she never spat them back in my face! Thank goodness she was not a picky eater. She did have a big appetite, so I had to find a wide variety of foods for her to eat throughout the day.

Taylor remained constipated, on and off, for six months. To see her in such agony, pushing and moaning, sometimes crying and screaming for days on end, was excruciating for me. I'm not sure if there is anything worse than seeing your child in pain. The memory of those months of suffering will never dissipate from my mind.

I continuously eliminated foods from her diet, replacing many with alternatives, all the while keeping a food and symptom diary. Each month, the number of days she was constipated diminished.

During that time, I took her to emergency, medical clinics and her doctor numerous times, only to be told each time, that constipation is a common childhood ailment. Laxatives, suppositories, and enemas were recommended time and time again. We tried many different laxatives on Taylor, but each one was effective only for a period of time. We simply couldn't get suppositories to work at all. Once in a while, when there seemed to be no other alternatives, we resorted to enemas.

If I had had a job outside the home during those six months, I would not have been able to keep it. I needed to be at Taylor's side each time she was in pain. I spent many consecutive days never leaving the house or answering the phone. Sometimes I never even got out of my pyjamas or brushed my teeth. I constantly tried to talk Taylor through her pain.

I remembered going on a hike with my Dad when I was a child and talking about our greatest fears, telling him that mine was being really close to someone that was sick and not being able to help. Here I was in just that situation.

My top priority, in terms of healing Taylor, was helping her have fun and relax. So, on days when she was well enough to venture out, we did just that. One time after Taylor had been through a very painful bout of constipation, I took her to the park. That day, there was another little girl who was about Taylor's age. I couldn't help but notice that she was so physically agile, making her way around the playground as though it was her second home. In comparison, I was simply so happy that Taylor had survived her bouts of constipation and so pleased to be at the park with her, doing a normal childhood activity. Taylor wasn't as physically agile as the other child but that was not surprising. Her body was usually so tense. Time spent running around was seriously curtailed with the number of days we spent indoors while she was in pain.

During those six months, I took Taylor to our family doctor, two pediatricians, three naturopaths and two cranial osteopaths in hopes that someone would come to our rescue.

One pediatrician told me to ignore her sensitivities and allergies. He literally instructed me to feed her cow's milk and take her swimming, stating that she would get over these reactions. Another pediatrician suggested we have Taylor X–rayed to see if there was anything wrong internally. This made me start to wonder if there *was* something wrong, physically. When we went to his office for the results, he told us that everything was fine with Taylor but that the X–ray showed that she was filled with stool. We talked about the foods I believed she was sensitive or allergic to and then he did an internal examination. The results were astounding–she was now clear inside! I was amazed and knew that it must have been the organic broccoli I had been pouring into her. At the end of the appointment, the doctor asked Taylor if she wanted a cookie. My husband and I looked at each other with concern, but we didn't believe that a doctor would give her something he had just heard me say she was reacting to. A few bites into the cookie, I asked him about the ingredients. His response was, "Those cookies are hypoallergenic; my nurse makes them. They contain baker's chocolate, not milk chocolate." Taylor was sensitive to the cocoa bean itself, as are many others. There were probably other ingredients in that cookie that were a problem for her. The pediatrician's words rang over and over in my head as Taylor writhed in pain in her crib that night. He also recommended putting Taylor on a laxative for about three months to see how she would be after that period. That was the last time I ever asked a medical doctor for help with Taylor's food sensitivities or allergies.

I had very good experiences with naturopathic doctors over the years and gained a wealth of knowledge from them regarding health. I decided to take Taylor to a naturopath to learn more about which foods would be good or harmful for her, to put her on some supplements that might help improve her digestion and correct any vitamin deficiencies she might have developed from her limited diet. I was already giving her some supplements that had been recommended by the professional staff in a heath food store in my area.

One naturopath prescribed liquid homeopathic remedies (UNDA drops). These particular drops were designed to cleanse her body. Within a few weeks of taking them, Taylor seemed able to handle more foods without reacting. But it wasn't long before she started having nightmares every night and her constipation began to worsen. It took me a while to determine the cause of her deterioration because the homeopathic remedies had been tested against her and were supposed to agree with her. When I finally called the naturopath and voiced my concerns, she told me that the alcohol content of these remedies must be the problematic factor. She had also tested a number of children's multi-vitamins against Taylor's hair and didn't feel comfortable recommending any one of them to us! She recommended that I take Taylor to a different naturopath who was trained in a number of modalities and was renowned for helping highly sensitive children.

We made the three-hour round trip to see this doctor. At the end of the appointment, we spent $400 and had been given some food ideas and eight or nine supplements to give Taylor three times a day. Some things were to be taken orally, some added to her drinks, and some rubbed on her skin. He showed me a technique for burning the alcohol off of some of the remedies that he had prescribed, which was very useful. I asked him if I should try the supplements on Taylor one at a time, to ensure that they did not constipate her. He said that wasn't necessary. I had heard great things about this doctor, so I was determined to try his approach on Taylor. After administering the numerous remedies, I felt that giving her so many things at once would make her feel like a "sick child" which might, in fact, make her more sick! Sure enough, after just one dose of each of these supplements, Taylor became slightly constipated. My faith in this naturopath was immediately lost.

I must tell you that, today, I believe that even though the naturopaths whom I consult are always able to provide me and countless others with assistance, there was a reason that they were unable to help my extremely sensitive child. I was meant to heal her myself, so that I could then help others do the same for their children.

The cranial osteopath appointments did make Taylor relax, even when she went a week without a bowel movement, but I still had to learn the physical causes of her constipation. Interestingly, one of these experts asked whether Taylor had had a bad fall or if something unusual had occurred during my pregnancy. When I stated that I had no knowledge of any problems having occurred, the cranial osteopath, as he continued to do his hands-on healing of Taylor, said that fear must have caused her body to become this tight. Subsequent to that appointment, I learned that fear is the emotional cause behind constipation. There is always a physical and emotional reason behind every physical ailment. I now had a mystery to solve. What was Taylor so afraid of? Her birth alone would have made her fearful, not to mention the reactions she experienced every time she ate.

By now, I was truly starting to lose it. I had eliminated all but 19 foods from Taylor's diet (the Interro test turned out to be, in the end, reasonably accurate in terms of the foods that caused the greatest problems for her). I fed her primarily organic fruits and vegetables, and continued with the supplements that seemed to make a difference. I had even converted all of Taylor's hair, skin, and dental care products to natural alternatives. Yet, Taylor was still becoming constipated but thankfully, nowhere near as much as she had been five months ago.

During this time, Craig and I were invited to attend a wedding in Nova Scotia. We left Taylor with some family members for four days. Within a day of our return, Taylor became very sick with a high fever and flu-like symptoms and was in pain from being constipated. She remained this way for several days. She was so ill that I didn't think she was going to survive. Only recently could I even admit this to myself.

One morning, soon after she started feeling better, I went to the health food store and told an employee, whom I had come to trust implicitly, everything that I was doing to help Taylor heal. Throughout my life, I have always been described as very strong emotionally. I was mortified to find myself crying when I asked this man what I was missing in helping Taylor. "What more can I do?" I asked. For the first time ever, his answer was, "Nothing". He added, "You've done everything." My frustration was completely overwhelming. My belief in myself was diminishing. My poor daughter was relying on me. I had told her I would help her, yet I was beginning to feel powerless.

Later that morning, I prayed. In the past, I had only thanked God for the bless-ings in my life but that day, I prayed for his help in discovering the missing link in healing Taylor. That afternoon, I sat with Taylor, listening to her moaning, watch-ing her body going into different contortions as she managed her pain. As though a light bulb went off in my head, I suddenly knew I needed to go to the bookstore. I couldn't wait until my husband came home from work. Our babysitter's mother, whom I didn't know well, answered the phone when I called, and as I started explaining things to her, I was ashamed to find myself crying again. A little while later, our babysitter came over.

I drove to the bookstore. I asked an employee where the books on allergies were. She directed me to a whole shelf of them. The first book that caught my eye was *Childhood Illness and the Allergy Connection* by Dr. Zoltan Rona. I picked up the book and read the back, noting that constipation was indeed a symptom of an allergic reaction. When I opened the book, I opened it right to the page on sec-ond-hand smoke and learned that a highly allergic child suffers more seriously from cigarette smoke exposure. I had my answer, the missing link. You see, the family members that Taylor stayed with when we went to the wedding were heavy smokers. She used to go there once a week and would often sleep over. I had noticed the link between her visits to their house and the onset of her constipation but didn't understand it. I knew they were only feeding her the food we provided for her. I'm sure most of you would never have even entertained taking your child into a "smokehouse". Let this be an example as to far I've come in my knowledge of health! I scanned the rest of the book and found that it discussed so many of the things I'd figured out for myself regarding sensitivities and allergies. I received the confirmation I needed that I was on the right track with the changes I had made to Taylor's diet and in healing her. I searched for another copy of the book, only to find that there wasn't one. I looked for other books on the subject and found that this was the only one there geared directly to children. A few months later, I learned the book was out of print. There isn't a doubt in my mind that this book was sent to me directly from God, as a result of my prayer.

When we called our family members to tell them about the link between Taylor's constipation and second-hand smoke, they were completely shocked –shocked that smoking could cause constipation and shocked that they could be making Taylor sick; their love for Taylor had always been obvious to the world. Less than a week later, on Easter Sunday, these family members told us that they didn't want to see us for a month. They defensively wanted to see if Taylor got better in that time. There is no describing the anger and hurt that Craig and I felt, after hearing their announcement. We needed their support at this time, not their withdrawal. That evening, after putting Taylor to bed, Craig and I fought. The frustration and stress of caring for our sick child had been eating away at us individually and as a couple for months now. Craig was saddened each time he came home from work to find Taylor in the throngs of pain and me, near frantic and even crying some days with the frustration of caring for her. Craig had been raised to revere the medical model, as are many, and he certainly didn't have much patience for my little food diary and proclamations that Taylor was getting better, when that was clearly not what he was seeing with his own eyes. He, being a male, wanted a solution. He wanted it NOW. That night, Craig told me to take Taylor to another doctor, to which I responded "Absolutely not". I told Craig that if he didn't read the book I found, we would never be on the same page and until he came to understand what I now understood, we had nothing more to talk about. I left the house in a fury.

When I returned home within half an hour (because I had forgotten my wallet and needed to go to the washroom!!!!), I tried to sneak in without Craig seeing or hearing me. He met me at the door, book in hand, and asked me if I had looked into our drinking water. Tears came to my eyes. I told him that I had read about the potential problems with drinking tap water but thought it was too far fetched to try changing our water. I knew everyone already saw me as "a freak" for the dietary changes I had made with Taylor. The next day, Craig called the water company in our town. We learned that our water had loads of chlorine and iron in it, more than the water in neighbouring towns, because our water was from a well. We already knew that Taylor was highly reactive to chlorine and that iron is generally constipating. Craig had discovered another missing link. We immediately stopped giving Taylor tap water, and bowel movements piled out of her for a number of days!

Then it was Mother's Day. I expected Taylor to have a bowel movement that morning, but she didn't. My mind began to spin. I wouldn't get out of bed. I felt that maybe I hadn't discovered all the culprits after all, that I failed Taylor as a mother and that I had just been spinning my wheels all those months. Then, Craig came into our room and said that she had just had a bowel movement. I knew I could get out of bed but that's all I knew for certain.

After the month was up, with Taylor on filtered water and no exposure to second-hand smoke, she was perfectly fine. She was a happy, healthy, bouncy little girl who had colour in her cheeks for the first time in her life. One month later, Taylor turned two. That summer, I spent every waking moment taking Taylor to playgrounds, amusement parks, on walks in the trees... well, you get the idea. I rejoiced in her every move. I was so happy that she was well. The pride I felt for myself and in my husband by healing Taylor and conquering yet another challenge is unsurpassed. I am not afraid to admit that I was really angry to have received so little help from the outside world. I was completely disappointed with the medical profession for their lack of knowledge regarding food reactions and their understanding of nutrition but it was their indifference to our plight, which truly maddened me. I received a considerable amount of comfort from reading "How to Raise a Healthy Child in Spite of your Doctor" and "What Your Doctor Doesn't Know about Nutritional Medicine May Be Killing You". As a result, I now understand why most doctors do not have knowledge in these matters but have full respect for their knowledge in other matters.

Today, Taylor is 10 years old. She can eat anything she wants in moderation, including dairy. I now do the majority of my grocery shopping at our local health food store, which offers numerous alternatives for Taylor and even has a restaurant. Even to this day, I am constantly trying new foods and recipes for Taylor so that she never becomes bored with her food choices, receives the nutrients she needs from having a well-rounded diet and doesn't develop new sensitivities. Isn't it amazing that at some point in the time when Taylor was sick, I discovered that her initials T.A.D. mean "God's gift"?

The very month that we sorted everything out with Taylor's health, I learned I was pregnant again! Two-and-a-half years after having Taylor, Craig and I gave birth to another daughter named Paige. Unlike her sister, she was in a rush to be born. I found that without all the interventions that go on in a hospital, labour can move along quite nicely. She was born in just under five hours, in our own home, with the assistance of a midwife.

Paige also had food sensitivities (*and* she was a picky eater!). I applied the lessons I'd learned from raising Taylor to caring for Paige and found that my knowledge was sound.

Of course, there are many more stories to tell but you'll have to read on to hear those!

Once I had two children who were reacting to foods, I knew my calling was to work with food and its effects, helping other parents face similar challenges. So, nine months after Paige was born, in October 2002, I started my own company, "The Resourceful Mother". A few years later, I tried to help some friends of ours with their autistic son. They refused to believe what I had to say about the impact of food, telling me that I was not a doctor or nutritionist. About a week later, a good friend of mine, who was a nutritionist, asked me to speak to a group of nutritionists and tell them our story and lessons learned. When these nutritionists told me that our story provided real life proof of the various protocols they learned in nutrition school, I was thrilled. I was so amazed and pleased that these experts *understood* me that I decided I wanted to join their ranks. The next day, I started nutrition school. The manager of the school told me that I looked familiar and asked if we had met before. I responded, "No, I was just meant to sign up for this program a long time ago." The two-year program filled in the gaps in my understanding of how food sensitivities and allergies come into being and cemented my confidence in what my daughters taught me about health. I now teach the Canadian School of Natural Nutrition's Pediatric Nutrition Course.

I have spent the last decade researching food sensitivities and allergies, through reading, attending nutrition school and seminars and talking to other parents. It is one of my greatest pleasures to assist other parents, individually and through seminars, in detecting, managing, and eliminating reactions to foods.

It was being **The Resourceful Mother** of two daughters with food sensitivities and allergies and learning the link between diet and disease that led me to find my calling. I will be eternally grateful to my daughters for helping me find the fulfilment I craved. Those who read these pages will probably be eternally grateful to Taylor and Paige, as well.

CHAPTER I

FROM REACTION TO PRO-ACTION

Recognizing and Making Sense of Common Food Reactions

"The incidence of diet-related problems is greater than the incidence of any other type of illness affecting mankind."[1]
Dr. James C. Breneman

All parents want the same for their children. Their good health is always our number one priority. Then what happens when our child is not well, not healthy, and not as we imagine they could be? Parents despair but then, full of love and determination, look for answers and a road to health. Parents, like you, take positive action. The first step in that action is knowledge. What you are about to read will arm you with the tools you need to *know better* and to *do better* by your children. There is no greater feeling than the satisfaction of bringing about health in those you love most.

Would you like your child to sleep soundly, behave well and concentrate in school? Does your child experience colic, constipation, eczema, recurrent ear infections or asthma? These are only some of the common health challenges facing the children of today. These health challenges are so prevalent that many of us have come to view them as "normal". *They are NOT normal.* If your child is not sleeping soundly, behaving well, concentrating in school, or is experiencing colic, constipation, eczema, recurrent ear infections or asthma, your child's body is signalling to you that aspects of their environment are not agreeing with them. These symptoms are your call to action.

Your starting point is to look at what your child is eating. If your child is eating the particular foods that fuel their body for maximum efficiency, they will not likely experience any of these health challenges. However, if your child is reacting to a particular food or foods, the earlier you can uncover the culprits, the better. Our bodies will keep communicating with us whether we listen or not. **When you ignore a reaction to a food, it becomes a "symptom". An ignored symptom** *becomes more ignored symptoms and more ignored symptoms turn into conditions. Then, often in adulthood, conditions turn into disease. The cumulative effect can be devastating.*

Anyone can react adversely to foods and the majority of people do. Believe it or not, most of you reading this book are probably suffering from physical, mental or emotional symptoms caused by undiagnosed, adverse reactions to food. It is not my intention to alarm you with this information. It is my intention to make you aware of the source of any health challenges that you or your child might be experiencing so that you may quickly restore health to the body!

You may already be thinking this is not the book for you. You may be skipping ahead and seeing the words "food sensitivities" and "food allergies" and seeing that many chapters are written to help the "food reactive child". You know your child is not reacting to food. All I ask before you put this book down is that you first read the list of symptoms, conditions and diseases that can be caused by food.

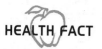

HEALTH FACT

Anyone can react adversely to foods and the majority of people do.

What are some of the symptoms, conditions and diseases that can be caused by food?

Over 200 symptoms and 50 conditions can be triggered or worsened by food. Those symptoms, conditions and disease include:

Abdominal bloating or fullness
Acne
Addiction to any food
Anxiety
Apathy
Arthritis (Childhood rheumatoid arthritis)
Asthma
Attention Deficit Disorder
Auto-immune diseases (e.g. Lupus, Multiple Sclerosis)
Autism
Backache
Bad breath
Bed-wetting in children over the age of three or four
Behavioural problems
Being easily frustrated
Binge eating
Bladder infections (recurrent)
Bloating
Bloodshot eyes
Blurred vision

Brain fog
Breathing difficulty
Brittle and splitting nails
Broken blood vessels under the skin
Bronchitis
Bruising
Burping
Canker sores
Celiac disease
Cold sores
Crohn's disease
Chronic fatigue
Clammy skin
Clearing of the throat repetitively
Clingy
Coated tongue
Colds or infections (frequent)
Colic
Colitis
Confusion
Conjunctivitis
Constipation

Coughing (chronic)
Cracked skin
Cramping of stomach, legs and feet
Dandruff
Dark circles, puffiness or bags under the eyes
Depression
Diabetes
Diaper rash
Diarrhea of unknown cause
Difficulty losing or gaining weight
Dizziness or faintness
Drowsiness after meals
Dry skin
Dyslexia
Ear infections (including inflammation,
    discharge or pain in ear)
Eczema
Epilepsy or seizures
Excessive hunger
Excessive mucus
Excessive saliva or drool in infants
Excessive spit-up in babies
Excessive thirst
Facial puffiness
Failure to laugh or smile often
Failure to thrive in babies
Fainting
Fast heartbeat
Fatigue (the #1 symptom caused by food)
Fever
Flatulence
Flushing
Food cravings
Forgetfulness
Fussy eating
Fussy in general
Gall bladder pain
Glazed eyes
"Growing pains" i.e. painful joints
Haemorrhoids
Hair loss
Handwriting changes
Headaches
Head banging
Hives
Hoarseness
Hunger all the time
Hyperactivity

Hypoglycemia
Irritable Bowel Syndrome
Inability to concentrate
Inability to return to sleep after being woken
Inability to speak
Indigestion
Insomnia
Irregular heartbeat
Irritability
Itchy skin, ears, nose, eyes or rectum
Learning difficulties or disabilities
Loose bowels
Low blood sugar
Mental dullness
Migraine headaches
Mood swings
Muscle weakness
Muscular and joint aches
Nausea
Neck ache
Nervousness
Nightmares
Nosebleeds
Nose picking (chronic)
Numbness
Obesity
Over-excitement
Pain of unknown cause
Pale complexion
Palpitations
Panic attacks
Poor comprehension
Poor coordination
Psoriasis
Rapid weight fluctuations
Recurrent infections
Red ears or eyes
Reflux
Restless leg syndrome
Ringing in the ears
Runny nose
Sadness
Schizophrenia
Shortness of breath
Skin rashes (around the mouth particularly,
    although the whole body might be
    affected)
Silly behaviour

Sinus congestion and headache
Sleep disturbances
Sneezing episodes
Sniffling (chronic)
Snoring
Sore throats
Speech impediments
Stomach aches
Stuffy nose
Sweating (excessive)
Swelling and wrinkles around the eyes
Swollen hands, feet, face
Tantrums
Tension
Throat tickle

Tonsillitis
Tourette syndrome
Twitching muscles
Vaginal discharge
Vaginal or scrotal itching
Violent behaviour
Virus
Vomiting
Vulgarity in speech and actions
Water retention
Watery eyes
Weak muscles
Weight gain
Wheezing
Whining

Are you as shocked as I was to learn that all of these can be caused by adverse reactions to food? This was groundbreaking information for me! I needed to know more. You, too, may now be wondering, is my child reacting adversely to food? If your child has one symptom right now, say a diaper rash, you may decide that you don't need to do anything differently in terms of feeding your child. If the diaper rash happens every once in a while and is not severe, I would agree with you. Now, say the diaper rash becomes more severe and is now raw and painful for your child and it is not going away. Would this be a time to look into things further? In my mind, absolutely! Say you decide to leave it and hope for the best. That rash may not go away and in fact, your child could start to become really fussy or have troubles sleeping and eventually, the diaper rash could become eczema on other parts of your child's body. This is what I mean when I tell you that symptoms, if ignored, often turn into more symptoms, which turn into conditions. Unfortunately, we all know people that have cancer or have died of cancer. Was cancer the first health challenge they ever experienced? In the majority of cases, the answer to that question is "No". They might have had recurrent infections or arthritis or health challenges of any kind, prior to being diagnosed with cancer. Their bodies were trying to communicate with them if only they had known what to do.

So, let's get back to our child with the diaper rash. I've already suggested to you that you look first at what your child has been eating in order to find your culprit. So now you think back….and you remember that a couple of weeks ago, you introduced rice cereal to your child. You know that rice cereal is the most hypo–allergenic food there is and it has been touted as the best first food for a child so that

HEALTH FACT

The biggest challenge I face in my work is helping others understand and recognize the link between what they are eating and how they are feeling.

couldn't be the culprit (Please see Chapter #5 for more information on rice cereal and healthier first foods). You're racking your brain but can't think of anything else you have done differently. ***Any food can cause an adverse reaction in a child, and any food can cause any reaction.*** Believe it or not, rice cereal is causing reactions in many children these days. You decide you had better remove the rice cereal to see if your child's diaper rash clears up. The rash clears up. It can be that simple. If you stay on top of your child's symptoms in this way, your child's symptoms will never multiply and your child will not have the health challenges that we are seeing in so many of those around us today. Does your child have a sensitivity to rice cereal? Yes. Can you make your child's body stronger so that rice cereal does not cause a reaction in your child? Yes, please read on. Can teething cause a diaper rash? Yes, but food can make the symptoms of teething worse. Can emotional challenges enter into the picture and cause physical symptoms? Absolutely, but that's a whole other subject for another time. Besides, it's easiest to address the physical causes of symptoms first, before exploring the emotional causes.

What are the most common foods (common allergens) that cause symptoms, conditions and disease?

Beef

Caffeine

Chemicals (additives, preservatives, food dyes)

Chocolate

Citrus Fruits (orange, grapefruit, lemon and
      lime)

Corn

Dairy (i.e. cow's milk, cheese, butter, sour
      cream, yogurt, cream cheese, ice cream)

Eggs

Gluten (the major protein found in wheat)

Peanuts or tree nuts

Shellfish or other fish

Soy

Strawberries

Sugar (refined)

Tomatoes

Yeast

Dairy (Cow's milk is the #1 leading allergen) and gluten are the top two perpetrators, followed by soy, sugar and yeast and they can be found in almost every item in a North American grocery store! There is a reason certain foods generate the most reactions. Simply put, common allergenic foods are commonly eaten foods that cause inflammation in the body and are mucus forming, when a child is lacking good bacteria (please read on to understand this better). The inflammation causes more bad bacteria to grow and eventually symptoms, conditions or disease can ensue. Please see Chapters #2 and #3 to learn more.

What are food allergies and sensitivities?

This book addresses all non life-threatening reactions to foods. You'll find that there are many differences of opinion among experts as to the meaning of the terms "allergies" and "sensitivities". I won't explain this controversy in detail but I think it's important for you to know that it exists. In one sense, it doesn't matter whether we use food "sensitivity", "intolerance", "allergy" or some other name; what is important is that physicians, other health professionals and parents realize that commonly eaten foods and other substances cause a wide variety of abnormal reactions or symptoms in children. Moreover, such symptoms often go unrecognized. Even the famous Dr. William G. Crook, MD, who has written numerous best-selling nutrition books, shared this opinion back in the fifties.

I will only share the most widely researched information with you. Please bear in mind, when you are comparing this book with other books or articles, that these same words may be used in entirely different ways.

Food allergies are adverse reactions to a substance involving the immune system i.e. classic allergy immunoglobulin IgE antibodies are formed. If a child only consumes a small amount of a food and has a reaction, he or she has an allergy to that food. Classic allergic (IgE) reactions are immediate, meaning that they occur within minutes and up to 2 hours from consumption, making them easy to detect. Foods like peanuts, shellfish, eggs and strawberries can cause immediate severe reactions such as hives, swelling, changes in breathing and anaphylactic shock. In babies, the most common symptom of an allergy is chronic diarrhea. Examples of others include vomiting, colic and constipation. Not all allergies produce severe reactions in children. Statistics vary as to how many children suffer from allergies but it is a much smaller percentage than those who suffer from food sensitivities.

"A Viennese physician, Baron Clemens von Pirquet, first used it (the word "allergy") in 1906 to mean, "Altered reactivity". (He) was a pediatrician and he felt the need for a new medical term to describe certain reactions in his young patients." "He was principally concerned with reactions involving the immune system, the set of cells that protect our bodies from infection. But he apparently intended his newly coined word to mean any altered response to the environment. In this context, environment means all the external things that can affect the body, whether in food or water, in the air we breathe, or in things that come into contact with our skin. Von Pirquet also introduced the word allergen to describe the substances that brought about these changed reactions."[2]

"After 1926, allergies were allergen–antibody reactions involving the immune system only. This decision was reinforced around 1967 when the immunoglobulin IgE was discovered. IgE was the first recognized antibody involved in immune–type reactions and became the classic marker for allergy. This historic decision severely limited the scope of allergy for the next 50 years."[3]

In 1965, Dr. Randolph Moss, along with other doctors, founded The Society for Clinical Ecology. These doctors recognized the link between food and many medical problems even though the IgE antibody did not show up in test results i.e. scratch tests. In other words, they recognized food sensitivities. The rest of the medical community did not endorse clinical ecology and this remains the case to this day, which is why you may not have heard of clinical ecology.

Decades later, European allergists narrowed down the definition of allergy to describe only the reactions that occur in *rapid* response to exposure to an allergen. The immediate or very near immediate nature of the reaction makes identifying the problematic food quite easy and the need for testing rather unnecessary.

Today, many physicians are aware of the existence of "delayed" allergies, involving the IgG antibodies but have no accurate way of testing for these allergies.

Food sensitivities, also called food intolerances, are adverse reactions to a substance that begin in the intestines and can affect any part of the body. Food sensitivities cause inflammation in the body but classic allergy antibodies are not involved in these reactions. When a child develops a rash i.e. inflammation 40 hours after eating cheese but a scratch test (performed by medical doctors, using needles in search of allergies i.e. IgE antibodies) for cheese comes up negative for the IgE antibody, then the rash, even if it occurs every time the child eats cheese, is not caused by an "allergy" to cheese. It is caused by a "food sensitivity".

HEALTH FACT

One could say that the number of people with some sort of food sensitivity is quite literally 100%.

The amount of time it can take for a delayed reaction to manifest itself is anywhere from a few hours to four days from consumption. Most reactions to food are delayed (95%, according to Dr. Carolee Bateson-Koch DC ND in Allergies, Disease in Disguise), making food sensitivities extremely difficult to detect and causing some children to suffer for years. If your child doesn't react to a small amount of a food but does react to a larger amount, your son or daughter has a food sensitivity. Food sensitivities often produce symptoms clinically indistinguishable from food allergies. An example might be congestion in the throat, lungs or nose.

I am convinced, along with many experts, that the majority of babies, children and adults today have food sensitivities and that food sensitivities are one of the greatest health challenges in North America. One could say that the number of people with some sort of food sensitivity is quite literally 100%. Who has not experienced some sort of adverse reaction to food, even a minor one, at one time or another? The late Dr. Arthur Coca of Cornell University, who was considered the dean of American immunologists, believed that as many as 90% of all Americans had one or more food sensitivities. That was 25 years ago! The situation has become so much worse since then.

Here's the good news: Food sensitivities and allergies are the body's attempt to make itself better. Food sensitivities need not be permanent. They usually disappear when levels of good bacteria are increased (Please read on). Sometimes problematic foods need to be eliminated from the diet for a short time and overall dietary habits need to be improved.

Here is the bad news: Food sensitivities can turn into food allergies over time.

Here is some more good news: We hear so much about allergies in the children of today. Are you afraid your child will become allergic? Fear begins when there is a lack of knowledge. Allergies are entirely preventable. It starts with preventing food sensitivities.

> Dr. Theron Randolph, a well-known allergist and immunologist, believed that "the population as a whole could experience a tremendous increase in well-being and productivity if food and chemical susceptibility were routinely considered in each case of chronic disease..."[4]

Food sensitivities—the great masqueraders

Food sensitivities, in particular, have been called "the great masqueraders." Usually, people do not suspect food sensitivities are the root of their problem or that of their child because most food sensitivities, by their very nature, are masked or hidden. Also, the term "food sensitivity" is much broader than the term "food allergy". It includes many types of problems that may be related to food: What do I mean by this?

1. **Different foods, different reactions**–Different foods cause different reactions in different individuals. Each person has his or her own biochemical individuality. We've all heard the phrase, "One man's meat is another man's poison" coined by Lucretius, the Roman poet and philosopher. You may be able to eat beef, but your best friend may get a migraine headache every time she eats it. Or you may be chronically fatigued by a sensitivity to milk but your son's milk sensitivity may show up as hyperactivity.

2. **Same food, different reactions**–The same food can cause different reactions in the same individual. A child has cereal with milk and suffers diarrhea shortly after eating and then, several hours later, suffers intense fatigue. Another common scenario is that a child may have consumed wheat for years, occasionally experiencing bouts of constipation. As a teenager, you notice that her skin starts to break out each time she consumes her favourite bread. Reactions to foods can start at any time and any age but often come about with repeated consumption of the same food. You can read more about this concept further on.

3. **Subtle reactions**–Reactions to foods are often subtle and can therefore remain hidden for months or years. Unfortunately, many of the 'symptoms' that babies and children experience are so commonly part of the childhood experience that parents do not know that there is even a problem. Diaper rashes, excessive spit up, gas, irritability, crying, and frequent colds or infections are perfect examples of symptoms of food sensitivities that many parents view as normal or attribute to other causes.

4. **Symptoms can be caused a number of ways**–A headache can be caused by a bump to the head, anxiety, exhaustion, lack of water or a magnesium deficiency to name a few. And many of the symptoms are those that can be produced by psychosomatic illness, in which emotional or mental distress evokes physical symptoms in the body. Thus the idea of food sensitivities being the cause of your child's symptoms seems even less credible.

5. **Delayed reactions**–Whereas classic food allergy reactions are immediate, there are no apparent immediate reactions with food sensitivities. In fact, the body's reaction to offending foods usually occurs in small steps. Each step leads to the next until the body reaches its breaking point– the final straw. At that time, the body reacts by developing one or more of a wide range of symptoms.

6. **Food frequency**–The development of sensitivities depends on exposure. The more frequently a person is exposed to a food, the greater his or her tendency is to become sensitive. Even with hundreds of foods available, most of us eat the same 15–20 foods in different combinations day after day. For example, dairy (milk, butter and cheese in particular) and wheat are eaten at almost every meal! When you eat milk products frequently, you're calling on specific enzymes to digest that milk. When this pattern continues, you create an enzyme deficiency for that food. A food sensitivity may well disappear if the problem food is not eaten for a couple of weeks or sometimes months but will likely return once the food is eaten regularly again.

7. **Food cravings and addiction**–Related to the last point, the foods to which we are most sensitive are the ones that we often have the hardest time living without. As humans, we have an unconscious tendency to protect the source of the problem from exposure. Our living and eating habits are routinely designed to feed addictions, not to break them. If your son has a temper tantrum when you tell him he's had enough goldfish crackers, you know that the crackers are a likely culprit for him! You can read more about this concept further on.

8. **Foods rarely eaten or disliked**–People can be sensitive to foods that they rarely eat or even dislike. Your child develops a rash on the rare occasions when he consumes cashews. Luckily, he doesn't even like cashews. This food would not be difficult for him or her to avoid, especially with all the nut free products that exist today.

9. **Hidden ingredients**–Many people think they are not consuming a particular food, when the reality is that they are having it every day. A good example is corn: your daughter may not eat corn as a vegetable very often, yet she eats it at practically every meal in the form of corn sugar (dextrose or glucose), corn syrup, cornstarch, corn oil, or as a hidden ingredient in other foods.

10. **Quantity**–With food sensitivities, there can be thresholds. A few strawberries cause no reaction in a child but a handful of the fruit sends them into a bout of hives. Remember: If a small amount of strawberries causes hives, your child is allergic to strawberries.

11. **Raw versus cooked**–People can be sensitive to raw foods but all right with the same food once it is cooked! You feed your son a stew containing carrots and he has no reaction. Then you feed him raw carrots and his cheeks turn red! This is because there is cellulose in raw vegetables that can be hard to digest for some people. Cellulose gets broken down in the cooking process.

12. **Cumulative effects**–Your son eats freshly baked bread every day for four days without reacting and then on the seventh day, he has a bad case of gas.

13. **Concomitant effects**–Your child is okay drinking a glass of milk but when he has it with wheat (i.e. a piece of toast), he reacts. For further confirmation on these last four points, read Dr. Lendon Smith's books!

14. **Other conditions**–Dysbiosis, candida, parasites, and low stomach acid increase reactions to food (You can read more about these underlying imbalances in Chapter #3).

15. **Food sensitivities are chronic, vaguely defined problems** that rarely respond to conventional medical treatment. The majority of medical doctors today have no idea how to recognize food sensitivities, never mind treat them. Millions of children are being prescribed drugs needlessly, hospitalized and even being operated on because the environmental cause of their health challenge is not understood. No drug or medical therapy can improve your child's health if you continue to bombard his or her body with their own personal poison.

What a conundrum! You may be asking yourself, 'How are these food sensitivities *ever* detected? Do they *really* exist? With this many variables, this is going to be way too difficult to get a handle on. Forget it! Ignorance is bliss.'

It is certainly not my intent to scare you away! Once you know what to look for, the process of detecting food sensitivities is not daunting. I assure you of this. The younger your child is, the easier it is to spot the culprit foods and, as you will see, there are tests performed by alternative practitioners that you can have done on, even newborn babies, which will guide you to detection.

We become addicted to the foods to which we react

I feel that it is necessary to discuss this concept further. A child who reacts adversely to a certain food may become addicted to that food. Often when a child eats a problematic food, stress chemicals like adrenaline, cortisol or endorphins are released, causing the child to feel pleasure for a short period of time after consumption. This makes it extra difficult for children to eliminate certain foods from their diets! Food addictions often occur with dairy and wheat, the two most heavily consumed foods in North America.

Foods are addictive because of:
- Sheer bulk of food—large amounts are eaten (2–5 lbs a day)
- Frequency—food is eaten daily, many times a day
- Duration of exposure—food stays in contact with the digestive tract for long periods of time. Fruit stays there for 30 minutes and more complicated foods, 6 hours or longer.

Three signs of addiction:
- Negative consequences ("I am sick without cheese")
- Denial ("I'm not addicted to cheese")
- Obsession ("I can't go without cheese for 3 days")

The easiest way to determine the food your child is reacting to is to ask yourself "What food would my child have the hardest time giving up?" or "What food does my child love the most?" Your answer to that question is usually your biggest culprit, the food causing the reaction. You will find that the food to which your child is reacting is a common allergen. It's very rare to hear anyone say, "I am addicted to broccoli!"

> "Let us say, for instance, that you developed an allergy to milk early in life. At first, this may have resulted in acute reactions, such as a rash or a cough. In time, if the allergy was not recognized and controlled, the symptoms may have become more generalized and less easily detected (the acute symptoms become suppressed because of the constant nature of the exposure, and the body has reacted by attempting to adapt itself to the problem). Since you probably went on drinking milk or eating milk products almost every day, one day's symptoms blurred into the next days. You developed a chronic disease, such as arthritis, migraine or depression. It never occurred to you that your daily dose of milk was the source of the problem.

In fact you were probably 'abusing' milk. You had become a milk junkie, a milk–o–holic. It is in the nature of this problem that a sudden loss of the craved substance can cause withdrawal symptoms. Since removal of milk brought on a particularly bad attack of the symptoms, you unconsciously learned to keep yourself on a maintenance dose. Milk in the morning with cereal, milk in your coffee, yogurt for lunch, a glass of milk with your dinner, and, of course, a platter of cheese tidbits before retiring.

Milk is just mentioned as an example. In fact, any food can be abused by overeating it. If a food is eaten in any form once in three days, or more frequently, it is being abused and may become a big problem for the consumer. Since it may take between 3 and 4 days for a meal to make its way through the digestive tract, the person in question is not free of that food before another dose is added to the stomach. Intolerance to this food may sneak up on the person who eats it after months, years or even decades of day–in and day–out ingestion."[5]

Why are food sensitivities and allergies so common these days?

As a group, our children are the sickest youth in the history of the human species. They are reacting to food and suffering from poor digestion, yeast problems, sensitivities and allergies like never before. All of these epidemics have one root cause— a lack of good bacteria in their intestines, also known as dysbiosis. Many of us hear the word 'bacteria', learn that it is in our bodies and immediately think "I have bacteria? Oh, that is bad. That shouldn't be." This is not true.

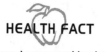

HEALTH FACT

We need more good bacteria than bad to ward off health imbalances.

The body is like a battlefield between good and bad bacteria. Good bacteria promotes good health. Too much bad bacteria causes infections and disease. We need more good bacteria than bad to ward off health imbalances. Lactobacillus acidophilus is the main strain of friendly bacteria in the body. It is found in the mouth and intestines of men and women and in the birth canal of women.

Even Health Canada recognizes that good bacteria:
- Removes bad bacteria or toxins (yeast, parasites etc) from the body before they enter into the bloodstream
- Protects the stomach lining and helps prevent leaky gut which is believed to be behind allergies (Please read further on)
- Aids in digestion by making the specialty enzymes like lactase and cellulase
- Prevents sensitivities and subsequently allergies
- Assists in the elimination of waste by improving the frequency and size of

bowel movements. A buildup of waste is the cause of 90% of symptoms, conditions and disease (Please see Chapter #4 to understand this more)
- Builds the immune system
- Stabilizes blood sugar

There are a multitude of factors that contribute to a lack of good bacteria (also called "poor intestinal flora"). Each one contributes to our toxic load, that is, the amount of food, chemicals, allergens and inhalant pollutants that a person can be exposed to before symptoms appear.

The following factors contribute to toxins or bad bacteria in the body of parents and their children, in turn. Eventually, when toxic load is reached, adverse food reactions occur (For more information on improving levels of good bacteria, please see Chapters #2 and #6):

1. **Genetics**–Every child is born with a certain toxic load. As parents, we pass on the propensity for our children to have adverse reactions to food, chemicals and/or the environment. For example, there seems to be a correlation between a family history of alcoholism, sugar cravings, and/or diabetes and children who are sensitive to sugar.

2. **Premature birth**–Premature babies have underdeveloped systems, making them more prone to food reactions.

3. **Birth by caesarean**–If a baby does not go through the birth canal, he or she cannot obtain as much good bacteria from mother as a baby that does. Whatever bacteria lives in the bowel will live in the vagina and then be passed onto babies.

4. **Vaccinations and immunization shots**–These injections leave the immune system in a weakened state and, therefore, more susceptible to allergens. You may find that your child's symptoms first presented themselves following an injection.

5. **Drugs**–Aspirin, Ibuprofen, Advil, Tylenol, asthma inhalers, antibiotics, birth control pills and recreational drugs lead to the overgrowth of bad bacteria in the gastrointestinal tract (bacteria, parasites, viruses, fungi). Drugs also disrupt the functioning of the cells along the intestinal walls, decrease liver function, increase chemical overload and destroy enzyme systems. The top 2 prescription drugs causing allergies are Penicillin and Aspirin.

6. **Frequent infections**–Bacterial, fungal (candida), viral and parasitic infections weaken the body, damaging the intestinal tissue, making it more susceptible to food sensitivities or allergies.

7. **Early introduction of potential allergens to infants**–Introducing commonly allergenic foods to children, before their digestive and immune systems have matured, causes many children to be unable to tolerate certain

foods. If a baby cannot digest a food, he or she has a greater chance of reacting to it. North American infant formula is based on cow's milk and soymilk, two common allergens.

8. **Undigested food particles**–These are formed from over-eating, eating too much of the same foods, not enough chewing, enzyme deficiencies (e.g. celiac disease, lactase deficiency causing lactose intolerance) or eating harder to digest foods (dairy, wheat, processed foods or those high in saturated fat etc).

9. **Nutritional deficiencies**–These often develop from eating too much junk food or too much of the same food. Vitamin or mineral deficiencies can result from diets high in sugar and refined foods (e.g. chocolate bars, sweets, cakes, white bread, fried foods etc). The more nutritional deficiencies that exist, the less digestive enzymes are made.

10. **Sugar**–A rapidly absorbed food, sugar fosters the growth of bad bacteria, encourages poor digestion and damages the immune system.

11. **Caffeine and soft drinks**–These are strong gut irritants and can be particularly dangerous for younger children.

12. **Chemicals**–Chemical dyes, preservatives and additives found in processed food, aspartame in drinks, fluoride in water, household cleaners and pesticides in the environment are big culprits.

13. **Alcohol**–Any liquor is rapidly absorbed, inhibits good bacteria and damages the intestinal wall.

14. **Cigarettes**–Smoking cigarettes or inhaling second-hand smoke make the holes in the intestine larger.

15. **Heavy metals e.g. mercury fillings**–Mercury and other metals are harmful to the immune system and block enzymes. This leads to food reactions often showing up as nervousness, anxiety and other neurological symptoms. There are healthy, although more costly, alternatives to mercury fillings.

16. **Stress**–Emotional and physical stress usually demand greater nutritional requirements, which are often not met. This, in turn, causes the organs and systems, particularly the immune system, to become stressed and lose their ability to work properly. Stress is a huge factor! And don't think that children cannot experience stress.

17. **Poor elimination**–Not having enough bowel movements (frequency or size) contributes to a person's toxic load.

18. **Age**–The older one is, the more food reactive they become because of a weakened immune system, organ degeneration and a greater toxic load. Often older people have nutritional deficiencies as well, due to a lifetime of the same eating patterns.

19. **Hormonal imbalances**–Thyroid imbalances, birth control pills and pregnancy can lead to an increase in nutritional needs as well as an overgrowth of bad bacteria that can be passed on to a child.

20. **Chlorinated water**–Chlorine, other chemicals and the bad bacteria in tap, bath and pool water increase one's toxic load through skin absorption.

21. **Air quality**–The quality of the air we breathe has deteriorated and increases bad bacteria in our bodies. Air pollution is caused by power plants, car exhaust, pesticides, and chemical cleaners to name a few. We keep the air conditioning or heat on all the time in our homes and schools, causing us to breathe in a lot of stale air. We also inhale the dust, mould and animal dander pumping through our ductwork.

22. **Radiation**–Computers, televisions, X-rays, and flying are some examples of electromagnetic radiation that increases our toxic load.

23. **Low stomach acid** (Please see Chapter #3)

24. **Hypoglycemia** (Please see Chapter #3)

25. **Allergic reactions or inflammation along the intestinal lining**–Reactions to foods, chemicals and the environment increase the toxins in the body.

26. **The typical modern diet**–This last factor requires further elaboration.

Our food choices are a major factor contributing to the preponderance of sensitivities and allergies that we see today. Our diets have degenerated considerably. If you look back to the beginning of the century, people ate whole foods and plenty of fresh foods. Children's treats were home made cookies instead of chips and other processed foods, laden with chemicals and dyes. The quality of their fruits and vegetables was even better than today. The soil their crops were grown in was more fertile, mineral rich, stronger and pest-resistant. There were no insecticides, pesticides, preservatives or dyes in the food, air or water of the older generations.

Today, the vitamin and mineral content of our foods has been sacrificed for longer shelf life and convenience. We eat far too many processed and refined foods like white bread, pasta and candy that lack fibre, vitamins and minerals. Even whole wheat bread now has five times more gluten than it did when it was originally made, just to make it lighter and fluffier. Humans have a difficult time digesting gluten! More fertilizers and chemical additives are being used than ever before that rob our bodies of vitamins and minerals and slow down the whole digestive system. As if that is not enough, our bodies also have to contend with genetically modified food. Our systems were not designed to take such assaults. Over the years, a poor diet causes a build-up of toxins that gradually poisons the body.

Everyone knows that cars require certain types of energy to run; ***the human race requires clean, natural, alive, good quality food to survive.*** The majority of children today are undernourished, overweight and suffering. In fact, food allergies and sensitivities themselves are forms of malnutrition. We, the adults, need to pay attention and help turn things around for our children and future generations.

The authors of *Your Hidden Food Allergies are Making You Fat* describe modern industrial life as "fast food, fast pace and less contact with nature". They state "Even though our lifestyles have changed dramatically over the past 5 or so generations, our genetic makeup has not." "We are Stone Age organisms living in an altered and artificial environment to which we have not adapted. And the more artificial the environment becomes, which most definitely includes our food, the less able we are to adapt to it and the sicker we become."

"In the last 50 years our diet has changed dramatically. The same digestive enzymes that were needed to digest only fresh fruits and vegetables and range–fed meats must now somehow deal with the huge amounts of preservatives, colourings, chemical fertilizers, insecticides and antibiotics in our foods. As our digestive enzymes fall short, our immune systems react to these substances to protect us from the toxic consequences."[6]

"The modern diet consisting primarily of processed and adulterated foods, contributes to food sensitivities in two ways: It introduces more unnatural and foreign substances into the body, and it does not provide adequate levels of nutrients necessary for proper liver detoxification." [7]

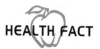

HEALTH FACT

In fact, food allergies and sensitivities themselves are forms of malnutrition.

Of course, this list of factors contributing to a lack of good bacteria and subsequently, food sensitivities and allergies is completely daunting. These factors surround us and pervade our lives. When I first came to learn the causes of food sensitivities and allergies, I remember I was sitting on the couch in my family room. The doom and gloom that took over my body was overpowering. I literally lifted my arms up to the ceiling and immediately dropped them in defeat. I wondered why we weren't being protected, why this knowledge wasn't getting out there and how it was possible to be healthy in this day and age.

In summary, a child's propensity for sensitivities or allergies depends on his or her genetic predisposition, environmental vulnerability, individual biochemistry, and toxic load at any particular time. I am here to tell you that my eldest was born with all of these factors working against her. She went from having problems with all common allergens to being able to eat *any* food. The body has an incredible capacity to heal. It is never too late to restore health to the body of a child.

Trust me, your child can live; I mean *really live* and enjoy life, even when he or she has the worst difficulties with food. Even if you are simply trying to keep your child healthy, there are ways to ensure that your child consumes healthy foods at restaurants, friends' houses, and amusement parks and travel anywhere in the world. I'm going to teach you exactly how to go about this and if needed, how to eliminate your child's challenges with foods all together.

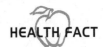

HEALTH FACT

It is never too late to restore health to the body of a child.

What causes food allergies?

All babies are born with a leaky gut, which means they have holes in their intestines. Their bodies were designed specifically that way so that mothers' milk, made up of nutrients and antibodies, can go through the leaky gut directly into the bloodstream, helping little bodies to grow and flourish! Within approximately four months, the holes in the intestine are supposed to close up.

When a child's intestinal lining remains or becomes more permeable (porous) than normal, it is referred to as leaky gut syndrome. Leaky gut syndrome, discovered by Dr. Theron Randolph decades ago, is believed to be the cause of allergies. It is a very common problem and is rapidly increasing.

If a food only partially breaks down (i.e. is not properly digested), bad bacteria (i.e. toxins) can be produced in the digestive tract. For example, sugar, caffeine, and prescription drugs upset the body's chemistry causing undigested food to get into the bloodstream. Abnormally large spaces present between the cells of the gut wall and allow the entry of toxic material–bacteria, fungi, parasites, undigested protein, fat and waste–into the bloodstream that would, in healthier circumstances, be repelled or eliminated. This means that larger than usual protein molecules now enter the bloodstream before they have a chance to be completely broken down. The immune system sees these molecules or toxic material as invading foreign substances and makes antibodies against them in an attempt to destroy them. This is called the immune response. ***Some of the toxic material migrates to tissues in the body causing symptoms, conditions and eventually, possibly, disease.***

Simultaneously, when the body begins to recognize a food as foreign, it immediately releases histamine in order to protect the body, causing inflammation in the gut lining and anywhere in the body e.g. hives, swollen or itchy lips, mouth, throat or eyes. ***The intestinal lining becomes leaky because of this inflammation.*** Anaphylaxis is severe swelling with difficulty breathing, which can cause death.

Dr. Zoltan Rona explains it well when he says, "If this immune response occurs in the respiratory tract, the end result could be asthma, bronchitis, sinusitis, or a middle-ear infection. If it happens in the joints, it can trigger (childhood) rheumatoid arthritis flare-ups. If immune reactions take place in the nervous system, the end result might very well be attention deficit disorder or depression. The genetic weakness of the individual is likely to determine the site of inflammation and eventual disease."[8]

Clearly, practically any organ or body tissue can be affected by food allergies created by the leaky gut. If we don't heal the intestines of our children, their bodies remain open to a constant bombardment of foreign invaders and their immune systems will become strained and overworked.

Leaky gut syndrome can also occur after a child experiences a critical illness, chronic illness, trauma, burn or major surgery. A child that frequently suffers from infections and is often on antibiotics develops a leaky gut. If a child regularly eats the foods to which he is sensitive or consumes junk food on a recurrent basis, a leaky gut will occur.

Dr. Michael Lyon says that, "One major junk food binge or a single course of antibiotics may create a leaky gut condition within hours. If the diet then lacks the proper nutritional support to repair the injured gut lining, or if the irritation continues, leaky gut syndrome can become a persistent problem."[9]

Once a child has leaky gut syndrome, you will find that he or she will react to more and more foods and it will become increasingly difficult to pinpoint the foods causing your child's symptoms.

A leaky gut and poor digestion, in combination, sets the stage for allergies. On the flip side, allergies can also *cause* a leaky gut and poor digestion!

What causes food sensitivities?

Health, in general, *depends* on the strength of the digestive system. **Food sensitivities are caused by a lack of good bacteria in the intestinal tract and poor digestion.**

We know that food sensitivities start in the intestine. The symptoms arise in the gastro-intestinal tract tissues because of repeated direct contact and long-term exposure; we're constantly eating. The intestine is where all the nutrients that are needed to sustain life are absorbed by our bodies. More than half the cells in the immune system are located in and around the gastrointestinal tract. If your child is born with the predisposition of weak digestive juices and lack of good bacteria or if your child's intestine is under enough stress from his or her food or environment i.e. your child continues to eat a food to which he or she is sensitive, nutrients cannot be absorbed and intestinal permeability will increase, eventually causing leaky gut, which will affect his or her immune system. When food affects the immune system, allergies ensue.

Nutritional deficiencies are simply assumed to be the result of inadequate intake of nutrients. Rarely is a person's ability to digest food looked at as a possible cause for nutritional deficiencies and subsequent ill health. Proper digestion of food is vital to the effective absorption, transportation and utilization of nutrients by the body!

As already stated, a woman with good bacteria in her intestinal system and birth canal, transfers it to her baby when he or she is born. If a mother does not have a lot of good bacteria herself and/or she has a caesarian section, she is unable to pass much good bacteria on to her newborn. As you can imagine, this is a common scenario.

Any genetic predisposition can be minimized, if not reversed, through diet and supplements (Don't let that word scare you! I'll explain everything!). If you work on your child's digestion and lack of good bacteria (Please read on), your child might be able to handle foods that he or she couldn't previously and be able to eat the same food every single day and not have a problem with digesting that food.

HEALTH FACT

Proper digestion of food is vital to the effective absorption, transportation and utilization of nutrients by the body!

You may be asking yourself "Is it the lack of good bacteria and genetic predisposition for poor digestion or the common allergenic foods that my child is eating that are causing the symptoms I'm seeing in my son? Is it my son or the food he is eating that needs my focus?" It is both. However, if you focus on increasing the amount of good bacteria in your son, in time, he'll be able to eat any of the common allergens or foods to which he reacts.

Technically, we are not really sensitive to foods, but to foods that we are not digesting properly. "To eat is human; to digest is divine."[10]

Taylor's violent reaction to her first bottle-feeding is a perfect example of her not having enough good bacteria to be able to digest cow's milk. It is also a perfect example of an allergy because she consumed such a small amount of milk, only one ounce, and had such a violent reaction. We stayed away from dairy, in all forms, for two years, increased the amount of good bacteria in her intestine, healed her intestine and improved her whole diet. To this day, ten years later, she has no dairy allergy. *For many of you, all you will need to do to heal your "food-reactive" child is increase your child's amount of good bacteria.*

Will my child outgrow their food allergies or sensitivities?

You recognize your child has food allergies or sensitivities. Many parents are told that their children will likely outgrow their allergies. In reality, this is rarely the case.

Dr. Dick Thom N.D. states, "They may indeed outgrow their childhood allergies only to develop more serious, "deeper" chronic problems later in life. For example, infantile eczema may later become bronchial asthma or some form of gastrointestinal problem."[11]

Dr. Skye Weintraub states, "The child may appear to "outgrow" the original condition, but what may be happening is that the response has changed as the child grew older and the symptoms just became masked. For example, the infant who reacts to drinking milk with diarrhea or colic may later have eczema. At age two there is a constant runny nose, ear infections, and dark circles under the eyes; at age four there is hyperactivity and bed-wetting; and at age twenty there is asthma. By that time, other foods, inhalants, or chemicals have complicated the original milk sensitivity."[12]

Some have said to me "Oh, that's great that Taylor outgrew her allergy to dairy!" I used to just fume inside when I heard that; the simple assumption was that it just went away with time, when we had gone to such great lengths to fix the situation. Now I realize how few people understand allergies, never mind sensitivities, and thus the need for this book.

A better question might be "Can we help our daughter overcome her allergies?" Yes, in the majority of cases, the answer to that question is a resounding "Yes!"

How to make the best use of this chapter's information

1. Look at the list of symptoms, conditions and disease and determine if your child is experiencing any of these health challenges. If not, you now know what to look for as time goes on.
2. Look at the list of common allergens and determine if your child eats any of these foods. Read more about these foods in Chapter #2.
3. Think of which food(s) you or your child cannot live without or the food(s) that you eat the most often—probably your child's biggest culprit(s) and likely found in the list of common allergens.
4. Review the list of factors that contribute to toxins or bad bacteria in the body and decide if your child needs to increase the amount of good bacteria in his or her body. Think about ways to avoid sources of bad bacteria. Read on to learn other ways.

UNDERSTANDING THE CULPRITS IN FOODS AND OTHER SUBSTANCES AND THEIR HEALTHIER ALTERNATIVES

"Don't be afraid of food. Food is a friend and ally—we cannot do without it. But we can abuse it, misunderstand it, and not listen to what our body tells us after we eat it. Only thereby do we turn it into an adversary."[1]

One of the most important steps you can take raising happy, well-adjusted children is to feed them healthily. Even if you are the best communicator in the world or the most imaginative parent alive and your child adores you, it is impossible for your child to grow up, reaching his or her full potential, without a healthy diet. However, we are conditioned to believe that particular foods are healthy and for many of us, they are not. If your child cannot digest wheat, he or she cannot get its nutrients and only experiences the repercussions from eating it.

HEALTH FACT

We are conditioned to believe that particular foods are healthy and for many of us, they are not.

It is true that there is nutrition in each and every food. Then what is it about certain foods that make them a problem for so many people to digest? What are the worst offenders? What are some of the characteristic symptoms caused by certain foods or food groups? Are there other names that manufacturers use for the problem foods to make you think you're getting something special? What are the healthier alternatives?

Remember: If your child has enough good bacteria and a healthy digestive system, he or she should be able to consume any of the foods discussed in this chapter without major repercussions. Once you understand better what is happening to our foods, the question is, do you want your child consuming the common allergens? The point is that if you simply avoid a food to which your child reacts, you will be treating the symptom rather than addressing the root cause. The wheat is not the cause of your child's symptoms although it may trigger his or her fatigue. Improving your child's good bacteria levels and the health of his or her digestive system is vital in addressing the root cause. It is only necessary to avoid the wheat until your child's intestinal and digestive tracts are healed and working properly. Once your child is healed and he or she eats the common allergens in moderation, your child will maintain balance and health.

You will find as you read this chapter that it is man's processing and use of foods that has created the greatest challenges for the human body. As a result, there are no universally safe foods. But, reacting to certain foods can create healthier eating. Let me explain why.

Dairy

Cow's milk is the number one food causing symptoms, conditions and disease in North American children, as well as adults. The majority of people's bodies are incapable of breaking down many of the proteins found in pasteurised cow's milk. Until the 1950's, you could buy unpasteurised (uncooked) cow's milk that contained 22 enzymes, making digestion of cow's milk a lot easier. Modern milk is pasteurised in order to create longer shelf life by destroying harmful bacteria. It also destroys friendly bacteria, enzymes, vitamins and minerals. Milk loses 50% of its available calcium, for example, during pasteurization. Homogenisation of milk makes the fat in milk nearly indigestible. Low fat and skim milk make calcium unavailable because fat is needed for the proper transportation and absorption of calcium. Most nutritional experts agree that unpasteurised, unhomogenised, raw dairy products are far healthier than what is generally available for purchase today.

The Tao of Detox provides a graphic description of the problem with pasteurization. It states, "Pasteurization kills the active enzyme in milk that is required to digest it. Since most people don't produce this enzyme in their bodies, the milk stagnates in the stomach and the indigestible protein putrefies into a slimy sludge that oozes through the digestive tract and plasters gummy layers of mucus to the intestinal walls, forming a tough, rubbery lining that increasingly binds up the bowels. The reason that babies froth at the mouth and regurgitate foamy white phlegm after being fed pasteurized cow's milk is because their newly functioning stomachs, which are genetically designed to digest human milk, cannot digest the bovine casein protein in cow's milk."[2]

Cow's milk contains at least 25 different proteins that may induce reactions in humans. There are three main proteins in whole milk: casein, whey, and lactalbumin. These milk proteins are found in all animal milks but in varying amounts. Most people have a hard time digesting one, if not all of these parts.

Cow's milk also contains lactose, which seems to be the component in cow's milk that is discussed the most. Lactase is the enzyme we need to digest the milk sugar (lactose) found in breast milk, cow, sheep and goat's milk. Lactose intolerance involves an inability of the body to produce lactase or enough lactase to digest the amount of lactose consumed. Symptoms of lactose intolerance include bloating, cramps, sharp pains, burning in stomach, nausea, diarrhea, constipation, dark circles under the eyes, achy joints, eczema, ear infections and bedwetting. Skimmed milk has the highest amount of lactose and whole milk has the least. Goat and sheep milks contain lactose yet are more easily digested. Cream and butter have hardly any lactose. The lactose in good quality yogurts purchased at health food stores have been mostly pre-digested by the good bacteria, so some children can handle yogurt but not other forms of dairy. Make sure that you buy the plain yogurt with no sugar or chemicals added and that the label says "active (or) living yogurt cultures". Yogurt that you can purchase at a regular grocery store is not properly fermented therefore the lactose is not broken down, which then impedes digestion.

The most common protein found in cow's milk is casein. Casein is not water-soluble and therefore, is hard to break down. Casein is a tough protein substance so strong and sticky that it is often used to make bookbinding glue and postal paste. Imagine what this stuff does to your bowels? Casein's molecular structure is nearly identical to that of gluten. **Here's the shocking piece of information. Casein is an ingredient used in all cheese substitutes! If you react to dairy and you decide to try the alternatives such as rice, soy or vegetable cheese and find that you are still reacting, it is because of the casein! Casein is a huge concern and simply has not been given the press that lactose has.**

Whey protein is water-soluble and is the most easily digested protein in milk. Whey is found in imitation milk products and other dairy substitutes, cream soups, soup mixes, many types of margarine, and pastries and cookies. Whey is added to many processed foods to improve their nutritional content. It is often used in protein shakes. It is a by-product of the cheese making process. Those that react strongly to dairy are likely to react to whey.

Lactalbumin or lactalbumin phosphate contains concentrated milk protein. This causes a strong reaction in those that are sensitive or allergic to milk.

Although pasteurized cow's milk is high in calcium, it is so difficult to digest that we really cannot consider it to be a good calcium source. It is also high in phosphorus, which binds to calcium, making it unabsorbable. The calcium is then lost in the urine. To prove that the calcium in milk is not being well digested, I invite you to consider this fact. In North America, we are the largest consumers of cow's milk and animal products. We also have the highest rate of osteoporosis in the world. ***There are far better absorbed sources of calcium than dairy (You will find those sources further on in this chapter).***

Today's cow's milk is also deficient in vitamins B1, C, E, and A. It prevents iron absorption. Given the ratio of calcium to magnesium, frequent milk drinkers can develop a magnesium deficiency. This deficiency causes children to have trouble sleeping, become constipated, irritable or anxious, and suffer muscle cramps, spasms or an irregular heartbeat.

Cow's milk is also **mucus producing**, causing mucus to build up in the body. Children that are full of mucus have recurring stuffy or runny noses, coughs, colds and flu, headaches, and ear and throat infections. This is also due to the improper ratio of calcium to magnesium in cow's milk.

As if that is not enough, cow's milk contains residues of growth hormones, used to ensure that cows produce five to six times more milk than untreated cows

> The *Tao of Detox* states, "…and in growing children these bovine growth factors can cause abnormal development, causing excessively rapid growth of tissues. Synthetic bovine hormones in commercial dairy milk, for example, have been indicated as a major factor in premature puberty in young girls."[3]

Girls as young as eight or nine are experiencing full breast development, sexual fertility, and pregnancy.

> Dr. Rona states, "Milk contains sixty percent saturated fat and is a major contributor to the development of atherosclerosis in young children."[4]

> Dr. Weintraub states, "Pasteurised and raw cow's milk contains antibodies of grass pollen, house dust mites, Aspergillus mold, and wheat proteins. There are enough allergens present to cause an allergic reaction in someone sensitive to these substances. The presence of these antibodies is probably because the cow is being exposed to the allergens in the feed: pollen and mold from grain, wheat protein from feed grain, and mites from barns or pastures. Sometimes, it even affects people who are not truly allergic to pollen, dust, mould, or wheat." [5]

An allergy to milk can cause gastrointestinal bleeding, leading to iron-deficiency anemia in infants due to a loss of blood in the stool. If the blood comes from high up in the intestinal tract, it will appear as dark or black and is not readily recognized. This blood loss can go undetected for long periods resulting in iron deficiency in the child.

Additional common complaints linked to the consumption of today's dairy products include acne, anger, irritability, body odour, colic, fatigue, headaches, hives, impaired digestion, obesity, and depression. Cow's milk has also been associated with more serious ailments such as tonsillitis, asthma, respiratory problems, gastrointestinal bleeding with iron deficiency anemia, migraine headaches, attention deficit hyperactivity disorder, Crohn's disease, insulin dependent diabetes, autism, epilepsy and more.

Dairy by another name

The most common dairy foods are cow's milk, butter, cream, sour cream, cottage cheese, cheese, ice cream, sherbet, and yogurt. Milk proteins are also used in food products under a variety of names such as milk solids, buttermilk solids, sour milk solids, milk derivatives, skim milk powder, casein, caseinates i.e. sodium caseinate, whey and albumin. Sometimes milk protein is found in processed meats. Obviously, dairy can lurk in the most unexpected places.

Healthier alternatives to dairy

Cow's milk–Enriched rice, almond, hemp, coconut or soymilk (please read on to learn about soy). If you can't give up cow's milk, please purchase organic cow's milk! If you can find unpasteurized raw cow's milk, even better!

Butter–Coconut oil (similar consistency to butter and doesn't taste like coconut), olive oil or flax oil (cannot heat flax oil). Butter is mostly milk fat and can often be tolerated by children who react to milk. Ghee, also known as clarified butter, is made by skimming off all the white protein particles (milk residue) from melted butter to produce a pure, clear "butter oil". This oil may be used for cooking at high heat without scorching the oil and producing free radicals.

Sour Cream–Sour cream made from soy.

Cream–Coconut milk can be used instead of cream.

Ice cream made from cow's milk–Ice cream made with soy, rice or hemp.

Yogurt made from cow's milk–Sheep, goat or soy yogurt. Kefir yogurt is the healthiest form of yogurt you can buy because the lactose has been broken down by the fermentation process; it also contains a high concentration of live good bacteria. Unfortunately, it is not well liked by most children! Fermented foods are generally high in enzyme and good bacteria content, which is one reason that they are easy to digest.

Cheese–The older and sharper the cheese, the more broken down the lactose and the better tolerated it is. There is also goat cheese (even mozzarella and cheddar) and sheep cheese that are well liked and are better digested than cow's milk cheese. If your child is sensitive to casein, almost all alternative cheeses (i.e.

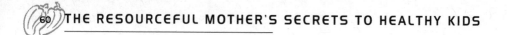

soy, goat, sheep and vegetarian cheese slices etc) contain casein. Many people with a dairy sensitivity can consume goat and sheep products without difficulty. However, both are still mucus forming. Remember: pizza does not need cheese as an ingredient!

Good sources of calcium (better absorbed by the body than dairy products)

Almonds, sesame seeds, dark green leafy vegetables, cauliflower, chickpeas, beans, lentils, brown and wild rice, carob flour, organic dried fruits, eggs, salmon with bones, oysters, grains, blackstrap molasses, and sea vegetables. Watch out for sugar and pop since they deplete calcium stores in the bones!

Red meat

Red meats, such as beef, pork and lamb, are a protein source. They are rich in vitamins B and D and minerals such as iron, zinc and selenium.

The downside of beef is that it can cross-react with milk; they're from the same source. Symptoms caused by consuming red meat are the same as those caused by consuming dairy products. Red meat is a particularly difficult food for humans, in general, to digest. Carnivores have an extremely short intestinal tract so that meat passes through quickly. Humans, however, are modelled after vegetarian animals; we have an intestine that is about 22 feet long. When we eat meat, it can stay in our intestines for up to three days, during which time, it can putrefy and harm our bodies. Over time this constipation can lead to all sorts of ailments. Fatigue is one of the first symptoms that results. Red meat is also inflammatory, full of saturated fat, cholesterol, and often nitrates, preservatives and countless other additives. As a result, red meat actually weakens the immune system.

HEALTH FACT

The downside of beef is that it can cross-react with milk; they're from the same source.

The major problem with virtually all animal products on the market today is the high quantities of drug and chemical residues they contain. Red meats, processed meats and luncheon meats are all treated with nitrates to preserve their red colours (ordinarily they would be grey). When nitrites interact with amino acids they create nitrosamines, which are cancer forming. Beef, pork, lamb and chicken are all heavily treated with antibiotics to stave off infection. Antibiotics stay in the meat when we consume it. Large numbers of hormones, tranquilizers and antibiotics are used to treat cattle and poultry. Hormones are used to make the animals hungrier so that they grow fatter and faster. They are also used to make cows produce more milk. It is common practice to inject certain animals with tranquilizers just before they are slaughtered and to dip certain foods (such as fish) in an antibiotic solution, to prevent them from spoiling. Animals are also fed antibiotics to prevent disease. Meat may be contaminated with sprays, which enter animals' bodies by way of the sprayed feed. In addition, the animals themselves are often sprayed to control flies and other insects.

Healthier alternatives to red meat

Poultry and fish are the very best options for children. If you are going to feed your child red meat, certified organic is best. Cutting the fat off prior to cooking can reduce some of the reactions to red meat.

Good sources of iron

While it is true that red meat is high in iron, there are healthier sources of iron. These include chicken, turkey, cod, flounder, salmon, tuna, almonds, beans, whole grains, broccoli, spinach and molasses. By the way, iron supplements prescribed by medical doctors are generally constipating. Healthier alternatives for children are Dr. Reckeweg's Ferrum Phos or Floravit yeast free liquid iron.

Wheat/Gluten

Most of the beneficial fibre has been removed from refined flour products such as donuts, pasta, cookies and bread so these foods move slowly through the digestive system and wreak havoc on a child's blood sugar levels. Society has caught onto the importance of eating whole grains i.e. whole wheat as opposed to refined flours. Whole grains are loaded with protein, fibre, vitamins (particularly Vitamin B) and minerals. What society hasn't caught onto is that wheat is the grain with the highest gluten content. Gluten is a tough protein substance that makes breads rise. It makes baked goods light and fluffy. There is five times the amount of gluten in wheat today than when wheat was originally grown. Gluten, just like dairy products (remember gluten's molecular structure is nearly identical to casein), is hard to digest and mucus forming. No wonder we are having so many troubles with wheat these days! Other grains that contain gluten are barley, oats, rye, triticale, bulger, and couscous.

Some families have found that switching to organic wheat products has resulted in their children's reactions disappearing. Wheat is one of the most heavily sprayed crops in the world. Recent studies have shown that children who react to wheat may actually be sensitive to the pesticide residues in wheat.

Years ago, a fungus attacked the wheat crops, causing farmers to change the way they made the wheat into flour and this processing of the grain causes reactions in certain individuals. The fact that chlorine and other chemicals are used to sanitize or bleach the flour is a perfect example of what processing can do to the health of a food.

Wheat causes numerous symptoms and conditions, some of which include bloating, irritable bowel syndrome, diarrhea, constipation, inflammatory bowel disease, fatigue, joint pains, headaches, nervousness, depression, ADD, dermatitis, psoriasis, acne, and bedwetting. Removing gluten helps celiac, chrohn's, colitis or any intestinal problems.

Wheat by another name

It really isn't easy identifying wheat in a lot of the ingredient lists of foods, drinks, body products and medicines. Wheat can be called all purpose flour, binder or binding, cereal, cereal binders, cereal protein, couscous, durham, edible starch, farina, filler, flour, food starch, gluten, graham flour, gum base, hydrolysed wheat protein, manna, modified food starch, modified starch, rusk, semolina, special edible starch, starch, thickener or thickening, triticale, white flour and anything with the word 'wheat' in it (except buckwheat which is a member of the rhubarb family and is perfectly safe).

Wheat can also be mixed with other flours such as rye or legume flour. Did you know that whiskey, beer, and other alcoholic beverages often contain wheat?

Healthier alternatives to wheat

Spelt and kamut flours—Ancient relatives of wheat. Spelt contains less gluten than wheat (5–6%) and therefore is more easily tolerated by most people. Kamut contains a different type of gluten, which makes it better tolerated. There is far more goodness found in these flours then in refined flours. Spelt flour is closest to wheat in terms of taste, use and versatility. It is full of fibre, protein and B vitamins. Kamut has a richer taste and is high in protein, amino acids, lipids, vitamins and minerals.

HEALTH FACT

Spelt and kamut flours contain less gluten and are more easily digested.

Brown rice—Unlike white rice, it retains its fibre, B vitamins and healthy oils. It contains no gluten.

Quinoa—Another ancient gluten–free grain that looks like a light brown couscous when cooked. It contains the highest protein and good fat of all the grains and is full of calcium and iron. The grain tastes a little nutty. Remember to rinse it in water before cooking it to get rid of a slightly bitter taste.

Sorghum—A gluten–free flour that generally has a neutral flavour and is sometimes slightly sweet. It is very high in fibre and iron, with a fairly high protein level as well.

Amaranth—A gluten–free flour with a sticky texture. It contains lots of fibre and iron and is great for baking.

Millet, buckwheat, arrowroot, potato, cassava and chickpea—Some of the other least allergenic and healthiest flours your child can eat.

Sprouted wheat breads—Healthier than breads made from the wheat grain. They contain more nutrients per unit than most foods. This is due to the fact that when a grain of wheat is sprouted, it retains all the original nutrients of the wheat berry and is therefore more easily digested than refined wheat. Only those with sensitivities to wheat can try these breads. Those with allergies or celiac disease react to sprouted wheat breads.

Sugar

In its natural state, sugar cane contains B vitamins and many trace minerals including chromium, which helps regulate the amount of sugar in the blood. The sugar to which we are usually exposed acts more like a drug in the body than a food because it has been refined and is devoid of its nutrients. You may notice that your child contracts the flu, cold or ear infections after holidays such as Halloween, Christmas or Easter, when a lot of sugar has been consumed.

> Dr. Zoltan Rona says that, "Sugar hinders the body's immune system and predisposes children to infections and allergies. The shape, activity, and number of white blood cells are adversely affected by heavy sugar consumption. Sugar is the single most underrated cause of immune system impairment." "Sugar is hidden in many commercially available foods. For example, a tablespoon of ketchup contains one teaspoon of sugar. Some soft drinks contain up to twelve teaspoons of sugar per eight ounces. Jellybeans and marshmallows derive one hundred percent of their calories from sugar. Even some unsweetened fruit juices contain the equivalent of ten teaspoons of sugar and should be avoided by diabetics, hypoglycemics, and those with high levels of triglycerides."[6]

> The *Allergy and Asthma Cure* says, "A teaspoon of sugar can suppress your immune system by 56%; 2 teaspoons, by 78%. There are more than 2 teaspoons of sugar in a glass of orange juice."[7]

Consuming sugar and sugar equivalents can cause hypoglycemia (blood sugar problems), which results in symptoms such as anxiety, panic, headaches, sudden fatigue after eating, mood swings, "spacey thinking", behaviour disorders (i.e. destructive and aggressive behaviour, ADD), hyperactivity and a craving for more sugar. Over time, this can lead to chronic fatigue and difficulties learning at school. Stiffness in bones, joints and tissues can also be caused by sugar. Acne, psoriasis or other skin problems can also be related to sugar consumption. Diseases such as diabetes and hypothyroidism come about after years of nutritional deficiency caused by high sugar consumption. Sugar feeds yeast and an overgrowth of yeast is called *candida* (Please see Chapter #3 for more information on candida). Candida and a leaky gut go hand in hand.

In one study, at the University of Sydney in Australia, it was shown that the consumption of dietary sugar contributed to the development of asthma. The children whose airways were hypersensitive to exercise ate 23 percent more sugar than those without breathing problems.

White sugar, white flour products, and candy are all lacking in minerals and must rob minerals from the body tissues in order to be metabolized. When we consume these foods, we lose B vitamins, calcium, phosphorus, iron, and other nutrients. Not only does bacteria touch our teeth but our teeth, storing places for calcium, become weakened as calcium is withdrawn from them internally and thereby become more susceptible to bacterial attack. This "siphoning" effect of sugar is also what lies behind the gnawing hunger it can produce in some people. They are hungry for what is missing—fibre, vitamins, minerals, protein, and water. It can provoke great binges as the sugar eater searches to satisfy it. Excessive sugar consumption is believed to be involved in a host of other very common problems: heart disease, high cholesterol, obesity (excess sugar is converted into fat in the blood), indigestion, crowding and malformation of teeth, dental cavities, lack of concentration, depression, and even violent criminal behaviour.

> In order to understand sugar cravings further, Dr. Skye Weintraub explains, "Diets that are high in sugar increase urinary chromium losses as much as 300 percent. A lack of necessary chromium will manifest itself in a sugar craving. This mineral is necessary to maintain a healthy blood sugar level and contributes to the proper use of carbohydrates and fats. The more sugar eaten, the more chromium the body loses, which makes the body crave more sugar, and so on."
> "A deficiency of protein may also contribute to sweet cravings."[8]

Especially when combined with starch, sugar also causes hypertension, violent behaviour and learning impediments in children. If a child is going to eat sugar, the healthiest way to eat it is to combine it with other foods, which are high in fibre. This food combining slows down the rate of digestion and consequentially its absorption into the blood. Some jam on bread or syrup on a pancake is better than a glass of fruit juice.

Sugar by another name

Sugar is hidden in numerous products that you would find in the grocery store. Even the rice in most sushi contains sugar; it helps to make it sticky. That is why it is important to *always* read ingredient labels. White flour products (white breads, cookies, cakes, donuts, pastries, pasta, pancakes) are not sugar themselves but are converted in the body to simple sugars. Sugar is also called evaporated cane juice, cane juice, dextrose, sucrose, fructose, maltose, lactose, brown sugar, invert sugar, and sorbitol.

Unhealthy alternatives to sugar

Artificial sweeteners are not healthy alternatives to refined sugar. Artificial sweet-eners such as aspartame, increase a child's cravings for sweets and fats. Aspartame is responsible for most of the adverse reactions to food additives. These reactions include headaches, dizziness, seizures, nausea, numbness, fatigue, blurry vision, hearing loss, obesity, diabetes, multiple sclerosis, lupus, mental illness and cancer.

Healthier alternatives to sugar

Healthier forms of sugar contain vitamins, minerals and phyto–nutrients that help regulate blood sugar levels.

Fruit juice–Organic 100% juice naturally contains sugar and is an excellent sweetener.

Organic maple syrup–Unfortunately formaldehyde is used in the processing of regular syrup.

Raw, unpasteurized honey–This pure form of honey has many healing qualities. It is an antiseptic, antioxidant and antibacterial.

Agave nectar–Great alternative to honey as agave nectar tastes and looks like honey. This nectar comes from the agave plant in Mexico and is rich in iron, calcium, potassium and magnesium. Agave is low on the glycemic index.

Date sugar–Made from dehydrated dates and is therefore high in nutrients. It doesn't dissolve in liquids.

Molasses–Unsulphured, black molasses is best. It is a by–product of sugar cane. It is rich in nutrients, particularly iron, calcium and potassium. It is helpful in healing sore joints.

Sucanat–This is evaporated cane juice. It has a low glycemic index score. It is darker than white sugar because it retains most of its vitamins and minerals. It helps baked goods have a crunchier consistency.

Stevia–A powdered or liquid extract from the leaves of stevia plants. It is the healthiest alternative and is suitable for diabetics. It has no effect on blood sugar and contains no calories. Many don't like the taste of it however, because it is so much sweeter than sugar.

Brown rice syrup–This is rice starch that has been converted to syrup. It is thicker and less sweet than other liquid sweeteners. It is best used in puddings.

Xylitol–This sweetener comes from fruits and vegetables and is suitable for diabetics.

Soy

Soy contains more protein than any of the other legumes (beans, peas, lentils and peanuts) and is low in saturated fat. Soy is rich in fibre, complex carbohydrates, vitamins and minerals, such as calcium and iron. Soy can reduce bad cholesterol and heart disease.

North America became really excited about soy in the 1960s and began using it in far too many products. Most people do not even know when they are consuming soy. It is often used in fillers and additives in processed foods. Genetically modifying soy caused many of the problems that arose from the food. Even if you purchase organic soy, it is estrogenic which means it can disrupt the hormones and is more harmful to boys than girls. Even children can end up with thyroid issues. Other symptoms of a reaction to soy include digestive challenges, bloody diarrhea, skin rashes, colic, ear infections, attention deficit disorder, premenstrual syndrome or endometriosis in teens.

> "Researchers in New Zealand found that soy beans can adversely affect hormonal development in infants and recommend caution using infant soy formula. Another study associated the development of autoimmune thyroid disease with soy formula."[9]

Asian populations, known to be very healthy, are reputed to consume a lot of soy. However, soy is consumed more as a condiment than as a replacement for animal foods and is usually in its fermented or really well cooked form, which is better digested and much healthier.

Organic soy products should only be consumed a maximum of two or three times a week. Important fact: Soy sauce contains wheat (unless labelled wheat–free)!

Healthier forms of soy
Fermented soy products such as tempeh and miso are easier to digest and are not estrogenic. Tamari sauce is soy sauce without wheat. Shoyeh is a newer soy sauce and is more pure than tamari sauce.

Yeast
Yeast is a type of fungus. Foods that rise often have yeast as an ingredient. Many children react to commercial yeast especially if they were born with candida (See Chapter #3) or acquired it over time.

Yeast is found in:
- Enriched flour, nutritional yeast, active dry yeast or any type of yeast
- Any edible fungi such as mushrooms, since they are molds themselves
- Any food that is fermented or contains a product of fermentation
- Any alcoholic drinks, brewed beverages, malted beverages or foods, Bovril, stock cubes,
- Overripe or moldy fruit i.e. melons (Cantaloupe also contains some of the same proteins as ragweed)

Grapes, in addition to being exposed to chemical pesticides, develop yeast on the skin that can stimulate yeast infection in the intestine!

Healthier alternatives to yeast
Eggs, baking powder, baking soda and sourdough culture (wild yeast as opposed to commercial yeast) are easier to digest.

Corn

Corn is a good source of fibre and builds bone and muscle. It is a brain food and is good for the nervous system. However, corn can be hard to digest. Today's corn is heavily sprayed with pesticides. It is also genetically modified, which changed it from an ear the size of your palm to the seed–bearing hulk grown on modern farms today. The processing of corn begins with soaking it in a sulphur dioxide solution to prevent fermentation. This tampering is what causes so many of the sensitivities and allergies to corn.

Corn is also used in over 130 products found in your grocery store at any one time and you know now that overuse causes reactions to foods. For example, there are many sugars that come from corn. Corn syrups are a result of using enzymes or acids on cornstarch to make it sweeter. Corn syrups are a major contributor to weight gain, particularly in the stomach area. Corn syrups are found in infant formula, maple, nut, and root–beer flavourings, ice cream, candy, and baked goods. Dextrose is corn sugar, which is often blended with white sugar and found in many artificial sweeteners. The fructose that is found in many food products comes from corn, cane or beet sugar, not from fruits, as you would assume. Glucose is commercially processed sugar derived from cornstarch. Since it is not very sweet, you could eat a large quantity without being aware of its presence in food. Glucose is a flavour found in ground–meat dishes, luncheon meats, and in maple syrup. Candy makers like to use glucose because it gives hard candies a clear appearance. One of the main sources of Sorbitol is dextrose. Even Xylitol, the latest "healthy" form of sugar can come from corncobs, peanut shells or wheat straw, all common allergens!

Reactions to corn include fatigue, hyperactivity, skin rashes, heart palpitations, joint pain, excessive gas, headaches, stomachaches and foot cramps.

Citrus fruits

Citrus fruits include oranges, grapefruits, lemons and limes. All of these fruits are stacked high in vitamins, minerals (including calcium) and fibre. These fruits are extremely healthy for us. However, the very large quantities of citric or acidic foods included in our diets and hidden in processed food, make us prone to their sensitivity.

Citric acid is most widely used. Its pleasant, sour, fruity taste makes it a perfect flavouring agent for drinks, candy and many other treats. Malic acid, the major acid in apples is second to citric acid in terms of its use. Both are found in pharmaceuticals as well. Non–organic citrus fruits are also fumigated for pest control.

Our digestive, metabolic and elimination processes sometimes don't deal well with citrus. Children who have stomach cramps may be reacting to the orange juice they are drinking. Those with urinary tract infections may want to avoid citrus fruits as they produce alkaline urine, which encourages the growth of bad bacteria. Citrus fruits can also cause headaches and worsen childhood arthritis.

There is also a condition called "pineapple mouth" or "citrus mouth". Pineapple mouth occurs when pineapple causes burning and redness of the lips and surrounding skin. Citrus mouth has similar symptoms and is caused when a child reacts to the oil (called limonene) found in the skin of citrus fruit, dill, caraway or celery. Limonene is a phyto–nutrient and is what make lemons good for detoxification.

Grapes

I mention grapes because I was really curious why my girls reacted to grapes. Grapes cleanse the body, increase energy, regulate blood cholesterol levels, lower the risk of cardiovascular disease and improve circulation.

Tartaric acid or tartrate, the main acid in grapes, grape juice, grape–flavoured drinks, wine and brandy can cause reactions in children such as headaches, hives, eczema, cramps, diarrhea and many others.

As previously mentioned, grapes are also highly sprayed and can grow yeast on the skin over time, which can cause yeast infections. The immune system of a plant becomes weak over time from always being sprayed with chemicals to ward off mold and fungus. It is a good fruit to buy organic.

High carbohydrate/starch/sugar vegetables and fruits

White potatoes, sweet potatoes, beets, peas, carrots, tomatoes, and corn contain the highest carbohydrate content. Children with candida (See Chapter #3) can react to these fruits and vegetables.

Nuts

Nuts are good sources of protein, fat, fibre, vitamins and minerals, and contain high levels of protease inhibitors, which prevent cancer.

Tree nuts include cashews, walnuts, almonds, macadamia, pecans, filberts, and pistachios, among others. Reactions to tree nuts are on the increase, perhaps because of their frequent use in processed foods and in foods that children like the most such as cakes and cookies.

Peanuts are actually legumes but you would probably expect to read about them in the nut section. Parents are really curious to hear why peanuts are as lethal to some children as they are. **Peanuts are specifically planted in fields where crops are heavily sprayed in order to clean up the soil. It's not the peanuts that are as much of a problem as the toxins that the peanuts absorb!** Also, peanuts and other tree nuts contain aflatoxins, a fungus, which comes about from the spraying of pesticides and fungicides. The spraying prevents the peanut plant from building its own protection against mold and fungus. These alfatoxins produce poisons and must be deactivated by good bacteria in the intestine. As well, the generation of parents whose children are so allergic or sensitive to peanuts, consumed peanut butter on a regular basis. Sandwiches made with peanut butter on its own, or with jam, honey or bananas were part of our staple diet in the seventies and eighties. The more we consume of a food, the greater the incidence of reactions to the food! Finally, peanuts contain saturated fat and lastly, they interfere with your child's essential fatty acid (See Chapter #6) metabolism.

Fresh, unroasted nuts are less susceptible to contamination. Ensure that you purchase organic peanut butter.

Eggs

Eggs are high in protein, vitamins and minerals. Although eggs are known for their cholesterol raising properties, eggs only raise cholesterol in hypersensitive people. Chicken can cross-contaminate with eggs, since they both come from chicken. Therefore a child can react to chicken and eggs.

> While most children react to the protein in the egg white, some react to the yolk protein. According to Dr. William Walsh, "It is best to eat the egg white with the yolk if both are tolerated." "If you purchase nothing else that is organic, please purchase and eat organic eggs when you can. There is a huge difference in the chemical composition between organic and non-organic. Organic eggs contain omega-3 and omega-6 fatty acids in the ratio that nature intended them to have: 1 to 1. Commercially raised eggs contain nineteen times more omega-6 fatty acids than omega-3s. That is what I believe makes commercially raised eggs unhealthy—not the cholesterol in them. If you buy organic eggs, your risk for contracting salmonella is decreased. Salmonella is the primary reason why commercially raised hens are given antibiotics and organic ones are not."[10]

The salmonella related to eggs and chicken is due to the unsanitary conditions the chicken is raised in. Organic eggs come from chickens that are raised healthily and, therefore, are far less prone to bacteria problems. Eggs can also be tainted by the chemicals and additives in chicken feed and by the chemicals added to ensure shell hardness and correct consistency and colour of the yolk.

Eggs are a mucus-forming food. For that reason, they should be limited to three or four a week.

Common adverse reactions caused by eggs include excessive gas, fatigue, joint pain and eczema.

Eggs by another name

On labels, eggs often appear as albumin, globulin, livetin, lysozyme, ovalbumin, ovoglobulin, ovomucin, ovomucoid, ovotransferrin, ovovitelia, ovovitellin, silici albuminate, simplesse, and vitellin.

Alternatives to eggs
Please see Appendix for baking substitutions.

Fish and shellfish
Fish is loaded with protein and good fats, which help prevent multiple symptoms, conditions and disease (See Chapter #6 for more information on good fats or essential fatty acids). However, not even fish is without drawbacks, unless it is a deep-water fish that is very fresh.

Mercury and toxic wastes build up in fish that live close to shore. The larger the fish, the more mercury it may contain because the larger fish eat the smaller fish. The safest fish to consume are pacific cod, herring, mahi mahi, pacific Pollock, tilapia, sardines, anchovy and wild Alaskan salmon. Canned tuna is made from young tuna so is considered safer than tuna steaks.

Many react to the protein in shellfish, called tropomycin. Shellfish may also contain high levels of mercury since mercury is a heavy metal and falls to the bottom of the ocean where shellfish live. The safest shellfish to consume are clams, oysters and scallops.

Fish are the second largest source of mercury toxicity in the world. Dental fillings are the largest source. Having said that, the health benefits of eating fish are too good to ignore. It is still a good idea to eat fish two to three times per week. High quality fish oils have had the mercury extracted and are recommended for every child.

Chocolate
Dark chocolate and cocoa powders are the healthiest forms of chocolate. They contain antioxidants, specifically flavanoids, which help protect the body against toxins and protect the heart. We are all aware of the mood elevating properties of chocolate since it increases serotonin levels in the brain. Chocolate also contains B vitamins and many minerals, particularly magnesium. Cocoa powder contains more magnesium than any other food.

HEALTH FACT

Chocolate cravings may also be a sign of a calcium or magnesium imbalance.

Chocolate contains caffeine, which can cause restlessness, headaches, dizziness, insomnia, and a rapid heart rate. In a child that reacts to chocolate, the food can cause mood problems such as depression, lethargy, and anxiety. As a result of the neurochemical imbalance that is created, a child can have strong cravings for chocolate. When a child becomes a "chocoholic" often his or her body needs more magnesium. If he eats candy bars and other chocolate-containing foods to get more magnesium, it will only create more imbalances. This is because chocolate contains an excessive amount of sugar, which leaches calcium out of the bones, ultimately leading to a greater imbalance of calcium and magnesium. It is better to give your child a calcium and magnesium supplement.

Healthier alternative to chocolate

Carob is a great alternative to chocolate and is available at most health-food stores. It comes from the fruit pod of a Middle Eastern locust tree. Carob contains no caffeine and is naturally sweet. You can purchase it in powdered form or as carob chips. Watch that the carob chips you purchase don't contain sugar or some other ingredient you are trying to avoid.

Raw cocoa nib has twice the antioxidants as regular chocolate. When mixed with honey or agave, it is very tasty. It does not have the bitter taste of roasted chocolate that you find with the semi-sweets or bitter sweets. Organic fair trade chocolate is recommended.

Food Groups

Mucus-forming or inflammatory foods

Most of the foods discussed in this chapter initiate or worsen symptoms by increasing mucus production or inflammation. The most common offenders are dairy and wheat products but some other foods that can make symptoms worse are eggs, chocolate, citrus fruits, seafood, caffeine, alcohol (I mention this because alcohol is found in children's foods!), animal protein, soy, strawberries, melons, chemicals in processed foods, sweets, spicy foods, salty foods and oily or fried foods. These foods can cause or worsen eczema, asthma, stuffy nose, colds, thirst, nausea, diarrhea, headaches or any symptom or condition involving inflammation.

Histamine-containing or histamine-releasing foods

There are certain foods found in regular grocery stores that cause histamines to be released in the body. They are cheese, egg white, milk, shellfish, tomato, chocolate, pork, pineapple, banana, papaya, strawberry, certain nuts, sausages, fish (i.e. tuna), spinach and alcohol (in food). Now you know why there are so many reactions to these foods. The symptoms caused by these foods i.e. nausea, diarrhea, skin rashes, flushing and headaches are indistinguishable from those caused by true food allergies. Therefore these foods are called "false food allergy" foods. If your child does not react to these foods and continues to eat them, it is advantageous to purchase the health food store versions.

> "Distinguishing between a false and true allergy isn't entirely crucial, as the consequences and the treatment are much the same. However, it appears that children with false food allergy may have some underlying deficiency that makes them more susceptible. For example, one study showed that 50 percent of patients with false food allergy are deficient in magnesium. It is also more likely that children will grow out of a false food allergy."[11]

Food Families

Nightshade family

All foods are divided into food families. Nightshade foods cause inflammation and include bell pepper, cayenne, chilli, eggplant, paprika, potato i.e. French fries, tomato, and tobacco. These foods can cause sensitivities, allergies, and sore joints in children and adults. Parents of children with arthritis may want to examine how often their child eats these foods. Again, lack of good bacteria is the underlying reason for a nightshade reaction. Solanine, found in the nightshades, damages the intestinal wall lining which then causes inflammation. The good bacteria protects the intestinal wall from damage and subsequent inflammation.

Cabbage family

Cabbage, cauliflower, broccoli and Brussels sprouts form the cabbage family of foods. These are the gas-producing foods that mothers are told to avoid when breastfeeding. Boiling well or fermenting these foods may allow your child to eat them if he or she reacts to them when they are uncooked but most children are fine with them.

Soft drinks

Soft drinks contain sugar, phosphates, and chemicals. Also, whenever a drink is carbonated, it leaches calcium and then magnesium from the body. Aspartame in diet pop causes 167 symptoms. It affects the nervous system, causes headaches, even seizures, and makes the large intestine more porous, allowing toxins to enter the bloodstream.

Chemicals, Colourings/Food Dyes, Additives, and Preservatives
(Anything on a product's ingredient list that you cannot pronounce!)

Every day, we are exposed to an overwhelming number of chemical contaminants in our air, water, food and general environment. Over 300 foreign chemicals have been identified in human fat. Fat is found in most organs and systems of the body, including the brain and nervous systems. Breast milk also has a high fat component. As a result, chemicals can be transferred to a newborn during one of the most crucial stages of development.

Since they are smaller and their systems are less mature, children are more susceptible to chemicals than adults. Chemicals go into and are stored in the fat of babies and most babies have a lot of fat! Studies indicate that children are not as capable of eliminating these toxins as adults.

Sceptics argue that the chemicals to which we are exposed have all been tested for safety and should have no ill effects. In fact, chemicals used prior to 1960 have never been tested. The tests that are performed are done with single chemicals, never with mixtures. With the mixture of 300 or more chemicals that we may encounter each day, "cocktail effects" could be very important. The way one chemical works with other chemicals in the body is not tested either. To test chemicals, animals are given increasingly larger doses to see how much of the chemical is safe. Scientists then take the average male's weight and extrapolate findings from the animals and apply them to men. Men can tolerate a higher toxic load than women or children because they're larger. Lastly, scientists do not test chemicals on people year after year but people consume chemicals year after year.

HEALTH FACT

Since they are smaller and their systems are less mature, children are more susceptible to chemicals than adults.

Chemicals are used to:
- Lengthen shelf life
- Create new foods i.e. increase variety
- Increase nutritional value with enriched products (synthetic vitamins)
- Improve the perception of flavour (i.e. MSG is a flavour enhancer)
- Make foods easier to prepare
- Make customers happier because products are more consistent

There are literally hundreds of additives used regularly in children's food. Manufacturers know that something brightly coloured, over–sweetened or processed to look like a favourite cartoon character is more likely to appeal to many children. Food additives are a major cause of health problems. They can wreak havoc with a child's immature digestive system, affecting growth, mood, concentration, sleep patterns and overall resistance to infection by overloading a child's system with toxins. This also results in children being more susceptible to sensitivities or allergies. Some children develop Multiple Chemical Syndrome where they cannot tolerate chemicals of any kind.

Most of the chemicals in our food are "anti–nutrients" meaning that they stop nutrients from being absorbed and used. These nutrients are the same ones that encourage healthy development and growth in children and prevent illnesses.

The good news is that the cleaner your child's diet is, the more your daughter or son will notice and dislike the taste of chemicals!

Pesticides

The FDA performed testing and found that the following 11 types of produce have the highest pesticide residue:

1. Celery
2. Grapes
3. Cantaloupe
4. Cherries

5. Peaches
6. Strawberries
7. Apricots
8. Sweet bell peppers
9. Apples
10. Spinach
11. Cucumbers

Washing and peeling can significantly reduce pesticide levels. Buying locally grown and in-season produce also helps as produce is often treated with fungicides for increased shelf life and long-distance distribution. Out of season produce is brought in from Mexico and other countries where the use of pesticides is not regulated. Pesticides like DDT, which have been banned here, are commonly used on their products in large doses.

Sulphites

Sulphur is a major contaminant of our food supply. Sulphur is used to enhance crispness, reduce or prevent spoilage and the discolouration of food during its preparation, storage and packaging. Sulphites are known for causing migraines and triggering asthma attacks in children.

HEALTH FACT

Produce is often treated with fungicides for increased shelf life and long-distance distribution.

A sulphur dioxide solution is used on French fries, potato chips and even freshly cut fruits and vegetables (common examples are apples, peaches and lettuce) in restaurants to stop browning and wilting. Sulphites prevent the black spots on shrimps that normally indicate staleness. Sulphites are also used in wine in order to prevent the fermentation of the wine and inhibit mold, yeast and contaminating bacteria. Even grapes have sulphites sprayed on to inhibit fungus growth on their leaves.

Sulphites are also added to non-organic versions of:
Avocado dip
Beer
Cider
Cod (dried)
Fruit (fresh and dried)
Fruit juices, purees and filling
Gelatin
Potatoes
Salad dressings (dry mix) and relishes
Salads (particularly at salad bars)

Sauces and gravies (canned or dried)
Sauerkraut and coleslaw
Shellfish and seafood
Soups (canned or dried)
Vegetables
Wine vinegar
Wine and wine coolers

MSG

One chemical that is very well known is MSG. It is used to improve the taste of foods. Some children experience headaches, chest pains, diarrhea, blurred vision, fatigue, flushing or stomach aches when exposed to MSG. MSG crosses the blood brain barrier and therefore can cause very severe reactions in children such as behavioural disorders, impaired intellect and brain damage with high doses.

MSG by another name

The following could contain MSG: protein hydrolyse, autolysed yeast extract, flavourings, glutamate, natural flavourings, bouillon, broth, stock, tomato paste, textured protein, whey protein, dried yeasts, yeast nutrients, hydrolysed vegetable or plant protein or hydrolysed soy and yeast. Even spice combinations, used for cooking, can contain chemicals including MSG!

Artificial Colours

Oranges, in particular, are frequently dyed because of the theory that consumers will not buy oranges with green speckles which is how they would look without dyes. As already mentioned, citrus fruits in general are covered in fungicides so it is tricky to tell whether a person is reacting to the dyes or the fungicides.

HEALTH FACT

Most of the chemicals in our food are "anti-nutrients" meaning that they stop nutrients from being absorbed and used.

Non–organic foods that are commonly dyed with artificial colours are:
Crème de menthe (occasionally used as an ingredient in chocolate)
Maraschino cherries and other coloured fruit
Jell–O and gelatin desserts
Mint sauce
Coloured ice cream
Coloured sherbet
Coloured candy
Cookie and pie frostings and fillings
Wieners
Bologna

Cheese
Butter
Oleomargarine
Oranges
Sweet potatoes
Irish potatoes
Root beer
Soft drinks

Cigarette smoke

Cigarette smoke is loaded with chemicals and harmful particles. North American cigarettes contain fungi, sugar and yeast! Second-hand smoke is far more dangerous than inhaled smoke!

> "Exposure to second hand smoke can produce a long list of acute symptoms including shortness of breath, asthma, pneumonia, bronchitis, headaches, fatigue, and irritation of the eyes, nose, throat, and lungs."[12]

Allergies and Holistic Healing cites a German study of 342 children revealing that food allergies are two times more common among children of smokers than among children of non-smokers.

Of course, exposure to cigarette smoke also increases a child's levels of bad bacteria, contributing to his or her overall toxic load.

Chlorine

Chlorine is found in swimming pools, some insecticides, detergents with Clorox, bleaching agents, bleaches and tap water. Chlorine and its chemical compounds can suppress the nervous and immune systems, damage the liver and kidneys, interfere with cell growth, deactivate vitamin C and many enzymes. It destroys good bacteria.

Chlorine can cause skin conditions, constipation, aggression, urinary tract and other infections, colds, and flu in children. It has also been documented as aggravating asthma, particularly in children that frequent public pools.

Fluoride

Fluoride is found in tap water and toothpaste. It can prevent enzymes from working, which means that the enzymes cannot protect your child's body from problematic foods. Fluoride can also deplete antioxidants (vitamins C and E, selenium, and others), which we know are necessary for good health.

Dr. Rona describes, "The case against fluoride:

1. Fluoride is deposited in the bone and soft tissues, where it has the potential to cause serious harm, such as brittle bones and cancer, in later years.

2. Fluoride causes a condition known as fluorosis, which can best be described as opaque white spots on the teeth and brown, ugly teeth. It is a visible sign of fluoride poisoning and indication of permanent damage to the teeth."[13]

He states "Several well-conducted studies show no correlation between the level of fluoride in water and cavities." He also says "The FDA considers fluoride an unapproved new drug with no proof of safety or effectiveness. It also does not consider fluoride an essential nutrient. "[14]

Symptoms caused by chemicals

Chemical exposure is one of the most hidden causes of physical and mental illnesses. Physical illnesses that can be caused by exposure to chemicals are middle-ear infections, sudden infant death syndrome, and damage to the nervous and immune systems. Mental and behavioural symptoms are very common with chemicals. Depression, excessive sleepiness, severe mental confusion, memory loss, learning disabilities, uncontrollable anger, clumsy behaviour, fibromyalgia, Multiple Sclerosis, Lupus, Parkinson's, and Epilepsy can all be attributed to chemicals. Benjamin Feingold and others point out the role of artificial colourings and flavourings in causing hyperactivity. As well, the hyperactive child craves food and drink often leading to obesity, diabetes and the like.

"In 1985, the *Lancet* (a medical journal) reported that of 76 hyperactive children treated with a low-allergen diet, 62 improved and a normal range of behaviour was achieved in 21 of these. Other symptoms such as headaches and fits were often improved. Of the 48 foods incriminated, artificial colourings and preservatives were the most common provoking substances. The study reported that benzoic acid and tartrazine had a bad effect on nearly eight out of the ten children involved."[15]

Something to think about when it comes to chemicals

Imagine you feed your child a Golden Delicious apple that you buy at your local grocery store. Your child eats it and has diarrhea within a few hours of consumption. Is your child reacting to the apple, the particular kind of apple or to the pesticides that were sprayed all over the apple? If your child tries an organic Golden Delicious apple and has no reaction, then you know that he or she has a problem with the chemicals on and inside the apple, as opposed to the apple itself. If the Golden Delicious apple is the problem then even eating an organic Golden Delicious apple will produce a reaction in your child. Don't make the mistake of thinking though that your child is sensitive to all apples. Try a Royal Gala apple on your child; there are more than a dozen different kinds of apples! Many children who react to fruits are not sensitive to the fruit itself but to the chemical pollution of the fruit. Once a fruit or vegetable has been sprayed with chemical solvents, there is no known way of removing the spray residue entirely no matter how much you scrub the fruit. Even peeling the fruit or vegetable doesn't get completely rid of the chemicals that went into the pulp itself. Some children who are not highly sensitive may be able to eat lightly steamed fruit but not raw, fresh fruit because some of the pesticides evaporate in the steaming process.

Remember: If you look at a product and it boasts "no sugar", there are usually chemicals inside.

Vitamins

At one time, vitamins prepared from food sources caused numerous reactions but in recent years, dairy, wheat, corn and sugar have been removed from most vitamins. This is not to say that your child won't react to a particular brand of vitamin. Certain brands of vitamins work better on some children than on others. If you read about vitamins in Chapter #6 and give one of them to your child and the vitamin does not help in the way it is professed to do, try another brand of that vitamin on your child.

Prescription Drugs

In 1928, penicillin was discovered and truly saved lives. Broad-spectrum antibiotics were introduced in the 1940s.

> Dr. Bernard Jensen discussed the challenges with prescribed drugs in his book. "No one imagined that strains of bacteria resistant to the new "wonder drugs" would develop. Nor was it even remotely suspected that uncontrolled use of these miracle medications would result in compromising of the immune system."[16]

In Chapter #1, I talked about antibiotics being the #1 contributor to the growth of bad bacteria, the weakening of the intestinal wall and the development of candida. When did our children become the sickest in history? Around the time antibiotics were introduced, our children started to become increasingly sick.

Some drugs have been highly useful, even lifesaving, but often have been misused and over-prescribed. Some of the more commonly used drugs deplete the body of important vitamins and minerals. It is generally well known that drugs can have serious side effects. Few people realize the complexity of most drugs or the number of ingredients they contain. Medications can cause symptoms such as intestinal upset, rashes, diarrhea, constipation, headaches and more. Aspirin can cause nausea, dizziness, ringing in the ears, and even asthma. A child taking aspirin may bleed more easily because the drug causes changes in the blood.

There are natural healthier alternatives to all of the commonly used drugs that do not deplete the body of good bacteria and nutrients or cause side effects. The quickest way to learn about the alternatives is to speak to your natural health practitioner or knowledgeable health food store employee.

Vaccinations

Many babies are born with no obvious reactions to foods. Then they are vaccinated and suddenly start reacting to a food. Your child's body can be doing just fine until his or her toxic load is surpassed and then all hell breaks loose!

HEALTH FACT

There are natural healthier alternatives to all of the commonly used drugs that do not deplete the body of good bacteria and nutrients or cause side effects.

Vaccinations are an extremely controversial topic. Many parents say to their adult children, "You were vaccinated. You are healthy. Why are you questioning vaccinating our grandchild?" And your answer would be that vaccinations are different today. They are combining vaccinations and giving more vaccinations than ever before without evaluating the side effects of doing so!

"In 1982, pediatricians were giving children 23 doses of 7 vaccines, including vaccines for measles, mumps and rubella. By 2007, the numbers of doses of vaccines the federal government recommended for universal use by age 12 years had more than doubled to 56 doses of 16 vaccines." "More than twice as many American children are suffering chronic brain and immune system dysfunction today than there were in the 1970s and 80s, when half as many vaccines were given to them."[17]

"Vaccines are the only product sold in North America that carry the risk of injury or death and which are legally required to be used by every healthy citizen. Until the late 1980s, few questioned the wisdom of this requirement. However, a growing segment of the population, including many in the alternative health care community, question the wisdom of injecting foreign proteins, aluminium, mercury derivatives, formaldehyde, unknown generic material, and possible contaminants into a child's bloodstream. They worry about the growing number of reports on the association between vaccines and hyperactivity, autism, seizure disorders, chronic ear infections, hearing impairment, diabetes, allergies, asthma, mental retardation, and auto-immune diseases."[18]

The grandson of U.S. Congressman Dan Burton became autistic after being vaccinated for mumps, measles and rubella. This forced the vaccine industry to remove the problematic mercury that was used as a preservative in vaccinations in the spring of 2002. It is my understanding that there are still vaccinations in distribution containing mercury but that all newly made vaccinations, with the exception of the flu and H1N1 shots, are mercury-free.

Other possible side effects of vaccinations include bowel blockage, high-pitched screaming, complete paralysis and death. In my opinion, the risk of your child developing side effects after receiving vaccinations is far greater than the risk that your child will contract one of the diseases that the vaccinations are designed to eliminate.

Your child can be vaccinated against mumps and still contract mumps. It is important to know that vaccinations do not provide permanent immunity from a disease the way contracting a bad case of the chicken pox, for example, does. Also, because vaccinations are injected directly into the body, bypassing the body's natural immune response, the body is deprived of developing its own immunity.

For those of you that believe that vaccinations are necessary for ending disease, how would you explain the fact that scarlet fever disappeared despite the fact that no vaccine or treatment was ever created for it? Epidemic diseases decreased throughout the 1800's, long before vaccinations were invented. Experts attribute the end of epidemic diseases not to mass vaccination, but to major improvements in sanitation.

Now, I am not suggesting that any parent not vaccinate their child without having a plan in place, in the event your child does come down with a serious illness. I am confident that my children's strong immune systems and my classical homeopath will be able to fight any disease to which my girls might be subjected.

If you do your own research on this subject and choose to vaccinate your child, I would highly recommend that you delay the vaccinations as long as possible. Waiting will allow your child's immune system to be stronger and better able to withstand the assault to their immune system that will occur when exposed to vaccinations.

Mothering Magazine is an excellent publication for naturally minded parents. In one of their issues, Barbara Loe Fisher, the cofounder and president of the National Vaccine Information Center (NVIC) and coauthor of an incredible book called DPT: A Shot in the Dark and editor of The Vaccine Reaction newsletter, wrote an article titled "In the Wake of Vaccines" and states "This human intervention is only about 50 years old. When you consider the evolution of human beings and our place in the natural order, an order that was created long before Edward Jenner came up with the idea of vaccination, 50 years is a very short period of time."[19]

Vaccinations are designed for children with healthy immune systems. We have a growing population of children who do not have healthy immune systems. The children who are likely to react adversely to vaccinations are the same children who are prone to allergies, ADD and autism. The children who are likely to react to vaccinations can often be spotted ahead of time. If one or more of the following factors is involved, there is an increased chance of vaccination reactions:

- Mother used antibiotics during pregnancy
- Child has had antibiotics
- Child has projectile vomiting of breast milk (sign of allergy development)
- Oral thrush and yeast problems in child or mother
- History of allergies in parents
- Smoking or alcohol use during pregnancy
- Poor nutrition in mother or child

Alcohol

I like the idea of discussing this because some people wonder why their children have such a problem with potatoes, corn, grapes, wheat, sugar or chemicals. Here are the most common alcohols that parents may have consumed and the foods from which they are made:

Vodka–Potatoes
Brandy–Grapes
Whiskey–Wheat, barley or corn
Beer–Nutritional yeast, sugar, chemicals
Wine–Nutritional yeast, sugar, chemicals and grapes

Alcohol increases holes in the intestine i.e. leaky gut. The types of alcohol that are most hazardous to our health are the fermented kinds, which are beer and wine–not the hard liquors. Not only is the processing of beer and wine unhealthy but all sorts of chemicals are added to these drinks. The distillation process used in making distilled liquor completely eliminates all of the toxic by–products of fermentation. So vodka and brandy, with a clear appearance, have higher alcohol content than beer or wine, but they are healthier and are generally consumed in smaller amounts than their alternatives. Also of note, the lighter spirits are less likely to cause hangovers than darker spirits!

If you or your spouse consumed a lot of alcohol over the years, your child can be born reacting to the foods that were used in the making of your favourite drinks. Also, because alcohol greatly contributes to but is never the sole cause of candida and/or a leaky gut, your child can be born with candida and/or a leaky gut if you or your spouse drank a lot of alcohol over the years. Alcohol itself can be an ingredient in children's foods as well, particularly in chocolate.

An important concept to understand

You've just read about all of the problems with the foods available at our grocery stores, problems that did not exist with food when our grandparents were being raised. You might be sitting there now trying to wrap your head around the idea that foods, considered nourishing for our bodies, are capable of producing such major illnesses. You may even blame the farmers, food manufacturers, government and who knows who else for the ill health of our nation.

HEALTH FACT

Experts attribute the end of epidemic diseases not to mass vaccination, but to major improvements in sanitation.

Whatever you do, do not blame yourself or even worse, your child, for the fact that he or she does not have healthy intestinal and digestive system. Remember, it is predominantly what is being done to food and other human interventions that have created the health imbalances in the children of today.

How to make the best use of this chapter's information

1. Read about all or just some of the common foods to which many North Americans are reacting.
2. You are probably becoming clearer on determining the foods to which your child is reacting or the foods you are going to start eating less of.
3. Now you know the healthier alternatives and can go to any health food store, that sells food, to learn more about these alternatives.
4. Read on to further develop your understanding of food's impact and how to integrate healthier alternatives into your family's lifestyle.

CHAPTER 3

THE DIRTY LAUNDRY LIST

Symptoms, Conditions and Disease Caused by Reactions to Food

"When health is absent, wisdom cannot reveal itself, art cannot manifest, strength cannot fight, wealth becomes useless, and intelligence cannot be applied." Herophilus[1]

Dr. Rona states, "When I first started general practice in 1978, childhood asthma, hay fever, hyperactivity and eczema were relatively uncommon... In the 1980's, however, I saw a growing number of children with chronic illnesses, recurrent infections and other puzzling health conditions such as chronic fatigue syndrome."[2]

It wasn't until the 1990's, that epidemics of altered immunity, food and chemical sensitivities, environmentally induced illness, depression, chronic headaches, joint and muscle disorders, diabetes, mood, behaviour and memory problems became rampant.

Simply because these symptoms and conditions are common does not mean we should view them as normal. Our children are suffering needlessly. These medical problems are usually preventable and treatable by consuming natural, alive and good quality foods. Food fights disease.

In this chapter, I am going to elaborate on some of the symptoms and conditions that can be triggered or worsened by lack of good bacteria and specific foods. Whole books have been written on each of the symptoms and conditions. Certainly, I have done far more research on most of these topics than what you see here. My desire is simply to alert you to the link between food and childhood ailments so that you can go on to do further research if you so desire.

You will notice that the main offenders for all symptoms, condition and disease are the common allergens previously listed! Chapter #6 will provide you with further detailed information on how to feed your child in order to reduce or eliminate all of the symptoms discussed in this chapter. You will also notice that a number of ailments can be caused or worsened by insufficient good bacteria/dysbiosis, candida, hypoglycemia, parasites and low stomach acid. There is a full description and methods for healing each of these conditions at the end of this chapter.

Remember, as long as children are reacting to foods, and we, as adults, pay attention and make the changes necessary to help them, society benefits as a whole.

Physical Symptoms

Chronic Ear Infections

"Middle ear infection affects two thirds of children in the United States by the age of two and is the most common cause of acquired hearing loss in children. Allergies to milk and other common foods and the frequent and indiscriminate use of prescription antibiotics are the root cause of most infections in children, especially middle ear infections." "Furthermore, infants and children who are frequently prescribed antibiotics for middle-ear infections have been noted to have a much higher incidence of both hyperactivity and autism."[3]

Mucus forming, inflammatory foods or foods to which your child is sensitive or allergic, all increase fluid in the ear by creating nasal congestion. The fluid from the back of the nasal passages should move easily to the ear but when there is enough congestion, it gets blocked and the fluid sits in the ear. Bacteria then starts to multiply and ear pain and fever eventually occurs. Children under the age of 6 are most susceptible to these infections because their Eustachian tubes are more horizontal than those of older children and adults, making drainage of fluids more difficult. Antibiotics increase the bad bacteria or yeast in the body and can, therefore, cause further ear infections. If your child does take antibiotics, probiotics (See Chapter #6) should be given to him or her at the same time and for two weeks after the course of antibiotics ends in order to put the good bacteria back into his or her body.

When common allergens (e.g. dairy, wheat, sugar and refined carbohydrates, peanuts, corn and eggs) are avoided, more times than not, there is a large improvement in the ears and hearing of children and the amount of fluid in the ears decreases significantly.

A natural remedy for helping ear infections: Put a couple of drops of olive oil with a little pureed garlic (the size of a pea) into your child's ear right before bed and let them sleep with this natural anti-inflammatory solution overnight. The garlic and oil penetrates the eardrum, settles the pain and kills infection.

Skin infections/Diaper rash/Eczema

Rashes are an attempt to get rid of toxins that are not properly eliminated by the body. The skin is an elimination organ. If the body cannot dispose of the toxins, the skin will break out in a rash in an attempt to rid the body of waste.

Eczema is a painful and itchy inflammatory skin eruption, which can occur on any part of the body. It often begins in infancy with dry patches or a rash on the cheeks, face and lower arms. It may begin as a diaper rash. As children get older, the inflammation spreads, affecting the hands, the wrists, and the creases in front of the elbows and behind the knees. The neck and ears are other affected areas. The nature of eczema is to change location on the body.

Remember I explained that symptoms lead to conditions? Eventually eczema can lead to asthma.

Food reactions are often involved with eczema and other factors can also play a role.

The most common causes of rashes/eczema include:
- Food sensitivities or allergies (e.g. wheat (#1), dairy (#2), soy, sugar (even the sugar in fruit can worsen chronic eczema in children), eggs, chocolate, nuts, strawberries, oranges, tomato, grapefruit, grapes, potatoes, soy, dark pop, peanuts, animal products)
- Environmental sensitivities or allergies (e.g. pollen)
- Coffee, tea and alcohol consumed by breastfeeding mothers
- Nutritional deficiencies
- Digestive abnormalities, including low stomach acidity, low enzyme levels, candida and insufficient good bacteria
- Stress and emotional factors

> "A study of more than two thousand children showed that feeding them cow's milk during the first nine months resulted in seven times more frequent complaints of eczema afterward."[4]

Diaper rash specifically, is often caused from the stool passing through the anus with a high concentration of allergens, causing irritation and burning of the skin. When there is only urine in the diaper yet there is a rash, this is a result of excess ammonia in the urine caused by incomplete protein metabolism or an overly acidic diet on the part of the mother or baby e.g. citrus fruits, tomatoes. Even if there is just a red circle of inflammation around the anal opening, it is usually due to a reaction to food or medicine.

The location of a rash is often important to determining the cause. If the rash is on the back of the arms and it never leaves the back of the arms, the cause is usually environmental. In contrast, red cheeks are caused from food.

To optimize skin health, your child needs to consume a natural diet. This includes no chemicals, processed foods, junk foods, caffeine or sugar. Animal products, including dairy and eggs, contain fats that aggravate skin problems. They may also be loaded with drugs such as antibiotics, steroid hormones, nitrates, nitrites and other artificial ingredients. Steroid creams, incidentally, can thin the skin and encourage the growth of candida.

Natural remedies for helping the skin: Aloe vera gel, a good quality calendula ointment and Candigen cream by Genestra can be applied topically. There is a natural alternative to cortisone cream called Derma Med that can be found at the health food store as well. Supplementing with probiotics and essential fatty acids (See Chapter #6 for more information) helps all skin conditions. Vitamin E ointment or oil prevents and heals scarring. Humidity and salt water are very helpful which is why eczema often improves in the summer. In winter months, humidifiers, solar lights, salt rinses and vitamin D can be of great help.

Colic/Excessive gas

In babies, colic appears to be the equivalent of indigestion.

The most common causes of colic include:
- Insufficient good bacteria
- Beginning of food sensitivities and/or allergy formation
- Mother ingesting cow's milk (Dairy, particularly cow's milk, is the leading problematic food)
- Nutritional deficiencies such as B vitamins, calcium, potassium or magnesium
- Calcium/Magnesium imbalance. Calcium (dairy) without magnesium can cause colic, especially in bottle fed babies (Mothers usually provide enough magnesium in their breast milk). If the body is low in magnesium, it upsets the calcium balance. This can cause muscle spasms in the stomach, causing colic.

As a rule, the baby experiencing colic after three months is suspect of food allergies, not just sensitivities. Others symptoms that would indicate allergies in an infant are acting hungry all the time, having excessive gas, spitting up, diarrhea or constipation.

Crying, colic and night waking are only a tiny portion of the range of symptoms that parents report disappearing after making dietary changes.

One aspect of colic that is difficult to explain is the fact that the symptoms tend to disappear or diminish around three months of age. One possibility is that the colic represents an initial "crisis" reaction as the child is exposed to cow's milk, and other ingredients in formula or foods consumed by mother and passed on through breast milk. The child later "adapts" to the problem foods and the colic apparently clears up but its sensitivity continues in the form of other symptoms, such as eczema, constipation or diarrhea.

According to Dr. Doris Rapp, if a mother smoked or smokes cigarettes or a baby is exposed to cigarette smoke, the baby will be more prone to colic.

Natural remedies for helping colic: Hyland's colic tablets and chamomile homeopathic pellets or tea.

Diarrhea

In diarrhea, soft, loose or semi-liquid stools are passed several times a day. There is usually a sense of urgency and often a child feels unwell. Diarrhea is basically a means of ridding the body of toxins, harmful bacteria or unwanted substances.

The most common causes of diarrhea include:
- Food sensitivities or allergies
- Infections
- Parasites or candida
- Poor food hygiene (food that has been kept for a long time causing "food poisoning")
- The natural laxative effect of some fruits (prunes, figs, rhubarb, avocado, pears)
- Celiac, crohns, ulcerative colitis, malabsorption, psychosomatic reaction, intense stress, or cancer.

For those with chronic diarrhea and no pain (one form of irritable bowel syndrome/IBS), food sensitivities are worth investigating, especially if there is bloating and gas as well. Again, it is muscle spasms that are behind diarrhea and cramps. Changing a child's diet usually alleviates the effects of a spastic colon. Some studies have shown that as many as 70% of IBS sufferers have food sensitivities. The IBS of some is made worse by eating bran, suggesting a sensitivity to wheat or other grains.

Multi-vitamins, mineral complexes and acidophilus (See Chapter #6 for more information) are paramount after diarrhea, in order to get the nutrients and good bacteria back into the body that diarrhea has washed away.

Foods for helping diarrhea: Bananas, rice, and applesauce.

Fatigue

Fatigue is the most common complaint that doctors hear today. In addition to feeling tired, symptoms of fatigue include headache, irritability and indigestion.

The most common causes of fatigue include:
- Food and chemical sensitivities or allergies are the #1 cause of fatigue, particularly to dairy, wheat, yeast and eggs
- Too many chemicals or too much caffeine
- Chocolate, sugar i.e. sweetened cereals and candy bars, white flour products

i.e. cakes and cookies and other junk foods. Refined carbohydrates weaken or shut down the immune system as early as one hour after eating them.
- Lack of protein
- Insufficient water intake
- Insufficient good bacteria, hypoglycemia, candida or parasites

Excessive tiredness that is not relieved by rest can be caused by depression, an infectious disease, anemia, under-active thyroid gland or a virus. It is often caused by food sensitivities especially in connection with migraines and IBS. Early morning tiredness is the most frequent problem. How food might produce fatigue is not yet known, but exorphins may play a part or it may be a side effect of some generalized immune reaction.

Natural remedies for helping fatigue: A multi-vitamin and mineral complex. As well, instead of reaching for sugar, encourage your child to reach for a protein source (See Chapter #6). Eating small portions every 2-3 hours and drinking more water can also make a big difference.

Headaches

We already learned that fatigue is considered the most frequent symptom of a food reaction. Headaches run a close second.

The number one cause of headaches and migraines is reactions to food. The most common foods reported to be involved in headaches and migraines are milk, cheese, chocolate, citrus foods, bananas, peanuts, pork, egg and caffeine. Any food or chemical sensitivity can trigger a headache or migraine.

Pre-headache symptoms in children include lethargy, loss of appetite and abdominal discomfort. Pre-headache symptoms and migraines are of shorter duration in children than in adults. However, nausea is more intense in youngsters and the frequency of attacks is much greater. As a child gets older, the abdominal discomfort decreases while the headaches intensify. At approximately 12 years of age, symptoms become more like those of adults. Does your child have allergic headaches? Look for wrinkling of the forehead, restlessness, holding or rubbing of the head and crying. During childhood migraines, a child may have a fever.

Migraines are related to blood vessel spasms in the head caused by inflammation. The resulting restriction of blood flow denies nutrition and oxygen to the brain and eyes. The subsequent decrease in energy and oxygen produces the vision changes and numbness that are commonly behind migraines.

Natural remedies for helping headaches: Cooking with a little cayenne pepper helps circulation. Magnesium and water helps. Magnesium helps to relax the muscles. Water hydrates the body and helps to keep toxins moving. Headaches are connected to an imbalance in the liver so increasing foods that are healthy for the liver i.e. lemon in water, berries and green leafy vegetables help open up the veins. The herb, white willow bark is a natural form of aspirin that relieves headaches naturally but does not address the root cause of the headache. It comes in capsules and can be opened into your child's food or swallowed with water.

Bloating
Causes of bloating:
- Food sensitivities (wheat and other grains are the worst culprits)
- Too much salt intake
- Not enough water
- Insufficient good bacteria, candida or parasites if the bloated area is the stomach
- Eating too quickly
- Poor food combining (See Chapter #5)

Natural remedies for helping bloating: Probiotics, aloe vera juice, peppermint tea and digestive enzymes (See Chapter #6 for more information).

Muscle aches and pains
Aches and pains in the muscles of the lower and upper back, neck and shoulders are especially linked to diet and allergic reactions. Enough said!

Natural remedies for helping muscle aches and pain: The homeopathic remedy Arnica or the herb white willow bark (purchased in powdered capsules that can be opened) can relieve pain on a temporary basis.

Joint pain
Inflammation or swelling of the joints is the cause of joint pain. The most frequent culprits for joint pain are dairy, wheat, egg, corn and pork. Sugar can cause pain in the knees and hands. Oranges can cause apprehension and depression followed by joint pain. Foods from the Nightshade family are other offenders (Please see Chapter #2 for a list of those foods). Lack of water contributes to joint pain as well. Joint pain may not appear for 42 to 72 hours after exposure to the problematic food.

Natural remedies for helping joint pain: The homeopathic remedy Arnica or the herb white willow bark (purchased in capsules that can be opened) can relieve pain on a temporary basis. Increasing foods that are healthy for the liver i.e. lemon in water, berries and green leafy vegetables also help alleviate joint pain.

Nausea
The most common causes of nausea include:
- A food sensitivity can cause nausea and indigestion although this is rarely the sole symptom. It seems that if the food affects the stomach in this way,

then it affects the digestive system as a whole, so there is usually diarrhea or other bowel symptoms, as well.

- Unwise eating habits are connected to nausea–eating too much, too quickly, eating while anxious, excited, angry, upset or tense, eating standing up, rushing about after a meal, eating late at night or having too much rich food.
- Second hand smoke
- Acidic food
- Spicy food
- Too much oil and fat
- Parasites
- Taking too many supplements at once or on an empty stomach

Natural remedy for helping nausea: Coccolus is the homeopathic remedy that helps eliminate nausea on a temporary basis.

Stomachaches

Stomachaches in children can be caused by:
- Food sensitivities
- High amount of carbohydrates (especially lots of juice)
- Calcium and/or magnesium deficiency (helps all muscles i.e. stomach)
- A certain make of probiotics not agreeing with your child or too much at once (See Chapter #6 for more on this)
- Parasites or candida

Natural remedies for helping stomachaches: Peppermint tea and a castor oil compress.

Sore throat (Pharyngitis, Laryngitis, Tonsillitis)

Whenever you see "itis" at the end of any word, it means "inflammation" or "swelling". If the swelling of blood vessels centers in the vocal cords, it can cause hoarseness and loss of voice. This can lead to a chronic cough and persistent throat clearing. If the swelling is at the back of the throat, it can cause a recurrent sore throat, swelling of the tongue, lips or membranes in the mouth, as well as nasal stuffiness.

Tonsillitis is a warning that the body is overwhelmed by the need to eliminate waste materials. When the tonsils become inflamed or enlarged, it is an indication that the body is trying to get rid of an overload of waste material. The tonsils excrete waste material into the pharynx area, where it is swallowed and then passed out with bowel movement, if all is working smoothly. Removing the tonsils compromises the elimination system in the body because it forces other excretory pathways to do the same job the tonsils once did.

Sore throat, difficulty swallowing, burning sensation, hoarseness, and loss of voice or Tonsillitis can all be caused by foods, particularly dairy and wheat.

Natural remedies for helping sore throats: Zinc lozenges, Vitamin C, warm water with honey and/or lemon, and chamomile tea reduce inflammation.

Bed-wetting

"Recent statistics show 20% to 25% of children are still affected by bed-wetting at the age of six."[5]

Bed-wetting is extremely common in children. When this occurs, it's time to look into matters further. The bladder is very sensitive to foods, especially proteins. Proteins cause swelling in the lining of the bladder (the overall size of the bladder remains the same), which decreases the capacity of the bladder and increases the frequency of urination and bedwetting.

A good percentage of these children have a case history of recurrent middle ear infections and have been treated repeatedly with antibiotics. Yeast infections or local infection of the urethra is also common in many children who bed-wet.

"In 1959, an exhaustive study of bed-wetting was conducted which showed that from 83% to 90% of all primary nocturnal (bed-wetting) could be controlled by the control of food allergens. In this study, the reactive foods in order of their frequency were milk–60%, wheat–20%, egg–20%, corn–15%, orange–15%, chocolate–15% and pork, tomato, peanut, seafood, and cinnamon–5%."[6]

Refined sugar products are other culprits.

Natural treatment for bed-wetting: Remove the foods that your child may be reacting to and then determine if your child has hypoglycemia and/or candida and treat (Please read further on).

Common Cold

This is the most commonly experienced sickness in children. As a result, catching a cold is the main way in which children build their immune systems. The common cold can be attributed to many factors. Children can pick up a virus from others. Children who are always coming down with colds or who have a hard time shaking colds are actually depleting their immune systems. These children are often eating foods to which they are sensitive or they have nutritional deficiencies. When a child's body in not eliminating toxins properly, the immune system tries to drain the body of excess mucus and toxins through coughing, a runny nose, sneezing and sweating from fever.

"Recurrent respiratory tract infections have been linked to the frequent ingestion of dairy products, wheat, artificial additives, and chemicals such as MSG."[7]

Mucus-forming foods are a major cause of colds and are responsible for their lengthy duration. In a child with a healthy immune system, colds should only last one or two days and then your child should be back at it!

When you give your child drugs such as antihistamines or decongestants, you only suppress their symptoms and prevent the elimination of toxins.

Natural remedies for preventing and treating colds include: Eliminating or minimizing the amount of dairy, wheat and sugar that your child is consuming. Adding Vitamin C powder i.e. ascorbic acid and bioflavonoids (See Chapter #6 for more information on why this works) to your child's all natural juice or adding zinc drops to your child's water. Lemon in water is also helpful, along with lots of fluids to flush out the toxins. Eucalyptus in your child's room at night helps too. You can help your child eliminate mucus and toxins further by giving them a green drink (See Appendix) or adding chlorella to his or her water. Drinking lots of purified water, herbal tea, and very diluted fruit juice also aids their recovery.

Asthma

When the airway muscle is functioning normally, it contracts and relaxes, calmly directing the flow of air. During an asthma attack, the airway muscle spasms and the blood vessels swell, causing the airway to narrow, restricting the flow of air through the lungs. This is what causes the wheezing, breathing difficulties, laboured breathing, shortness of breath, panting and excess bronchial mucus that characterize asthma.

The inflammation causing these symptoms can stem from reactions to foods or chemicals. Dietary improvements can control muscle spasms the same way they control the blood vessel swelling in the lining of the airway. If your child seems to develop wheezing within one to four hours after eating a certain food (especially if it happens on more than one occasion), it is not a coincidence!

"The link between allergies and asthma has been completely substantiated. It is very hard to discuss one without the other...78% of all those diagnosed with asthma have allergies."[8]

Irritants that may trigger an asthma attack include:
- Foods (e.g. Dairy, wheat, oranges, bananas, sugar, eggs, shellfish, nuts, chocolate and other inflammatory foods)
- Chemicals i.e. dyes, sulphites, preservatives, MSG

- Children's aspirin or other drugs
- Air pollution
- Aerosol sprays
- Perfumes
- Animal dander
- Dust mites
- Molds
- Pollens
- Cold outdoor temperatures
- Exercise
- Heredity
- Obesity
- Respiratory and sinus infections
- Viruses
- Cigarette smoke
- Stress
- Thunderstorms

Natural remedies for helping with asthma: Children with asthma need to consume enough good fats, such as flax seeds or fish oils, which are anti-inflammatory. Probiotics are also essential for reestablishing a healthy balance between good and bad bacteria. Limiting sugar is essential to counteracting candida and boosting the immune system. Minimizing saturated fats and animal products is helpful because of their inflammatory properties. Vitamin C with bioflavonoids, along with onions and garlic are natural antihistamines and antioxidants. Quercitin, often combined with the Vitamin C, stabilizes mast cells. Magnesium relaxes the body. Asthma attacks are highly correlated to lack of magnesium, which breaks down mucus. Lots of filtered water loosens the stuffiness.

Having eczema as an infant is a strong indicator of asthma risk as a child or an adult.

Overweight/Obesity

"26% of Canadians aged 2 to 17 are now overweight or obese–more than double the rate 30 years ago."[9]

There is a large percentage of overweight children and adults in our society. Many are severely overweight. The North American diet typically consists of over-processed, nutrient-deficient foods. Children who eat a diet of pre-prepared, chemical laden, and low fibre foods, are often overweight and at risk of heart disease, as well as, many other degenerative diseases. Obviously, children lacking in proper exercise are even more at risk.

Common causes of overweight children include:
- Food sensitivities i.e. dairy, wheat, sugar
- Poor digestion and malnutrition
- Water retention
- Eating too much junk food
- Overeating healthy food

'Eating the wrong foods' is the phrase I use to encompass all of these causes of obesity. The next paragraph details what I mean by this. Of course, lack of exercise and stress are other major contributors to obesity.

Being overweight, malnutrition, cravings and food sensitivities are all intertwined. Here is why:

1. Some children, who are lacking certain nutrients or are malnourished, eat more than usual because their bodies are continually searching for the vitamins and minerals their bodies need. If the foods a child is given are lacking in vitamins and minerals, this pattern will continue until a child is given nutrient rich foods.

2. If the foods that a child is given are foods to which he or she reacts, he or she cannot absorb the vitamins and minerals from that food and the child will keep eating in hopes of obtaining those nutrients.

3. A malnourished child will often lack energy so he or she might crave sugar or baked goods made with white flour, subconsciously knowing that these foods will get the blood sugar levels up fast. The more sweets a child consumes, the greater his or her nutritional deficits become. The more sensitive a child becomes to the sugar, the more sugar he or she craves. Therefore, the more the child eats, the more overweight they become. A child could crave any food; sugar and refined carbohydrates are the biggest culprits for overweight children and that is why I used them as examples. Eating whole foods in the natural state has been shown to be the fastest way to eliminate cravings.

4. Food sensitivities can be responsible for edema or swelling in the hands, feet, stomach, face (particularly around the eyes), ankles or the whole body. This buildup of liquid can be erroneously perceived as excess fat. Some adults can diet and not lose much weight. When this happens, often the individual is continuously eating a food to which they are sensitive. Removing problematic foods from a child's diet may cause a child to lose weight. Wheat or other glutenous grains, as well as chemicals, are two of the biggest causes of edema.

5. When the body is reacting to food, the metabolic rate of the body slows down, compromising thyroid and adrenal function.

6. Here is the final blow. White refined flour and sugar will over–trigger the release of the hormone insulin. When excess insulin is secreted, it is stored as fat. Cell receptors eventually become insensitive to the amount of insulin released and the body will secrete more and more insulin to deal with the glucose from food. Again, more insulin equals more fat storage. The state of insulin insensitivity is the first step toward the development of obesity and Type II diabetes. Please read the diabetes section further on in this chapter for more on this.

You may understand all of this but ask, "How does a child overeat healthy food?" Children are born knowing when they are hungry and when they have had enough to eat. One of a parent's most important jobs is to ensure a child always pays heed to these signals. Telling a child to finish what's on his or her plate is the first step to overriding your child's ability to listen to his or her signals. Please don't fall into this trap! One serving of poultry, fish, legumes, eggs, grains, fruits or vegetables is only the size of your child's palm.

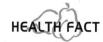

HEALTH FACT

Children are born knowing when they are hungry and when they have had enough to eat.

If a child does eat too much, the stomach lining stretches. This stimulates the cells to secrete hydrochloric acid, which puts the body into an acidic state. Similarly, fried or fatty foods cause the food to stay in the stomach for a longer period of time, leading to an acid build up. All food, if eaten in too great a quantity for the digestive enzymes to process, can lead to the production of toxins.

Celiac Disease

We already know that there can be diarrhea or other symptoms caused from eating certain food without any major damage to the gut. With celiac disease, the lining of the small intestine shows clear signs of damage when examined under a microscope.

In this disease, there is just one type of food at fault–gluten, the main protein found in wheat and related grains (rye, barley, oats). The symptoms are very specific. In babies they consist of pale, foul–smelling stools, gas, bloating and poor growth. These symptoms usually develop a few weeks after cereal has been introduced into the diet. In older children, symptoms include diarrhea, pain, bloating, weight loss, not feeling well, irritability and weakness. In rare cases, constipation may be the main symptom. Often a child with celiac disease ends up reacting to other foods as well. This is because the damage done by celiac disease to the gut lining makes it much leakier. Other food molecules are then able to get through, into the bloodstream, paving the way for food allergies.

Unfortunately, medical tests don't catch all cases, so the best confirmation is, as always, the elimination diet (See Chapter #5), where foods containing gluten are removed from a child's diet and then returned, watching for a reaction.

Non-inflammatory bowel disease
Irritable bowel syndrome (IBS)

IBS is the most common intestinal disorder diagnosed in North America. It is now appearing in 6 year olds! IBS is caused by a problem in bowel functions wherein the number and strength of contractions of the intestinal tract changes all the time. When the waves are fast and strong, diarrhea can result. When the waves are slow, constipation usually follows. IBS can lead to crohn's disease or ulcerative colitis and it mimics other disorders, such as appendicitis.

The causes of IBS are unknown but it may be related to:
- Food sensitivities or allergies (particularly dairy and wheat)
- Processed foods
- Insufficient good bacteria, candida or parasites
- Stress

Inflammatory bowel diseases (IBD)
Crohn's disease and Ulcerative Colitis

If the body's antibodies end up attacking the lining of the gut itself, the result may be Crohn's disease or Colitis. In the past few decades, these digestive disorders have increased dramatically.

> "The main difference (between these two diseases) lies in the area of the intestinal tract affected. Crohn's disease affects the entire lining of the intestinal wall and can occur anywhere from the mouth to the anus. Ulcerative colitis affects only two layers of the intestinal wall ...and typically occurs in the colon."[10]

The main symptom of both is diarrhea, containing blood and mucus. A stool sample is taken and examined under the microscope to assess the degree of inflammation in the gut.

The two common medical approaches for treating IBD are medication and surgery. However, crohn's and colitis are commonly caused by food, especially when they affect children under one year old. Dr. Peter Milla, of the Institute of Childs Health in London, made a special study of infant colitis and found that the symptoms were caused by food in about 75% of the cases. There are clear signs of immune-system involvement, so this is, in fact, a food allergy. This condition is known as food-allergic colitis or FAC and most babies suffering from it are bottle-fed. Some are breastfed infants responding to foods that the mother is eating.

The common causes of IBD include:
- Food allergies (particularly the common allergens)

- Fast foods, refined foods, sugar and a deficiency of fibre
- Antibiotic exposure
- Autoimmune disease
- Candida or parasites
- Genetic predisposition

Stress can worsen any digestive difficulties. The main role of the intestinal tract is nutrient absorption. As a result, malabsorption syndrome and malnutrition are of great concern for children suffering from these conditions.

Juvenile Diabetes

Juvenile Diabetes affects nearly two million children and young adults in North America. This condition was once, almost exclusively, a disease affecting adults over 45 years old! Now one quarter of all children is showing signs of Type 2 Diabetes.

Early symptoms of diabetes include a frequent need to urinate, excessive thirst, fatigue, and weight loss. If diabetes is not diagnosed and addressed in its early stages, it causes high blood pressure and severe hyperglycemia. Left untreated, it leads to blindness, kidney disease, leg amputations, heart attacks and stroke.

Sugar is the most obvious offender in childhood diabetes. However, most people don't realize that when consuming white flour, it immediately gets converted into sugar by the liver. This greatly increases blood sugar levels without actually eating sugar. Sugar depresses the immune system and acts as an appetite stimulant; the more sugar one eats, the more one is likely to eat, in general. It increases the body's loss of chromium through the urine and is linked directly to glucose intolerance (i.e. diabetes and hypoglycemia). Sugar is hazardous to diabetics and perpetuates the disease. Even the smallest amount of sugar should be eliminated from a diabetic's diet.

Evidence continues to mount that another trigger of childhood diabetes or insulin–dependent diabetes is a sensitivity or allergy to cow's milk albumin and possibly gluten, as well.

According to Dr. Rona, several studies indicate that just increasing the fibre content of a diabetic child's diet to 40 grams a day, while eliminating refined sugars, lowers insulin requirements by as much as 30%. Increasing fibre intake helps slow the release of sugar into the bloodstream and improves glucose uptake by cells and tissues.

Diabetes is preventable through dietary changes. A little effort goes a long way toward the treatment and prevention of diabetes naturally.

Mental symptoms

"The effect of food allergy on the central nervous system (the brain) is perhaps the most difficult subject to discuss because it is surrounded by uncertainty and controversy. Many doctors and lay people do not accept the idea that food chemicals can impair brain function or be responsible for the many symptoms our patients suffer. They believe that anxiety, depression, and other mood disorders are more likely to be the root of these problems. I disagree. In our modern diet, we found that certain components are known neurotoxins that can generate allergic disease through injury to nerves."[11]

Interestingly, Dr. Skye Weintraub states, "In 1971, the first mental illness program was established to detect brain allergies. These doctors found that 90 percent of patients admitted to institutions had this problem. Wheat and milk proved to be major factors triggering allergic brain responses. Any food, inhalant, or environmental chemical could provoke these severe symptoms."[12]

The mental symptoms most often mentioned in connection with food sensitivities are aggression and depression. Other reported symptoms are dizziness, confusion, inability to concentrate, tension, nervousness, insomnia, emotional instability, mood swings, tantrums, mental exhaustion, learning disorders, poor memory, irritability, hyperactivity and other behavioural challenges.

Autistic spectrum disorder (ASD) is a group of developmental disorders that I was interested to learn are all related.

Here is the list of them in order of severity from least to most severe:
- Attention Deficit Disorder
- Attention Deficit Disorder with Hyperactivity
- Dyslexia
- Asperger's syndrome
- Hyperlexia
- PDD
- Autism

Moodiness/bad temper/depression/anxiety/aggression
Causes:
- Food sensitivities or allergies (particularly gluten)
- Chocolates, cakes and other refined carbohydrates, sugar and lack of fibre
- Intake of sugar-rich foods, sugar depletes the body of B vitamins, especially vitamin B1, which can bring on depression
- Frequent consumption of caffeine (e.g. pop, chocolate)
- Oranges can cause anxiety and depression followed by joint pain
- Insufficient good bacteria, hypoglycemia, candida or parasites
- Insufficient protein

- Insufficient essential fatty acids
- Vitamin or mineral deficiencies (e.g. iron, calcium/magnesium)
- Dehydration
- Hypothyroidism (if it's sub clinical, it can almost always be reversed by eliminating sugar and refined carbohydrates, according to Dr. Rona)
- Insufficient sleep
- Heavy metal excess (e.g. dental fillings)
- Emotional or social factors

Foods that specifically prevent depression are fish, meat, eggs, nuts and chamomile tea (contain tryptophan).

Medical doctors such as Dr. Doris Rapp and Dr. William Walsh explain that food allergies directly affect the body's nervous system by causing swelling of the brain, which can then trigger aggression. Dr. Rapp says that some children hit and punch their mothers repeatedly when they eat the wrong foods.

Fuzzy thinking and learning disabilities

Causes of unclear thinking include:
- Food sensitivities or allergies (particularly to dairy and wheat)
- Insufficient good bacteria or candida
- Lack of Essential Fatty Acids (Please see Chapter #6 for more information on EFAs)
- Vitamin or mineral deficiency i.e. zinc deficiency has a large impact on short and long term memory ("no zinc, no think"), thinking and IQ. (Please see Chapter #6 for more information on zinc)

Attention Deficit Disorder (with or without hyperactivity)

As you saw earlier, ADD/ADHD is within the autistic spectrum. ADD affects infants, children, adolescents and adults. It is thought that children are usually affected by ADD before birth and, left untreated, continue to suffer from the condition into adulthood. It shows up as abnormalities in behaviour such as hyperactivity, short attention span, learning disorders, aggression and communication problems in early childhood. It affects more boys than girls by a ratio of 3:1.

Other conditions that occur in many ADD children include eczema, asthma, chronic infections, hay fever, headaches, stomachaches, and fungal infections of the scalp, skin and nails.

Medical doctors usually consider ADD to be of unknown causes. Complimentary medicine lists the causes of ADD as being:
- Reactions to chemicals (particularly artificial colours and flavours, aspartame), dyes, inhalants and other irritants in food or the environment

- Reactions to sugar
- Food sensitivities or allergies (particularly dairy, wheat, corn, soy and eggs)–
  Dr. Michael Lyon states in "Is Your Child's Brain Starving?" that food sensi-
  tivities are always the underlying cause of ADD
- Hypoglycemia–blood sugar drops and a stress reaction ensues
- Toxic heavy metals (lead or cadmium excesses)
- Protein deficiencies
- Poor digestion (digestive enzyme or stomach acid deficiencies) causes
  inflammation, which can disrupt neurotransmitter balance.
- Residual bacteria, fungi and parasites from chronic infections
- Hormonal imbalances
- EFA, magnesium, zinc, iron, B vitamin or other deficiencies
- Repeated use of antibiotics and other drugs
- Trauma in pregnancy
- Genetics

ADD has been diagnosed for decades but has become more prevalent in recent
years due to the increased use of processed and refined foods, as well as chemicals in our environment.

Dr. William G. Crook wrote *Can Your Child Read...Is He Hyperactive?* and stated that
hyperactivity could be detected long before school age, even in infancy. He
believed that hyperactive infants require more than the usual amount of holding,
touching and soothing.

> He wrote, "And I've found that a number of my patients were able to
> discontinue the Ritalin after changing their diets. In some of these
> patients, the hyperactivity improved dramatically when a specific
> food the child was sensitive to was avoided. Other children improved
> when carbonated beverages, sugar–coated cereals, snacks and the like
> were replaced by a diet consisting of 5 or 6 feedings a day of quality
> nutrients...." [13]

Dr. Crook identified wheat, sugar, and corn or corn products as the "common
troublemakers" for hyperactivity and listed citrus foods, peanut butter, potato,
pork, beef, egg, food colouring and other additives as other culprits. Potentially, a
child can react to any food with hyperactivity.

Autism

> "Autism is the most common neurological disorder affecting children
> and one of the most common developmental disabilities affecting
> Canadians. Autism, once considered a rare disorder, has increased

dramatically in recent years–about one in 200 children in Canada has Autism. In the past six years, there has been a 150 percent increase in the number of reported cases."[14]

Autism shows up in the first 30 months of life. Autistic children live in their own world and are disconnected from other people, unable to develop social relationships or to use language to communicate. They seem to be out of touch with reality and unable to learn from experience or to modify their behaviour to fit changes in their environment. Repetitive rituals mark their behaviour.

Some of the many theories are that autism is a syndrome linked to:
- Environmental, food or chemical allergies (particularly to casein, gluten and soy)
- Toxic heavy metal reactions (particularly mercury and aluminum which is found in vaccinations, amalgam fillings, deep–sea fish including tuna, and air emissions resulting from burning coal, cement plants and gasoline combustion)
- Protein deficiencies or imbalances
- Candida and parasites
- Poor digestion
- Deficiencies of vitamins (B6), minerals (magnesium and zinc) and essential fatty acids
- Congenital or genetic defects (1%)

Jenny McCarthy, author of *Louder than Words*, has been on Oprah multiple times, giving voice to the story of her autistic son. He is now in recovery due to the removal of dairy and gluten from his diet.

When the autistic child makes dietary changes, there may be initial withdrawal reactions such as upset stomach, anxiety, clinginess and temper tantrums. These are actually good signs. They will gradually change over a period of 3 months, often eventually resulting in the reversal of some, or a large percentage, of the symptoms of autism.

"The Autism Research Institute has been evaluating various biomedical treatments of autism since 1967....Mercury detoxification was rated helpful by 73 percent of parents, with the gluten-free/casein–free diet coming in second with 63 percent."[15]

Epilepsy

Children with severe migraines sometimes suffer from seizures, probably epileptic in nature. Epilepsy is a chronic seizure disorder that affects approximately 2 percent of children in the United States. Often, other allergic conditions show up in epileptic children, such as asthma, allergic rhinitis or eczema. Studies have shown that eliminating certain foods can help these children. How foods might provoke a seizure is a mystery but they may affect the blood vessels supplying the brain, as they are thought to do in migraines. Chemicals, especially in food, are a major cause of seizures. Aspartame has a well-known link to epilepsy. Refined, fried and salty foods are other culprits. Heavy metals, particularly from vaccinations, are another major cause of epilepsy.

> Dr. Rona writes, "According to Dr. Harris Coulter, author of two books analyzing the impact of mass vaccinations, the incidence of epilepsy and seizure disorders increased in 1945, at around the same time that the United Sates started its mass vaccination program. A study of 500,000 children by the Centers for Disease Control and Prevention in Atlanta reported that the seizure rate among children given the MMR shot rose 2.7 times within four to seven days, and increased to 3.3 times within fourteen days."[16]

Genetics, malnutrition, hypoglycemia, head injuries, lack of oxygen, infection, and meningitis can also be linked to epilepsy.

A special diet called the ketogenic diet has helped to control epilepsy in some children. This high fat, low protein and low carbohydrate diet was often used in treating seizures in the 1920s before anticonvulsant medications were available. When a child does not respond to anticonvulsant medications, this diet is often recommended. There is a window of time in which this diet can work. A qualified health practitioner needs to supervise the implementation of the ketogenic diet.

In summary: Well-documented case histories lend support to the idea that food sensitivities and allergies can, sometimes, be at the root of serious mental illness. No one is suggesting that the mental hospitals are full of food-reactive individuals who simply need an elimination diet to set them free from their illnesses. However, reactions to foods, drugs or chemicals can definitely play a role.

There are a few conditions whose symptoms mimic, cause or worsen food sensitivities and allergies. Everyone has these conditions in varying degrees, unless they have been doing things differently than the rest of the population, in terms of their health i.e. consuming different foods or supplements. They are:
- **Insufficient good bacteria/Dysbiosis**
- **Candida**
- **Hypoglycemia**
- **Parasites**
- **Low Stomach Acid (hydrochloric acid (HCl))**

Your priority is to identify and eliminate foods that are causing reactions in your child. Once that is done, you can then determine whether you need to address any of these conditions that are causing or worsening reactions to food.

Insufficient Good Bacteria/Dysbiosis

Dysbiosis is the name of the condition in which one has insufficient good bacteria but yeast has not overgrown. This condition, along with the causes of bad bacteria, was detailed in Chapter #1.

Children can be born with dysbiosis or acquire it over time. A child with dysbiosis will have digestive problems and produce fewer enzymes. When a child is lactose intolerant, he or she is lactase deficient, a dysbiosis condition. Everyone who is lactose intolerant is lacking in good bacteria.

Symptoms of insufficient good bacteria or dysbiosis in children are:
- Abdominal pain, distension, bloating
- Change in bowel movements
- Gas
- Fatigue
- Food sensitivities
- Foul smelling stool
- Headaches
- Hives
- Indigestion
- Malabsorption
- Weight loss
- Nausea

For those of you that are reading this book while pregnant, I encourage you to start taking probiotics (i.e. acidophilus) to build your store of good bacteria and re-read the list of causes of bad bacteria so that you know what to avoid. Luckily for you, a lot of the causes of bad bacteria are prohibited for pregnant women i.e. alcohol, drugs, x–rays etc.

For those of you that have a newborn and know that you have lots of bad bacteria (after reading the list of culprits) and maybe even had a cesarean, your breast milk will provide your child with good bacteria. You can always give your baby extra probiotics on the tip of your finger. Please see Chapter #6 to learn more about probiotics and other supplements.

For those of you that have a child with dysbiosis, you simply need to give him or her probiotics and help him or her to follow the "steps to optimal digestion" in Chapter #5 and the condition should go away. You should also notice your child reacting to foods less.

Candida

Candida occurs when one has insufficient good bacteria and yeast has overgrown. Candida albicans is a yeast that normally lives in our intestinal and vaginal tracts and mucus membranes ie. mouth, along with friendly or good bacteria. Its excessive growth (to at least 60 yeast and fungus type organisms) creates an imbalance in multiple systems in the body.

Frequent use of antibiotics (don't forget these can be the same antibiotics that are given to animals) is considered the #1 cause of depleted populations of gut flora, both good and bad, and the weakening of the intestinal wall, subsequently causing candida.

Symptoms of candida begin in the intestinal tract and eventually lead to intestinal permeability and allergic reactions. Remember, earlier you read that 99% of the time, when there is candida, there is a leaky gut or allergies. Dr. William Crook wrote a wonderful book on the subject called *The Yeast Connection*. Twenty-five years later, only a few medical doctors know about candida.

Definitive symptoms of candida in children are:
- Athlete's foot
- Excessive earwax
- Fungus, often in damp areas such as between the toes
- Genital itchiness or jock itch i.e. yeast infection
- Itchy ears, nose and anus
- Oral thrush and white-coated tongue
- Repeated bladder infections

Other commonly reported symptoms of candida include:
- Aching joints and muscles
- Asthma
- Cravings for sweets
- Eczema
- Headaches or migraines
- Irregular heartbeat
- Irritability
- Poor concentration
- Psoriasis

If a mother has candida, she'll pass it on to her child. Candida crosses the placental barrier in utero. If a child gets thrush, he or she has candida. If a child has yeast infections, lots of bloating and gas, or discharge, he or she clearly has an imbalance of bacteria, probably candida. The bloating and gas are caused by the yeast fermenting the food, which then produces carbon dioxide as a by-product.

Constipation and diarrhea are often symptoms of candida, which worsen the absorption of nutrients, allow yeast to proliferate and usually make a child tired. Often when a child craves and/or reacts to fruit or vegetables (high starch ones), you will find that candida is the cause; the body is saying no to sugar even in the form of fruits and vegetables!

Eliminating candida and replenishing good bacteria in children is not difficult. Simply follow these steps:

1. Remove refined carbohydrates and sugar from his or her diet, as refined carbohydrates quickly convert to sugar in the body and sugar feeds yeast.
2. Eliminate foods with high yeast, mold or fungus content from your child's diet i.e. cheese, mushrooms, melons
3. Give your child Probiotics (See Chapter #6)
4. Ensure that your child's colon is eliminating properly (See Chapter #4) so that it can eliminate the dead bacteria (sounds lovely, I know)
5. Teach him or her the steps to optimal digestion (See Chapter #5)
6. Give your child the homeopathic remedy called "Candida albicans" 30 CH for extra support, as directed by your homeopath (optional)
7. Change your child out of wet bathing suits quickly and be careful of lengthy stays in hot tubs because yeast proliferates in wet environments

In summary: The Candida Protocol is to destroy yeast, vacate the colon (with lots of water and fibre) and repopulate with good bacteria. The key to eliminating candida is to restore the levels of good bacteria in your child's body.

It is easier to heal children of candida because there is less of an imbalance than exists with adults. If all you do is change your child's diet (first 2 recommendations above), your child's digestive system may improve to such an extent that their candida symptoms may disappear without needing to follow the next steps.

However, a 10-year old child can have systemic candida, which means that following all of the above steps eliminates candida for only a short time but it always returns. You see, as yeast grows, it turns into fungal form and eventually enters the bloodstream through a leaky gut. From there, it circulates throughout body, suppressing the immune system. Candida albicans produces 80 known toxins that impair the immune system!

Once candida is in the bloodstream, you need to kill the yeast with probiotics and potentially other supplements. Diet alone does not eliminate it. The supplement to give your child with systemic candida is Grapefruit Seed Extract (GSE) in drops or powder form or Oil of Oregano in capsules (has a strong taste otherwise!), in addition to following the steps above.

If you are not convinced your child has candida, see if probiotics and digestive enzymes (see Chapter #6) get rid of his or her symptoms e.g. bloating, pains, and increased food sensitivities. If the symptoms do not disappear then you will need to treat them for candida and/or make dietary changes.

Removing candida does not eliminate allergies. It is, however, a huge piece of the puzzle in restoring a healthy immune system, which is needed to eliminate allergies. Removing candida, removes bad bacteria, allowing the inflamed gut to heal. A healed gut will no longer permit the passage of undigested food particles, so food sensitivities or allergies can be prevented. When I say "removing candida", I mean bringing its numbers into balance with the other normal inhabitants of the colon, remembering that candida is a normal inhabitant of the intestine.

There are symptoms that might be caused by candida or hypoglycemia. They are:
- Sugar or bread cravings
- Brain fog
- Irritability
- Memory loss
- Mental confusion
- Depression or anger without reason
- Anxiety or panic attacks
- Inability to concentrate
- Phobic/Compulsive behaviours
- Lethargy
- Mood swings

These symptoms and the definitive symptoms of candida sound very similiar to the symptoms of food sensitivities and allergies, don't they? By eliminating candida, you can start to control your child's symptoms as well as their reactions to food.

We now know how to clear up the candida but what is hypoglycemia and how do we get rid of it?

Hypoglycemia

Hypoglycemia is "low blood sugar". Again, this is extremely common in children and adults! According to Dr. Lendon Smith, approximately 80% of people with food sensitivities have hypoglycemia.

Dr. Mary Ann Block, the author of "No More Ritalin" says, "Low blood sugar, or hypoglycemia, is the most significant underlying problem I find in children who exhibit behavioural problems."[17]

She lists the behavioural symptoms of hypoglycemia as "The child who is agitated or irritable when he or she wakes up in the morning or before meals and then is better after eating. " And "the child with Jekyll and Hyde behaviour, who is sweet and fine one minute and then for no apparent reason is agitated, angry, and irritable the next."[18]

When you see a child that is calmly playing and suddenly spirals out of control, consider hypoglycemia. It is best to read through the symptoms of hypoglycemia though, as not every child with hypoglycemia spirals out of control.

As with dysbiosis and candida, infants can be born with hypoglycemia, and very often are.

A child who awakes screaming or yelling is hypoglycemic. Thank you Taylor for teaching me that fact!

People with candida also have hypoglycemia. People with hypoglycemia do not always have candida. If you treat hypoglycemia first, you will help your child eliminate his or her sugar or bread cravings. This is necessary for abolishing candida. You can always treat both conditions simultaneously. Unfortunately, hypoglycemia, left untreated, leads to diabetes.

To stabilize blood sugar, children need:
- Smaller meals more often, with fibre (If your child's blood sugar drops too low and he or she doesn't eat, the adrenal glands are being stressed, which means your child is stressed!). Make sure your child never gets hungry.
- Protein and/or complex carbohydrates at every meal. Complex carbohydrates alone will only help stabilize blood sugar if you have enough of them. Protein and carbohydrates together are really good for kids to sustain energy (See Chapter #6 for protein and complex carbohydrate sources).
- Elimination of refined carbohydrates and sugar such as candy, cakes and pop.
- Removal of caffeine from the diet (Pop, chocolate, and no coffee or tea for breastfeeding moms)

Cinnamon, almonds, spirulina, onion and garlic are foods that help stabilize blood sugar. You can also give the supplement chromium to children over 5 years old, to help regulate blood sugar levels.

Dr. Rona suggests feeding your child more of the following blood sugar-controlling foods, provided these are not foods causing reactions:

Chromium-rich foods: whole grains, mushrooms, grapes, raisins, cucumber, string beans.

Foods high in water-soluble fibre: flaxseed

Complex whole-grain and legume carbohydrates: whole rice, yams, squash, celery, peach, blueberries, peas

Foods rich in other trace minerals such as iodine and silicon: sesame
  seeds, seeds and nuts, apples, celery, cherries, onions, beans, legumes
Omega–3 and omega–6 fatty acid–containing foods: vegetable, nut, and
  seed oils; salmon, herring, mackerel, sardines, walnuts, flaxseed oil, evening
  primrose oil, black currant oil
Spices: cinnamon

When people eat, it takes 20 minutes from the time they stop eating to feel full
and it takes 2 hours for their blood sugar to rise. This is why people eat sugar right
after a meal, to bring the blood sugar up sooner. To help children counteract this
challenge, follow the steps to stabilize blood sugar and refrain from serving dessert
after each meal so your child doesn't get into this bad and unnecessary habit.

Dysglycemia is a condition of irregular blood sugar function. Swinging blood
sugar levels even within the normal range can cause symptoms. As well, food sensitivities and allergies mess with blood sugar levels, so the problematic foods need
to be detected and avoided.

Parasites

Parasites are "organisms that derive food, nutrition and shelter by
living in or on another organism and do not contribute beneficially
to that organism."[19]

Parasites impede digestion and damage the intestinal lining on which they
attach. They are potentially one of the biggest causes of food sensitivities.

Allergies, Disease in Disguise states, "Probably no other factor has been so
overlooked by doctors in North America as the incidence of parasites."
"(It) is far more common in N.A. than previously suspected." "Parasitic
infection (causes) toxicity, tissue damage and immune system
suppression."[20]

"The incidence of parasitic diseases in North America is skyrocketing
because of increased international travel, contamination of the water
and food supply, and the overuse of chemicals, mercury, and
prescription antibiotics."[21]

The most common parasites in North America are pinworms, whipworms, round-
worms and hookworms. E.coli and malaria are others we're increasingly hearing about.

Common symptoms of Parasitic Infestation:

- Abdominal cramps
- Anemia
- Bedwetting
- Bloating
- Blood in stools
- Blurry or unclear vision (especially when bending over or standing up)
- Brain fog
- Burning sensation in the stomach
- Carsickness
- Chest pains or heartburn
- Chronic fatigue
- Chronic dry cough
- Constipation
- Damp lips at night, dry lips during the day
- Diarrhea
- Drooling while asleep
- Distended stomach
- Eating more than normal but still feeling hungry
- Excessive appetite
- Excessive weight loss
- Excessive gas
- Fast heartbeat
- Fatigue
- Flu-like symptoms, coughing, sore throat, fever
- Food sensitivities or allergies
- Grinding teeth at night
- Hair pulling
- Impaired memory
- Inflammatory bowel disease
- Irritable bowel syndrome
- Itchy rectum, nose, and ears
- Joint pain
- Loss of appetite
- Muscle aches and pains
- Nausea
- Nervousness
- Numb hands
- Pain in the back, thighs and shoulders
- Pain in the navel

- Pimples above cheeks
- Rash
- Shortness of breath
- Sleep disturbances
- Slow reflexes
- Unclear thinking
- Yellowish face

Parasites eat the food in your child's intestine, so your son or daughter will lose nutrients and subsequently feel very tired. An itchy anus is a common symptom of parasites in children, as is constant hunger. Parasites cannot always be found in testing because many are cyclic, going through dormant and active phases. This is why having a list of symptoms to look for is so helpful.

Children acquire parasites from:
- Consuming food (fruits, vegetables, pork products i.e. bacon, ham, hot dogs, cold cuts, pork chops or beef (cows fed the dried dead flesh of other cows often have parasites), sushi, tap water or other contaminated material
- Skin contact with contaminated soil (a hookworm burrowing into a bare foot in the sand) or pools, hot tubs, gyms
- Crossing the placental barrier
- Injection of infective material (a mosquito bite producing malaria)
- Animals ie. dogs, cats, horses
- Inhalation ie. dust

Eliminating parasites in children can take up to 3 months. Eliminating parasites is not a fun subject to discuss. Here's why. You need to pay attention to the full moons. The eggs of parasites hatch at full moon! There is a reason for all the stories of craziness during a full moon! You want to ensure you start treatment just before or on the day of a full moon. It may take a few full moons before you see the eggs in your child's bowel movements; they look like pieces of broken up popcorn. If you are unable to see all of your child's bowel movements, (for example, if they are in school) do not fret. You will see your child's symptoms start to diminish. Once you see the eggs or your child's symptoms start to dissipate, you should keep your child on the protocol for one more month just to make sure you got all the little critters!

Wormwood and black walnut are the herbs of choice for eliminating parasites but I'm not sure how to get these foul tasting remedies into your child. I recommend Dr. Reckeweg's parasite formula #56 along with the homeopathic remedy Cina 30 CH.

In terms of food cures, cloves are toxic to parasites, weakening them so they can't survive for long. Grate or crush the cloves and put them in smoothies or protein shakes. Garlic is anti-parasitic (particularly with pinworms) but is not strong. You can add it to food to keep parasites at bay. Also pumpkin seeds (slice the tapeworms!), oregano oil and grapefruit seed extract are anti-parasitic.

Naturopaths often recommend giving children a parasite cleanse or using some of these natural remedies twice a year for prevention. This is because a stool analysis brought into your medical doctor's office does not always reveal a parasite.

> According to *Allergies, Disease in Disguise*, "When organisms such as candida and other parasites are eliminated or brought under control, it is not unusual for 80% of the allergies displayed by the patient to be improved..."[22]

Low Stomach Acid (hydrochloric acid or HCl)

Stomach acid (hydrochloric acid or HCl) is essential to digesting proteins and absorbing nutrients. In fact, low HCl is one of main causes of poor absorption of minerals. It is suspected that about half the population of North America has low stomach acidity.

Children can have low hydrochloric acid, which means that the stomach cannot easily push food through to the intestines. This can result in burping, abdominal bloating, excessive gas, constipation or diarrhea and weak, peeling or cracked fingernails. Digestive problems such as these can lead to or be caused by food sensitivities that can harm the intestines. Children with low stomach acid often have increased parasites, bad bacteria or yeast growing in the intestines, which increases sickness in general.

HCl digests proteins in the stomach. If HCl is low, then proteins that are not completely digested pass into the intestine. If the intestine is too porous or leaky, undigested protein molecules can move into the bloodstream setting up an immune response in the body.

More serious disorders being associated with too little stomach acid include asthma, celiac disease, chronic autoimmune disorders, food allergies and intolerance, acne, chronic hives, undigested food in stool, chronic candida infections, iron deficiency anemia, diabetes, eczema, psoriasis, seborrhoea dermatitis, vertigo, and tooth and periodontal disease.

What causes low stomach acid?
- Genetics: A child can be born enzyme deficient or acquire it over time.
- Iron and/or magnesium and/or zinc deficiency (See Chapter #6 for more information)

- Low thyroid function: Children can have low thyroid function. One of the causes is the frequent consumption of soy. Sea vegetables and coconut oil are natural thyroid enhancers that can be fed to children.
- Stress: Stress diminishes HCl production and weakens digestion. When children are stressed, their reactions to foods become worse.
- Drugs: Drugs inhibit enzymes, which are needed for the formation of hydrochloric acid.
- Eating allergenic foods repeatedly: This can damage the lining of the stomach, leading to low or nonexistent production of hydrochloric acid. This is particularly true with those who are heavy consumers of milk and other dairy products and wheat.

You can choose from one of the following to put the acidity back into your child's stomach and aid in digestion:

- Vitamin C (ascorbic acid)
- Lemon juice
- Apple cider vinegar

You simply need to add one of these ingredients into your child's water and have him or her drink the water 20 minutes prior to mealtime. If you do this for two weeks and you don't see an improvement in your child's reactions to food, the reactions are probably not related to stomach acid.

Don't lose sight of the fact that increasing your child's vegetable consumption helps increase his or her stomach acid too!

As you can see, nearly identical symptoms link dysbiosis, candida, hypoglycemia, parasites, low stomach acid and food sensitivities or allergies. A child may have only one of these conditions at a time or they may have all six. Children that are the sickest have all six.

In Conclusion

The entire physical healing process is engineered by the immune system. This brilliant system is our main defense against viruses, fungi and bacteria. A properly functioning immune system is the vital foundation on which we build well being. Consuming the vitamins, minerals and anti-oxidants that come from food is the number one way in which to strengthen our immune systems and avoid symptoms, conditions and disease.

"You are doing your children a lifetime of favours by giving them a strong nutritional foundation. You will strengthen their immune system, eliminate allergies and sensitivities, achieve and/or maintain a healthy weight, improve their emotional well-being, enhance their performance physically and academically and at the same time, teach them discipline and self respect. Your children will be happier to be healthier."[23]

"We live in a fast-food, fast-paced society, where meals can be obtained in under five minutes and solutions found by the end of an hour-long television show. We've come to expect that if we feel really, really strongly about something, we should be able to fix it–and fast. We don't like waiting. Once we've identified a problem, we want it to go away quickly. This isn't going to happen without significant, long-term lifestyle changes. They are by nature difficult to alter. They require time, patience, and perseverance–a little like parenting in general."[24]

The foods that I recommend you feed your child in Chapter #6 help improve, if not eliminate, every symptom, condition and disease. I was amazed to learn that when Taylor was unable to eat any of the common allergens, she was decreasing her chances of contracting all of the symptoms and sickness discussed in this chapter!

How to make the best use of this chapter's information

1. First, I would recommend looking up your child's particular symptom or sickness and reading the root causes behind it. Remember: Addressing your child's diet is the first step to eliminating symptoms, even if there are other root causes.

2. Then skip down to the end of this chapter and read about insufficient good bacteria, candida, hypoglycemia, parasites, and low stomach acid. The majority of today's children have these conditions, in varying degrees. Gradually, work on feeding your child the healthier alternatives and then you can address these conditions e.g. eliminate dairy (pasteurized) from your child's diet. After one or two weeks of being dairy-free, give your child acidophilus (See Chapter #6) to put the good bacteria back into their body. Replace dairy with healthier calcium sources. Then, see if these other conditions need to be addressed or not.

3. If you do feel at this point that you need to eliminate a food from your child's diet, read Chapter #4 to see what you need to look for in terms of your child's bowel health and then read Chapter #5 to determine how to detect food sensitivities and allergies for certain.

4. Then, look up your own symptom and condition in this chapter and learn the root causes.

5. As you go through life, you will realize that these symptoms, conditions and disease, are very common and you can look them each up when you need to or read about them all now if you're as flabbergasted by this information as I was.

CHAPTER 4

GOOD RIDDANCE! THE IMPORTANCE OF THE ELIMINATION OF TOXINS

There may be people who quickly glance at the title of this chapter and say to themselves "Good, I can skip this one". Please don't! *I specifically made this the subject of its' own chapter because it is so important to understand. Insufficient elimination of toxins is a far more common problem than you realize. If left untreated, your child suffers immeasurably.*

The three *most* important nutritional ways in which to raise a healthy and happy child are to:

1. Remove foods to which your child is reacting
2. Feed your child healthy food
3. Ensure that your child is eliminating enough toxins

The trouble is, that parents think they are doing all three and they are not. I know because it happened to me. Unfortunately, most parents do not discover their lack of knowledge in these matters until their child starts having symptoms. Don't blame yourself for not knowing–move forward and read on.

Over 90% of human ailments begin with a congested colon. It is the build–up of waste or bad bacteria in the body that is behind most symptoms, conditions and disease.

Dr. Bernard Jensen was a chiropractor and nutrition pioneer who received numerous prestigious awards and honours for his research and teachings in clinical nutrition and the healing arts. He was the person that made it clear to the world that the bowel is the most important organ in the body.

> Dr. Jensen stated "I believe that the number–one source of the misery and decay we are witnessing in our society today is autointoxication– self–poisoning caused by micro organisms, metabolic waste, and other toxins in the body."[1]

You see, if waste is not eliminated and accumulates in the body, bad bacteria grows and digestion deteriorates. In essence, the body cannot function with half-digested nutrients. When digestion deteriorates, the body starts reacting to food. As the body becomes increasingly toxic, proper oxygen cannot reach the tissues. Without oxygen, the body loses energy, and the tired body continues heading downhill until sickness and disease set in. If there is a problem in the body and you take care of the bowel, every other organ's health will improve.

Long ago, people understood the importance of bowel movements and their relationship to good health. People were taught how to care for the bowel. Mothers ensured that their children had bowel movements every day and never let the children leave home without first having their fibre rich breakfast and spoonful of cod liver oil (essential fatty acids)! If a child became sick, he or she was given an enema! Somehow over the years, bowel wisdom became lost, and the bowel has become a subject that is rarely discussed. **We need to raise our bowel consciousness again.**

A child who is constipated will often simultaneously experience a realm of other symptoms, such as:

- Aggression, which can result in a small child hitting others for no apparent reason
- Anxiety or depression
- An unusually small appetite
- Asthma
- Bad breath or body odour
- Bowel cancer
- Brain fog
- Fatigue or exhaustion
- Fears that may be many, unwarranted and of unwarranted severity
- Frequent illness e.g. colds, bronchitis, flu
- Gas or bloating
- Headaches
- Heart trouble
- Hemorrhoids
- Irritability, whininess or moodiness
- Lower back pain
- Obesity
- Rashes or eczema
- Skin, hair or nail problems
- Sleep problems such as trouble falling asleep, staying asleep and/or sleeping soundly
- Stomach aches, cramps or hernias
- Vitamin and mineral deficiencies

There is no end to the symptoms that emerge when a child is not eliminating their toxins properly. Toxins from bowel bacteria and undigested food particles may play a role in the development of:

- Candida
- Colitis
- Diabetes
- Meningitis
- Migraines
- Thyroid disease

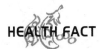

HEALTH FACT

Children, as well as adults, should have one large bowel movement each day, preferably two or three.

Ideal elimination

The digestive system holds the whole body together. It is responsible for absorbing all vitamins and minerals and for eliminating waste. Children, as well as adults, should have one large bowel movement each day, preferably two or three. Ideally, bowel movements are soft, light brown or golden, and cause no pain or discomfort when being expelled from the body. The length of your child's arm, from his or her wrist to elbow, is the ideal size of a bowel movement. The same goes for adults. Note: that length is much greater for adults than it is for children!

> "Normal healthy stool should leave the body easily, settle in the water and gently submerge. If there is not enough daily fibre in the diet (30–40 grams), the stool will quickly plummet to the bottom of the toilet. If the stool floats, the likely reason is too much undigested fat."[2]

Please don't panic if your child's bowel movement is floating or sinking. This is where there is the most disagreement among experts. Far more important is the frequency, colour and consistency of your child's bowel movements.

Bile is a liver secretion that helps us digest our food. A golden bowel movement has enough bile. If your child's bowel movement is consistently yellow (other than when they are newborn), there is too much bile or food is passing through his or her body too quickly. Clay coloured stools represent lack of sufficient bile. To increase bile, you can give your child lemon with his or her water.

Dark bowel movements or pain in expelling a bowel movement means the movement is dehydrated, so you know to increase your child's water consumption. Dark or black bowel movements can also be caused by supplements. Another reason for this colour is that blood coming from high up in the intestinal tract is entering the bowel movements. This blood loss can go undetected for a long time and eventually cause a child to become iron deficient. Cow's milk is the biggest cause of this bleeding!

When your child is having lots of bowel movements (5 or more in a day) or loose stools, it means that your child is not digesting his or her food in the stomach or small intestines. Loose stools indicate an irritant, allergen or virus. A diet deficient in good fats can also cause this condition. A child will become nutrient-depleted if his or her bowel movements remain this way for longer than a few days.

> "People from primitive cultures who live totally apart from modern civilization and consume a diet of pure, whole, natural foods—foods unprocessed and seldom cooked—usually have a bowel movement about one-half hour following each meal."[3]

Common Bowel Problems

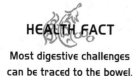

HEALTH FACT

Most digestive challenges can be traced to the bowel.

As you have already learned, most digestive challenges can be traced to the bowel. Bowel problems range from slow transit time for waste to insufficient bile secretion. The most common bowel problem, by far, is constipation.

What is constipation?

Almost everyone experiences constipation at one time or another. Some have only fleeting episodes. Many more suffer on a regular basis. Constipation is so widespread that it is considered normal. People who are constipated often do not even know they are!

> Dr. Jensen explains, "Constipation is often referred to by those who have studied it as the "modern plague." Indeed, I consider it the greatest present-day internal danger to health. Intestinal toxemia and autointoxication are direct results of intestinal constipation. Constipation contributes to the lowering of the body's resistance, predisposing the body to many acute illnesses and the initiation of many degenerative and chronic processes. Constipation indirectly cripples and kills more people in our country than almost any other single disease condition having to do with deficient function."[4]

Constipation is one of the least understood symptoms. Even the term "constipation" has many definitions, depending on your source! It can be defined as "a lack of regular and easy defecation on a daily basis". However, many believe that it is not necessary to have a bowel movement every day. Your doctor might state that constipation is common in children and that it is not something to worry about. They might say that exclusively breastfed babies do not need to have regular and frequent bowel movements. They also may say that lots of children grimace and need to work very hard to expel a bowel movement. Think of how you feel if you haven't had a bowel movement in a day, in two days, or say, a week.

Think of how you feel when you have to struggle to push one out! *Without a doubt, your child needs to have at least one large, soft, but formed bowel movement a day.*

Constipation actually means that a person is not eliminating as much as his or her body needs. Well, no wonder this is the least understood symptom. 'What does *that* mean?' or 'How much is enough?' you might ask. This is where it gets tricky. Your child might be having one large bowel movement a day or your child might be having one to three bowel movements a day, yet he or she is still experiencing some of the symptoms caused by constipation. The likely cause is that your child does not have enough good bacteria (See Chapter #1 for more information) and therefore, is not having bowel movements that are large enough or frequent enough for his or her needs. The only way to know for certain whether they are eliminating properly, is to observe them and watch their patterns, keeping an eye out for the symptoms. Every child is different. Taylor usually has one bowel movement a day and often, two. She has colour in her cheeks, is happy and displays none of the symptoms of constipation. For a long time, I worried that she wasn't having two bowel movements every day, never mind three. Then I came to learn that, for her, one to two bowel movements a day was enough.

In general, if your child is bloated or is experiencing discomfort, wanting to go and not being able to, then they really are constipated. A healthy bowel feels healthy. There is regularity to the pattern. It is not erratic. There is no sense of pain, either before or afterwards, and the movement feels complete and not as if there is still some feces left to pass. You can discuss this with your older child if you are uncertain as to whether your child is constipated.

Interestingly enough, diarrhea can be a form of constipation. It is a condition in the intestinal tract in which bowel movements are so badly clogged that only the eliminative liquids are able to pass through.

What are transit and reaction times?
Transit time
The time it takes for a food to be eaten, travel the length of the intestinal tract and be eliminated is called the bowel transit time. Bowel transit time should be less than 24 hours. Constipation slows the transit time down. When transit time is slower, putrefied material stays in the colon longer. Subsequently, the waste enters the bloodstream through the intestinal wall. This can cause auto–intoxification, which is what leads to the previously mentioned symptoms and conditions.

In addition, the build–up of waste in the intestinal walls caused by the slow transit time prevents the body from properly absorbing vitamins and minerals. Once I had determined all of my eldest daughter's sensitivities and she was eating the healthiest foods available, I learned that she was deficient in many vitamins and minerals! You can just imagine my shock! It was because of the long and frequent bouts of constipation in her past. I finally understood why she was more tired during the day than other children; her body was deprived of the nutrients needed for energy and vitality due to all the constipation she had experienced!

So what does transit time mean to you and your child? If your child has a food that agrees with his or her body, your son or daughter will have a bowel movement within 24 hours of consuming that food. If your child is not sensitive to corn, you can use corn to test the length of your child's transit time. Simply feed your child some corn and see how long it takes to see it come out in his or her bowel movement.

Now you probably understand the importance of speeding up your child's bowel transit time and want to know how to accomplish this task. Simply feed your son or daughter high–fibre foods such as fruits, vegetables, legumes, and whole cereal grains! Vegetables are largely made up of complex carbohydrates, so they do not produce nearly the amount of putrefaction waste that high protein foods do.

At the Mayo Clinic in the 1930s, doctors studied the effects on the colon of a high–fibre diet. They found that fibre prevented the bowel from becoming flaccid and lazy. Natural, alive, and pure foods can help develop bowel tone. As a result, proper diet was introduced as a viable alternative to surgery.

Reaction time

This is the tricky part. When your daughter consumes a food to which she is sensitive, she may have a bowel movement the day she consumes that food but not the next day. She may have one the next day and the day after but not the next day! You see what I mean about the detective work? Luckily for you, this change in reaction time occurs gradually. Your baby may miss a bowel movement the day she consumes the offending food or the next day. Your older baby may miss a bowel movement two days after consuming the offending food. Your toddler may miss a bowel movement three days after consuming the food to which she is sensitive. As your child's constipation becomes less frequent and her bowel becomes healthier, the reaction time will decrease one day at a time until it is back to where it should be. Another thing to consider is that your child may go without a bowel movement for more than just one day, just from eating one offending food. When Taylor was younger, she would eat a food to which she was sensitive and 2 days later not have a bowel movement and remain constipated for 2 or 3 days. You can see where a food and symptom diary is absolutely vital to understanding what is really going on with your child. Once you maintain that diary, it is possible to determine exactly why your child misses a bowel movement each and every time. The body is that easy to read if we just learn how to read it.

So now you may be putting all the pieces together but you want to know what has caused the constipation to begin with.

What are some of the well-known causes of constipation?

- Lack of fibre e.g. whole grain breads, pastas and cereals, vegetables, fruits, legumes, seeds & nuts. Fibre triggers healthy bowel contractions.
- Lack of fluids–water provides bulk to stools
- Lack of exercise–stimulates lymphatic flow and bowel
- Consuming certain foods that are constipating such as white rice and bananas
- Iron supplements from anywhere other than a health food store
- Stress/depression

I feel the need to elaborate on the final point. Few people realize the benefits of a relaxed and peaceful lifestyle. They are often unaware of the mind's ability to impact the body. When our children experience fear, anxiety, anger, depression or stress, it upsets the delicate processes of the body, in particular those of digestion and elimination. For example, a tensed colon may respond with diarrhea or constipation as the nerve impulses carry the message of fright to the bowel. The bowel remains affected until peace returns to the mind.

What are some of the lesser-known causes of constipation?

- Food, chemical and/or environmental sensitivities
- Lack of good bacteria
- Certain prescription and over-the-counter drugs (i.e. Children's Triaminic and Tylenol)
- Chocolates, cakes, white flour products, white rice etc. Sugar and junk foods are generally constipating
- Heavy cow's milk consumption
- Lack of good bacteria i.e. probiotics/acidophilus (See Chapter #6)
- Lack of essential fatty acids (efa's) which lubricate the intestinal system i.e. flax seed and fish (See Chapter #5)
- Magnesium or other vitamin/mineral deficiency (See Chapter #6)
- Insufficient amounts of digestive enzymes (See Chapter #6)
- Misalignments or subluxations of the spine, requiring your child to see a chiropractor (See Chapter #9)
- A change in your child's lifestyle or physical condition (i.e. teething in babies, sickness, travel)

Most people are aware of the fact that diarrhea can be caused by an adverse reaction to a food or chemical or drug. What most people don't know is that constipation can also be caused by a food, chemical, drug or environmental sensitivity! It used to be that whenever Taylor ate or was exposed to something to which she was sensitive, she became constipated.

Over-the-counter drugs, chemicals, tap water, cigarette smoke, teething and sickness

I found that my eldest daughter had problems with every cold medication I tried on her, which sent me on a long journey of learning about natural remedies. Did you know that there is a natural remedy out there for every single ailment? As a result, my youngest daughter has never had a drug in her body, other than those present in non-organic meats or poultry.

Over the years, both of my girls have become constipated from eating junk food or any of the common allergens. For periods of times, neither of my girls could handle chemicals in their foods. It bears repeating that when your child tries a food, it may be the chemicals or pesticides that have been added to the food that they are reacting to and not the food itself.

My eldest became constipated from our tap water, due to the large amounts of chlorine, other chemicals, heavy metals and iron (generally constipating) present in it. When we changed her water source, bowel movements piled out of her for days.

You learned in the "Our Story" section that my eldest daughter also became constipated from spending long periods of time in a cigarette smoke infested house. Who would guess that one could become constipated from cigarette smoke? A cold, sore throat, bronchial infection or asthma, yes…. but constipation? *If constipation is the way a child's body reacts to a problem in his or her environment, then he or she will become constipated from cigarette smoke or any other seemingly unrelated triggers.*

Both my girls developed constipation whenever they were teething. As well, when they had colds or were sick, they would go a number of days without bowel movements.

How do you eliminate your child's constipation?

Review the causes of constipation. Remember to look at your child's levels of good bacteria and diet first when trying to determine the triggers of his or her constipation. Then consider the environmental factors to which your child is exposed. If you are exclusively breastfeeding, your child may be constipated from the foods that *you are consuming.*

Please try to stay away from laxatives, suppositories and enemas. These methods might clear up the symptom in the short term but they do not address the cause of the problem or solve the problem for the long term. Laxatives, suppositories and enemas are physically harmful to your child and their invasiveness can cause them serious emotional harm. Prolonged use of laxatives can damage your child's large intestine and cause lazy bowel syndrome, which creates a dependency on laxatives.

HEALTH FACT

Prolonged use of laxatives can damage your child's large intestine and cause lazy bowel syndrome, which creates a dependency on laxatives.

So...what exactly do you do?

You do everything possible to soften the bowel movement within your child so that when it comes out, it doesn't hurt. Here are some ideas for softening bowel movements:

- First and foremost, stay away from any foods or environmental aspects to which your child is reacting.
- Feed your child fruits, vegetables and fibre that, you are certain, agree with your child (See Chapter #6 for more information). Remember, bananas and white rice are generally constipating.
- Put probiotics, vitamin C, and flax oil or ground flax seeds in his or her sandwiches, drinks, soups or whatever you can sneak them into. These are three supplements that benefit all children. (See Chapter #6 for more information).
- Give your child laxative foods or juice. For example, prune juice, either on its own or mixed with something else e.g. another kind of juice or water, Other examples are pectin-containing fruits such as figs or pears. Grapes, cherries, licorice and spinach are other laxative foods.
- Give your child a green drink or chlorella diluted with water.
- Give your child herbal tea that is nourishing and contains gastro-intestinal stimulants such as ginger, peppermint, elderberry, cinnamon, or dandelion root.
- Provide your child with a homeopathic remedy, preferably a constitutional remedy chosen specifically for your child by a Classical Homeopath (See Chapter #9 for more information).

Methods for cleansing your child's body

Simply improving your child's good bacteria levels, eating healthy foods and staying away from the foods, chemicals and environmental factors to which your child reacts, helps keep your child's body free of toxins. In addition to those methods that we've discussed so far and those in later chapters, there are many other ideas for cleansing your child's body of toxins.

Please choose one idea from this list of ideas and incorporate it each day:

- Detoxifying foods include beans, eggs, garlic, onion, green powders, flax seeds and organic fruits and vegetables.
- Detoxifying vitamins and minerals: C, A, zinc are examples that you can read more about in Chapter #6
- Water (See Chapter #5)
- Exercise (See Chapter #5)
- Epsom salt baths (about a cup per bath)
- Homeopathic pellets or drops prescribed by a Naturopath or Homeopath (See Chapter #9)

- Infrared sauna–a newer type sauna where one can remain inside, sweating for a long time without suffering ill effects

For those children with conditions or disease, naturopathic assisted chelation or intravenous therapy removes heavy metals along with other toxins.

When your child is "holding in" bowel movements

This action begins with a child either being afraid, too busy or so focused on what they are doing, that they do not want to have a bowel movement. And the longer a child holds the bowel movement in, the more impacted the bowel movement becomes and the harder it is for the child to pass.

The main reason that a child becomes afraid of having a bowel movement is that he or she thinks it will hurt when it comes out. Why do children think it will hurt? Past experience–they already felt the hard bowel movement trying to come out the last time. How does it become hard? From eating the wrong foods....not foods that are wrong for everyone...but foods that are *specifically* wrong for your child.

I spoke earlier about how emotions impact the bowels. Some children live in fear, due to their life circumstances. Therefore, fear can become the emotional reason behind their constipation. Hmmm, remember the story I told you about Taylor's arrival on earth? Any reason she might be filled with fear? Absolutely. Fear can stem back to a baby's delivery or even as far back to the time spent in the womb.

1. If you are not confident that what you have tried has, indeed, softened the bowel movement, explain to your child that when the bowel movement comes out, it may hurt but that once it's out, they will feel a lot better. You may also want to point out to him or her that the longer the bowel movement stays inside them, the harder it will become and therefore, the more difficult it will be for them to expel it. You may find that when the bowel movement is expelled, you will see the end of it is soft. This means that you have accomplished the task of softening your child's bowel movement. Alternatively, you may also discover that it is the second bowel movement that comes out soft.

2. If you are confident that your attempts have softened the bowel movement, there is another issue with which to contend. Your child's bottom may be sore from holding in the bowel movement. Also, they very likely could have hemorrhoids inside or out. If your child is sore, he or she will not want to let the bowel movement out and risk hurting the area further. All you need to do is purchase some fast acting natural cream and apply it to the area. A good quality calendula cream works very well. The best plan is to apply the cream before bed so that it can take effect over night. Your child will be ready the next morning to push the already soft bowel movement out.

3. If some of the bowel movement comes out and you see that it is soft yet your child will not push anymore out, you know one of two things. Your child's bottom is still sore and it hurts when the bowel movement comes out or you know "It is all in your child's mind", meaning that your child will not, under any circumstance, want to let that bowel movement out. This is a force to be reckoned with, let me tell you. Here is what to do:

a) Know that the bowel movement will come out eventually and that there is no rush.

b) Realize that the very best way to help your child, at this point, is to relax him or her and yourself. Try to:

- Give your child a tummy massage (moving your hand or a tennis ball in a clockwise motion around the belly button) or rest your hand on your child's tummy until you feel heat.
- Rub your child's foot from heel upwards, in a circular motion.
- Apply hot water bottles or hot towels on the tummy
- Prepare Sitz baths with Epsom salts, particularly cold–water baths and hot–cold contrast baths stimulate circulation in the pelvic area and increase nerve activity. The mornings are the best time for your child to have one. Sitz baths are wonderful for cleansing the body and help with bladder problems too!
- Take your child for a walk
- Read to your child
- Tell your child funny stories
- Make your child laugh
- Turn on his or her favourite calm television show or movie
- Show your child how to breathe and encourage him or her to listen to the breathing. Feel your child's legs and arms and make sure they are not tensed.
- Talk to your child about visualizing the bowel movement coming out of his or her bottom and filling either a diaper or the toilet bowl. Talk about the relief your child will feel when the bowel movement is no longer inside him or her, about the running around and playing she or she will be able to do when no longer filled with feces.
- Know that it is not uncommon for children between three and seven to be scared of having bowel movements. We've talked about the pain that sometimes accompanies bowel movements. Other children are confused about the origin and destination of their bowel movements. They might be afraid that flushing them down the toilet is losing a part of their bodies. Still others are fearful of being flushed down the toilet themselves! To help children understand, you can draw pictures of food going into the mouth, getting chewed up and

digested, being absorbed into the body as nutrients, and then being expelled as waste. Often children love drawing the pipes that carry the waste away from their home to waste treatment plants!

- If your child uses or will use a potty, don't be shy about moving the potty to a location they are comfortable in, whether that be outdoors, in their own bedroom or in the toy room.

You get the idea. The important part to remember is to always be patient with your child. If you show your impatience or your frustration, use negative language or threaten your child in any way, your child's fear will worsen and the constipation will persist.

4. If, over time, there is still no bowel movement, your child might be relaxed, while still holding the bowel movement in. Try breathing deeply and squeezing your buttocks in simultaneously. Another point to consider is that a child might think they are pushing a bowel movement out but in fact he or she is squeezing the bowel movement in! Try asking your child to push a bowel movement out. If they think a bowel movement has come out and nothing has come out, you know your child is confused about this.

5. If you've tried all of the above and your child has had no luck expelling a bowel movement, you and your child are now most likely exhausted and probably bewildered. It is important for you to understand that taking one or all of the above courses of action should, in most cases, nip the problem in the bud. However, if you have a child anything like mine, there comes a time when emotions govern all logic. You must decide what you want to do at this point, depending on how many days you've devoted to this, and how you, your child and the rest of your family have been handling the stress of all this. If you've decided you've all had enough, there is one final approach to try.

You may decide to rest a castor oil pack on your child's tummy to encourage a bowel movement or give your child some kind of enema, preferably a homemade one. In this case, you would use an empty enema container that you purchased from the drugstore and fill it with warm filtered water with a teaspoon of sea salt and insert it into your child's rectum. If you decide to go this route, I do not advise using the enema as a threat to your child in hopes of getting him or her to go to the washroom independently. We, as adults, could never imagine the fear that a child experiences when he or she simply sees an unknown apparatus that is going to be inserted in their body.

Experience has taught me that enemas are *never* necessary once you determine the root cause of your child's constipation.

Toilet training your child who is or was chronically constipated

It's pretty tricky, let me tell you. My eldest daughter, who experienced so much constipation, got to the point where she fully understood what was needed of her and what her body's cues were, yet wanted to expel her bowel movements in a diaper. For months, she would ask me for a diaper whenever she knew she had to have a bowel movement. She was more comfortable having her bowel movements in a diaper. Many children are like this. The important thing to know is that toilet training a child who was or is chronically constipated, may take longer. I simply had patience and waited until Taylor was ready to surrender her diapers. If someone were to ask me today how I toilet trained my girls, my answer, in both cases, would be "I have no idea. They did it themselves, when they were ready."

Some of you might say "Well, that doesn't really help me! What do I do?" Here are the steps I followed with both my girls:

1. You can read a book on the topic or simply explain to your child that the idea is for them to eventually urinate or have a bowel movement on the toilet.
2. Start changing your child's diapers more frequently so that when they urinate or have a bowel movement, you are able to point it out to them so that they become aware of what it feels like to go the washroom.
3. Then ask your child to tell you when they think they have urinated or had a bowel movement in their diaper.
4. Check for accuracy and congratulate them when they are right, suggesting that next time they go on the toilet.
5. Once your child is aware of when they are going to the washroom, start asking your child every once in a while if they need to use the toilet. No stress, no pressure, no rush.
6. As soon as your child uses the toilet correctly, ensure that you congratulate him or her!
7. Putting pull-ups or underwear on your child prematurely is a waste of time and money and frustrates everyone. Save the pull-ups until your child has gone to the toilet successfully a few times, for example, in case of accidents while sleeping at night.
8. Accidents simply mean a child is not ready. There is no need for a negative word to be uttered when they occur. Negativity, frustration or added stress towards your child could inadvertently slow down or stop the training process. Rest assured your child will go to the toilet when ready.

Coping with your child's painful symptoms

There are many symptoms, in addition to constipation, that cause pain in children. Examples include colic, stomach aches, headaches or migraines, backaches, neck aches, sore throats, fevers, muscle or joint pain, rashes, eczema, psoriasis and ear, bladder or kidney infections. A number of sections of in book will help you get to the root cause of these symptoms or conditions. There are also sections of the book that explain how food, natural treatments and alternative therapies help to heal these ailments. In the mean time, you may be faced with the challenge of having a child who is in pain. It is my intent, in this section of the book, to give you some ideas as to help you and your child cope with pain.

First of all, it is important to realize that pain serves a purpose. When an infant or child is experiencing a health challenge that we cannot see with the naked eye, it is pain that alerts us to the fact that something is wrong. We need to take action in order to help our child overcome his or her particular challenge.

Babies have the same pain sensations as adults but lack the ability to avoid its source or to understand the pain. Babies benefit physically and emotionally each time they are able to alert their parent, without the use of words, to any discomfort or pain they are experiencing and each time a parent can put an end to their suffering.

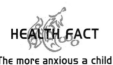

HEALTH FACT

The more anxious a child feels, the more pain a child feels.

When you have child who is in pain, it is important that you listen to your child's words, observe their behaviour and then interact with them. Here are a number of ideas for helping you deal with your child most effectively if they are in pain:

- The more anxious a child feels, the more pain a child feels. Babies and younger children rely heavily on the adults around them for cues about how anxious to be. It is important that you know that your child looks up to you and expects you to protect and comfort them in times of fear, pain or distress. When you don't minimize or overreact to your child's experiences, you will help your child remain in safe reality. When you can help your child's nervous system remain calm, it is less likely to send emergency pain signals to the brain. Absence of anxiety is not a cure for pain, but it changes its intensity.

- It is helpful to let your child describe where it hurts and maybe have them explain how the sore part of their body feels. The louder your two-year-old expresses distress, the more pain they are most likely experiencing. When your child verbally explains his or her pain in your comforting presence, it can bring relief. One of the best books that I read and drew from on this subject is *Soothing Your Child's Pain* by Dr. Kenneth Gorfinkle.

    He states, "Research shows that the sooner a child talks about a painful or frightening event, the less likely he or she will develop an emotional problem." [5] He also says "You can help your child enrich his "pain/feeling vocabulary" with the use of colour, shape, and metaphor. Pain can be red or orange, pointy or bumpy, scratchy or achy, loud or quiet, big or little."[6]

- When you respond to your child's expressions of pain, just the sound of your voice can be a tremendous healing therapy for them. Try to talk to your child using positive words that they understand. One of the hardest things to do is answer your child's questions when you yourself do not have the answers. In this situation, just be honest and say that you don't know all the answers but that you are working hard to determine the cause of your child's pain.

One of the most important aspects of Taylor's recovery was her trust in me. When I continually told her the following, she believed me:

HEALTH FACT

Each time a child exerts some control over his pain, they experience less anxiety and ultimately less pain.

"Mama is going to help you get better."

"You are going to get well. It won't be long now. I promise you that."

"Mom is reading books and talking to others all the time, trying to get help."

"Mommy loves you." "Do you know how much I love you?"

"God made your body this way so that we could learn from it."

Reassure your child that he or she has done nothing wrong. Your child might say "I hurt because I did something wrong." As a supportive and understanding parent, you can easily dispel these feelings. More ideas as to how to communicate with your child and others can be found in Chapter #7.

- Each time a child exerts some control over his pain, they experience less anxiety and ultimately less pain. You can help your child retain a feeling of control by suggesting that they draw pictures of the pain or how the pain feels, maybe even using colours to show you how it hurts. You can also prepare them for a visit to the chiropractor, for example.

- Involving your child in creating ways to ease or avoid his discomfort is another way to help your child feel in control and make a big difference to your child's emotional and physical wellbeing. When my youngest had joint pain at 4 years old, I told her I was going to get my books to help us come up with a solution. After reading a few sections, we arrived at some solutions that we tried and found to work. The next time Paige was in pain, *she* asked that I get the helpful books.

- Suppose you give your child a remedy and they feel better in 3 minutes, obviously too quickly for the remedy to have taken effect. The remedy gave him hope that relief from his pain was around the corner. Hope is a powerful analgesic. Giving your child something to look forward to is another way to impart hope.

- Touch, soothing actions and empathy are other analgesics. Every time you pick up your baby or child and carry them, rock back and forth, and stroke them with your hands, you are providing comfort and pleasure. You will find that when you hold, hug and empathize with your child, their tummy ache feels better. A child will tell you that a lack of empathy will make his pain worse. When you tell your son or daughter that they are being very brave and that crying is normal and okay, you are being empathetic and allowing your child to feel whatever they truly feel. You can also explain that your hug is helping them to feel better. These kinds of discussion are in no way trivial, as they help you and your child master fear, danger, trust, and care each time your child is faced with new challenges.

- Any time that you leave your child's side, when he or she is in pain, let him know that you are leaving, what you are doing and when you will return. This will lower his level of anxiety and confusion.

Nancy Cain states in *Healing the Child*, "There is no question in my mind that the greatest fear of all young children is separation from their parents."[7]

She further explains, "It's not the illness or injury itself that is most traumatic for your child. It's the separation from you that causes your child the greatest pain."[8]

- Many mothers have observed the overall euphoric and sedating effect their breast-feeding has on their distressed babies.
- At any age, babies and children can ignore some pain when something else captures their attention. The more deeply absorbed you can help your child to be, the more effectively distracted he or she will be.

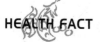

HEALTH FACT

Many mothers have observed the overall euphoric and sedating effect their breast-feeding has on their distressed babies.

A good way to distract your child is to use imagination and fantasy. You can use your own creativity to come up with ideas and images that instill calm in your child. If your child has a headache with a fever, you could encourage them to imagine pumping their legs on a swing, propelling higher and higher, while a cool wind blows against their face. Soothing music, a guided taped children's meditation or prayer are other useful ways to help your child ease his anxiety, stress and pain. Once you teach your child these various methods, your child will know how to use the concept of "mind over matter" by themselves.

- Blankets, stuffed animals, soothers, and your baby or child's thumb provide critical comfort. You may see your baby or child sucking his thumb, while stroking her skin with the corner of her special blanket; your child has learned to comfort herself, a necessary skill to have in life!

- Some children have irrational fears about their bodies. When you ask your child to point to where it hurts, they may be reluctant to do so in case it makes the pain worse or they discover something horrible like a hole or blood. For these reasons, some children find it easier and less threatening to point to the part of a doll's body that represents the place where they are experiencing pain. Dolls, stuffed animals or puppets make very effective tools for easing children's fears and talking about physical or emotional problems. You can even use dolls and drawings to explain the human body and how it works to your child.

- Sometimes you need to ask for and accept help. You may be worried that if you admit that you cannot cope, you'll be subjected to judgment by others. Remember that anyone that judges you has never been in your situation. If you are a stay-at-home mom, others may make you feel as though you have all the time in the world; your only job is to raise your child so how could you dare ask for help? The stress of raising a healthy child is extremely high but the stress of raising a child who is suffering is so much greater and much more exhausting, both physically and mentally. The saying 'It takes a village to raise a child' really is true. Unfortunately, most of us do not have this benefit in this day and age but we usually can find at least one person to help us when we are in need.

- Determine some techniques to preserve your sanity. If you are losing sleep night after night, you may have to ask for help from your spouse or some-one else occasionally. You may decide to go for a long drive early in the evening in order to refuel for the anticipated long evening ahead. Please refer to Chapter #7 for other ideas about taking care of yourself.

- Your child's chronic pain can actually cause you emotional damage because it can make you feel trapped. If it continues for months or years, it feels like there is no end to the pain. A growing feeling of hopelessness and even depression can ensue.

  Healing the Child says, "As a parent, you think you can protect your children from anything. You can make them feel better when they hurt. You can comfort them when they are scared. You can cheer them up when they are sad. But when your child becomes seriously ill or is fighting for his or her life, you feel helpless."[9]

I used to get so worked up inside when Taylor was in pain with her colic and subsequently, her constipation. **If you, the parent, have undergone physical or emotional pain in childhood, you can relive that pain every time you see your child suffering.** This often leads a parent to go above and beyond the call of duty in trying to prevent or end their child's struggles. The fact that I was allowing these constipation episodes with Taylor to paralyze our household for up to 4 or 5 days, demonstrates this point nicely.

Looking back with hindsight, in my mind's eye, the situation seemed far more desperate than it really was. I needed more laughter and more perspective from others so that I could just lighten up. To give my situation perspective, I meditated, got out of the house on my own, journalled, drove my car in silence and listened to music. I found that solutions came to me and in turn, peace overcame me. Once I determined the causes of Taylor's pain, helping other parents became a large part of my emotional healing process. I often see myself in other struggling parents and when helping them to cope, I heal.

- Sometimes it is helpful to let your child take risks, endure the painful consequences, and learn from the experience. Paige's joint pain came about from eating cheese. One time she was at a party and wanted to eat the cheese that was being served. I told her what would happen if she ate the cheese but it had been so long since she had felt the pain that she decided to eat the cheese. She enjoyed many slices of cheese, had excruciating joint pain the next night and truly learned from the experience!
- You are your child's number one advocate. If he or she is in pain, take responsibility for getting their pain under adequate control. Please don't ever give up!

How to make the best use of this chapter's information

1. Is your child having at least one large bowel movement every day—from their wrist to their elbow? If not, please read this chapter more carefully. There are many parents that tell me that their child is not reacting to food but later, realize that their child is not having frequent or large enough bowel movements.
2. Read how to cleanse your child's body on a regular basis so that the bad bacteria or toxins do not build up in their bodies and make them sick.
3. If your child is holding in bowel movements, getting ready for toilet training or in pain of any kind as a result of symptoms, you will benefit from the information discussed in this chapter.
4. Remember: Implementing a healthy diet is the first step to improving you child's bowel and overall health. Read the next chapter to learn more about preventing, detecting and eliminating all symptoms caused by food.

CHAPTER 5

THE SECRET'S OUT

How to Prevent, Detect, Minimize and Eliminate Reactions to Foods

---

There are a number of methods you can implement in order to prevent the onset of food reactions and improve your child's digestion. There are also a lot of discrepancies in this area, but the methods I am sharing with you are ones proven to work for my family and the families that I assist.

Preventing and minimizing reactions to food

Pre-pregnancy

Some have the good fortune of being able to plan their approximate time of conception; this section is written for those parents–to–be. Being tested by a naturopath (See Chapter #9) a year prior to conceiving and, subsequently, following the naturopath's protocol, will get both of your bodies into the best shape possible to conceive, carry and grow a healthy baby. In that year, you and your spouse can detoxify, get rid of candida, improve your digestion and good bacteria levels, stabilize your blood sugar and elevate your nutrition overall. As it takes at least 100 days for a sperm to develop, it would be ideal if both parents–to–be could eat as healthy as possible at least three months prior to conceiving a child.

In Utero

It is most important for you to know that the strength of your unborn baby's immune system depends on the quality of nutrients he or she receives in the womb. As well, a baby can be exposed to allergenic foods through the placenta when in utero, therefore:

- If sensitivities or allergies run in a mother's family, it is wise for the pregnant mother to find alternatives and refrain from eating the foods that cause adverse reactions for her.

- If both parents react to numerous foods or if they already have one child with many food sensitivities or allergies, it is recommended that pregnant mothers eliminate those foods causing the most adverse reactions from their diets.
- It is key that a pregnant woman eat a variety of foods so that she does not create a sensitivity to any one food in her unborn child.
- Processed foods should be avoided.
- Peanuts should not be part of a pregnant woman's diet; it is simply not a food with which to mess around.
- Supplement with probiotics or good bacteria (See Chapters #1 and #6).

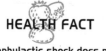

HEALTH FACT

Anaphylactic shock does not happen from one taste of a food.

The reason these steps are relevant is this: If your child has never been exposed to a food, he or she is less likely to be sensitive or allergic to it. Anaphylactic shock does not happen from one taste of a food. Thankfully, everyone has warnings. So, if a mother can eliminate problem foods or potential problem foods from her diet, parents are guaranteeing that their child will benefit. This does *not* mean that you must begin scrutinizing every label and eliminating foods whose labels read "may have been in contact with peanuts" if neither you, nor your husband, has ever had a problem with peanuts.

"According to a study in the June 1995 issue of the *Journal of Allergy and Clinical Immunology*, high-risk infants who do not consume cow's milk, eggs, and peanuts during infancy and whose mothers also avoided those foods during the perinatal period had a reduced incidence of food allergy and eczema in the first two years of life."[1]

It is vital that a mother-to-be take all necessary steps to increase her good bacteria and improve her digestion. This means staying away from the factors that contribute to the preponderance of sensitivities and allergies, many of which already need to be avoided in pregnancy (i.e. smoking, prescriptions drugs, pop and others listed in Chapter #1).

Consuming a good quality acidophilus, along with digestive enzymes (you can learn more about these products in the Supplement section of this chapter) would certainly help a mother create healthy intestines for herself. You would think that if a mother took extra good care of her intestines, it could only bode well for her baby...and you would be right!

"If your mother smoked while she was pregnant, you have four times the risk of anyone else for developing an allergy whether or not you also have a family history of allergy."[2]

While breast feeding or formula feeding your child

(I'll be addressing mothers in this section but if you are a father or other loved one, please pass on this information on to mother.)

What do you need to know about breastfeeding exclusively?

You've heard it a million times, breastfeeding your child is best and it's true. It is the number one way in which you can help your child develop to his or her full potential, physically, mentally and emotionally. Breastfeeding helps reduce the risk of allergy, as it provides antibodies that strengthen the immune system. Breast-feeding for a child's first year means that he or she never needs to go on allergenic formulas (more on this later in this chapter). Mother's milk is also filled with essential fatty acids, acidophilus and other beneficial nutrients that create healthy intestines in babies. I have written more about the contents of breast milk further on.

Let's say you are able to exclusively breastfeed your baby. I mentioned earlier that your child might react to what you eat, through your breast milk. If your child experiences any symptoms, think of what you're eating first before exploring other options. If you are not yet committed to the idea of keeping a food and symptom diary, try eliminating the following from your diet and replacing these foods with healthier alternatives (See Chapter #6):

1. **Dairy**–If dairy is the culprit, your baby's symptoms will improve within a couple of days; baby's bodies are very responsive. If your baby's symptoms are better but not gone, then try eliminating:
2. **Wheat**

You've just eliminated the top 2 common allergens from your child's diet. If that improves some of your baby's symptoms but your baby is still experiencing other symptoms, you are beginning to see the power of food before your very eyes. Take the next step. Explore this further and keep a food and symptom journal and/or start a more comprehensive elimination diet (more information can be found further on in this chapter).

I knew that it would be helpful for me to stay away from all the common allergens when I was pregnant with Paige. I also knew that I would need to give up these foods when I breastfed her. I determined that I would have too hard of a time cutting all these foods from my diet for such a lengthy time frame. So I decided to give up the problematic foods for the time in which I breastfed her. I stayed away from all of the common allergens and gas producing foods i.e. onions, garlic, broccoli, cauliflower, brussels sprouts, a very difficult task, to be sure. When she was about three months old, I had ribs (containing sugar, chemicals etc) for dinner at a restaurant. Paige spent about two hours that night crying, filled with gas and discomfort. I had my confirmation that I was doing the right thing, staying away from all the common allergens. After six months, I found that I could no longer deprive myself of many of the foods that I loved. I'm being totally honest, admitting that to you! I stopped breastfeeding and knew that I had done the best that I could have personally done. Everyone's experience is unique. All your child asks is that you do *your best* by them, whatever that may be.

You need to be comfortable with whatever decision you make. If you decide that you do not want to breastfeed your child at all or can only handle breast-feeding your child some of the time, that is your own decision. It doesn't matter what you read or what others tell you. You may be one to go crazy from lack of sleep or become completely stressed from breastfeeding. If this is the case, your baby, and other family members, will not only feel your pain but will be negatively impacted by your stress. When it comes to breastfeeding, I believe it us up to you and you alone to decide what is best for yourself and your family.

What should you do if you cannot breastfeed your baby exclusively?

You may be like me and cannot breastfeed exclusively (I found out with my second child that I had tubular breasts, which made breastfeeding exclusively impossible). What should you do?

Just one ounce of breast milk, added to your baby's bottle of formula can decrease, if not eliminate, your child's reaction to their formula. I know it's hard to believe but I know it to be true.

When I knew I wouldn't be able to breast feed my second daughter exclusively, I imported an organic soy formula from the United States. At the time, the world was only aware of the problems caused from genetically modified soy. I felt that if I fed my child organic soy formula, that I was circumventing the problem with soy. Not too much later, the world became aware of the estrogenic qualities of soy, which certainly made soy formula an unappealing option.

About every three hours I breastfed Paige and then topped her up with the formula. Paige developed eczema all around her neck and occasionally around her mouth. Where did the formula dribble when I was feeding her? Around her mouth and down into the folds of her neck. Eventually, she developed another symptom that alerted me to the fact that the formula was a problem for her; she starting going without bowel movements for up to a week at a time. I was told this was normal and not to worry about it. I had already learned all about healthy bowel movement frequency from Taylor and Paige had two or three bowel movements a day in the beginning, so there was no way that I was falling for this line. By this point, I had stopped breastfeeding Paige prior to each bottle. I noticed that when I breastfed her at night, after the breast milk had had a chance to accumulate, Paige had a bowel movement the next morning. I tried this a few times and the same thing happened. I went to my parents' meeting and told everyone my experience. My doula was there and said studies show that just one ounce of breast milk added to formula, can improve a child's digestion and lessen reactions to formula!

I rented an electric breast pump from the hospital and started pumping my breast milk in between feeding Paige and found, interestingly enough, that I could only ever pump one ounce of breast milk at a time, no matter how long I tried. I added that milk to Paige's formula and continued to ensure that I breastfed her prior to each bottle. She began having regular bowel movements. When Paige got older and started losing patience with breastfeeding, I simply added the one-ounce directly to her bottle and all was well. Breast milk is truly liquid gold.

For those of you that *cannot* breastfeed exclusively, I would strongly advise you to consider feeding your baby the breast milk that you have or pumping your milk and adding it to your child's formula.

That said, if you are breastfeeding and formula feeding, it is tricky to determine if it is something you are eating or your child's formula that is causing your child's symptoms. It is up to you what one you want to tackle first: maintaining a food and symptom diary for yourself or trying different formulas to see if a new formula makes a difference.

It is important to know that the **primary ingredients in infant formulas are dairy, soy, sugar and corn—all common allergens.** I must admit that I have not found one perfect formula to recommend you feed your baby. You will need to do your own research as to what you feel comfortable feeding your child and then watch them closely to see how they react to your choice. Do not be afraid to try different formulas!

Different formula types

HEALTH FACT

Breast milk is truly liquid gold.

In Britain, a lactose-free goat's milk formula is sold which is ideal for many babies. I look forward to the day that we can purchase the same in Canada.

There are two formulas in North America that have been around for years, which are hypoallergenic, named Alimentum (Ross) and Nutrimagen (Mead Johnson). These formulas can be found at drug stores and are more costly than those found at grocery stores. They are both based on cow's milk but the cow's milk protein is hydrolysed i.e. treated with digestive enzymes so that the cow's milk is broken down to such a degree that many babies can handle the formula. Alimentum contains soy but no corn. Nutrimagen contains no soy but contains corn. Recently, Enfamil came out with a hydrolysed cow's milk formula called Gentlease A+, which contains both soy and corn. Even the formula makers are recognizing the link between cow's milk and symptoms and describe hypoallergenic infant formula as "clinically proven for the dietary management of babies with cow's milk protein allergy symptoms, including colic, rash, eczema, and wheezing."

The company I ordered the organic soy formula from also make an organic cow's milk based formula, which may bode well for some babies. You can explore the ingredients and order it from www.naturesone.com. As well, there is organic cow's milk formula being sold at health food stores and The Real Canadian Super-store.

Lastly, in Dick Thom's book *Coping with Food Intolerances*, he lists recipes for making your own baby formula if you have the comfort level to do so. I have added two of them to the Appendix.

If you think your child might be reacting to his or her formula, you can add two supplements to the formula to help them digest it better. They are acidophilus (increases your child's good bacteria) and essential fatty acids. Both of these are found in breast milk. Essential Fatty Acids (EFAs) are often added to formulas by the manufacturer but are not as easy to assimilate in the body as adding EFAs yourself. Please read Chapter #6 for more information on these supplements.

When introducing solids

Dr. Lendon Smith states in *How to Raise a Healthy Child*, "A patient of mine was fed egg at 3 months to increase her iron intake; she promptly developed hives. When egg was reintroduced at 9 months, she reacted with swollen lips, cramps and diarrhea. Egg at 18 months caused anaphylactic shock, with pallor and a collapse in the floor. I am convinced if the egg had initially been served after her first birthday, she would not have developed the allergy at all."[3]

Dr. Dick Thom states, "If you are exposed to cow's milk any time in the first six months of life (including breast milk if your mother was drinking cow's milk), you're more likely to be sensitive to it than someone who had no exposure in those early months of life. In fact, in Sweden's hospital nurseries, nurses are not permitted to give cow's milk to infants without a doctor's prescription!" A baby is more likely to be sensitive to any of the common allergens if they are introduced in the first six months to one year of life!"[4]

There is a different order of introducing solids to children than previously recommended, in order to minimise the onset of food sensitivities and allergies and improve digestion. We all know the method that most doctors touted for years. Feed your baby cereal at 4 months. Now many of them are recommending cereal at 6 months. Ironically, Health Canada is now saying that cereal should not be a baby's first food. Better to start with fruits and vegetables. Even though Health Canada is on the right track, there is much more to learn about the order of introduction of solids!

Understanding your infant's body

This section is intended to explain some of the background as to why it is best to feed your baby fruits and vegetables from 6 months on.

Your baby is born with immature digestive, intestinal and immune systems.

It is not until 3 months after birth that the immune system even begins to protect a newborn. Luckily, a newborn still has his or her mother's antibodies to augment their defences during the first three months. These antibodies continue to protect newborns for longer periods of time if breastfed. In the early years of your child's life, they will be exposed to many different bacteria and viruses and probably contract numerous colds, fevers and other illnesses. This is how the body builds the immune system. The immune system can take at least 7 years to be considered fully developed!

A healthy intestinal system is important to a child's immune function because there are millions of immune cells lining the intestines, providing a line of defence against bacteria and other invaders. A weak intestinal system will leave a child more exposed to colds, flu and autoimmune disease. If your child is under 7 years old and has recurrent colds, infections or a condition, you may want to look at your child's levels of good bacteria, foods or environment a little more closely.

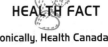

HEALTH FACT

Ironically, Health Canada is now saying that cereal should not be a baby's first food.

Research very clearly shows that leaving first foods as late as possible will help to ensure that your child's digestive, intestinal and immune systems are mature enough to cope. Common sense dictates that the less work these systems have to do in terms of digesting food, the more time and energy the systems can put into growth and development!

> *Eating Alive* says, "If the stomach and intestine are treated with care, it is extremely difficult for the rest of the body to have disease."[5]

Porous intestine or "leaky gut"

In Chapter #1, we discussed the fact that your baby is born with a porous intestine, commonly referred to as a "leaky gut". This means that there are small holes in the lining of the intestines, which allow important nutrients, like the macromolecules and antibodies in mother's milk, to pass through the intestinal wall. These holes close up at around four months of age, which is why doctors, for the longest time, recommended introducing solids at this age. These days, there are so many sources of bad bacteria, (discussed in Chapter #1), preventing the holes in the gut from closing. That makes another good reason to delay the introduction of solids until at least 6 months old.

Small stomach size

When your baby is born, he or she has a stomach about the size of a chickpea! This means that there is not much room for any quantity of food; a baby's body is designed more for absorption than digestion.

At around 6 months old, your baby's stomach grows to the size of a walnut; again, this is not very large! That's okay though, because until a year old, milk is the most important food for your baby. Solids are only experiential.

Few teeth, if any

The more teeth your child has, the better he or she is able to digest solids. More teeth means more saliva and more saliva means more salivary digestive enzymes!

In summary, the longer you wait to introduce solids, the better. Wait until your child's digestive, intestinal and immune systems are better able to handle small amounts of food and their tummy and teeth grow!

Order of Introduction

> Prescription for Dietary Wellness discusses the fact that white rice cereal is stripped of nutrients and high in starch. It states, "Until they are at least one year old, babies do not have the ability to digest starches (starches are not present in breast milk). Feeding starchy foods such as wheat cereals, turnips, and potatoes, and highly processed foods to babies before their digestive systems are able to break them, can lead to a variety of childhood illnesses and food allergies."[6]

The best first foods to offer your child in order to reduce stress on their bodily systems is a selection of steamed fruits and vegetables. **Fruits and vegetables are closest to breast milk in terms of their consistency and digestibility. They are also the least likely to cause reactions.**

Experts disagree as to whether fruits or vegetables should be introduced first. They also disagree about *which* fruits and vegetables should be introduced first. You now know the symptoms that can be caused by food, (See Chapter #1) so if your child experiences one or more of those symptoms, you know to stop the introduction of that food and try again in a few months or longer, depending on the reaction. If you find that your child is mildly reacting to fruits or vegetables with a high amount of carbohydrates, such as peaches, sweet potatoes, or carrots, this is an indication that your child has candida (See Chapter #3). All you need to do is give your child acidophilus and retry the problematic fruits and vegetables in a month's time. Until the problem is corrected, simply feed your child foods with fewer carbohydrates, such as broccoli, cauliflower, string beans or turnip. Strawberries, tomatoes, and citrus fruits are some of the common allergens that should be avoided until your child is at least a year old.

After introducing fruits and vegetables, there continues to be dispute among experts. Some say that around 9 months, nuts (other than peanuts) and seeds can be introduced.

Some say no nuts or seeds until after two years old. It *is* agreed that once your child becomes one year old, you may start to introduce harder to digest foods and some of the common allergenic foods. Remember that, at one year old, milk is no longer the most important source of nutrients and your child needs to receive protein, fats and carbohydrates from other sources.

Harder to digest foods can be introduced in this order:
- Legumes i.e. green peas, chick peas, lentils, and beans
- Grains (no/low gluten grains are easier to digest than grains with gluten)
- Proteins i.e. eggs, meat, poultry and fish
- Common allergens (see Chapter #1)

Honey should not be given to a child until after the age of one, as children are more prone to botulism before then. Chocolate and peanuts should not be introduced until at least two years, or some say, three years of age.

> "The cautious approach has been proven through a variety of different studies aimed at helping to prevent allergies and intolerance in susceptible children. For example, Dr. Zeiger's investigation followed 165 children from birth to age seven that were at high risk of developing allergies because of their parents' allergic conditions. He concluded: "Avoiding the early introduction of potentially allergenic foods is the basic step in the primary prevention of food allergies in children who are at high risk, but some infants may still become sensitized or allergic to a food. Signs of food allergy in infants include eczema, hives, wheezing, or vomiting from formula. Fortunately, early detection of a food allergy can help reduce its severity."[7]

Method of Introduction
The first day you feed your child solids should be a day when he or she is happy and healthy (i.e. they should be well rested, not have a cold or be in any pain from teething). The reason for this is that you want to be able to determine if your child is reacting to the food he or she just tried or if there is another contributing factor to their symptom.

The best time of day to introduce solids is in the morning or early afternoon, so that if your child does have a reaction, you are lessening the chances that you and your baby's night's sleep will be ruined! Solids should be fed in between breast-feedings or bottles. You don't want your child to be so hungry that they fill up on solids and not have an appetite for their milk.

I highly recommend using *organic* fruits and vegetables when introducing them to your child for the first time; this ensures that if your child reacts, he or she is reacting to the food itself, not the insecticides or pesticides in the food. Please read further on in this chapter to learn other reasons to choose organic.

Once you've found a food that your child likes and doesn't immediately react to it, offer the same food for four days, watching for any reactions. As we discussed, it can take up to four days for your child to react to a food. If there is a reaction, stop feeding the offending food to your child and try it again in a few months, depending on the severity of the reaction.

If there is no reaction, on the fifth day, you can introduce another fruit or vegetable. You can feed this food for breakfast. The food that you already tested on your child can be their lunch. In this way, you can build up the variety of foods that your child consumes each day.

Ensuring that your child eats a variety of foods each day increases their chances of obtaining the nutrients they need and minimises the chances of them being sensitive to any one food, as different enzymes are created to digest each new food. ***Never introduce more than one new food in a four-day time span (it's called the four-day rule) because you need to know which food causes a reaction, if any.***

I have shared the most important information about introducing solids to your child. For more information on introducing solids and feeding babies and toddlers, please refer to my website and have a look at the classes I offer.

Once your child is able to chew his or her food
In addition to choosing foods that are easy to digest and ensuring your child stays away from the sources of bad bacteria, the very best way to help your child digest their food better is to follow these steps:

Steps to Optimal Digestion
A large percentage of digestion occurs in the mouth, believe it or not!

Encourage your child (and yourself!) to:
1. Chew his or her food until it is a paste. This is the most important thing one can do to improve digestion.
2. Relax while eating (no television or computer or eating on the move). Sit quietly for a few minutes before and after each meal.
3. Try not to drink any liquids while eating as liquids dilute the enzymes and hydrochloric or stomach acid (See Chapter #3 for more on this) needed to digest food. Little sips of warm liquids are okay (i.e. herbal teas with a meal are acceptable, if needed to help with the chewing process). If you can get your child in the habit of drinking about 20 minutes before or after a meal, it is easiest on the digestive system. Warm water with lemon juice is a wonderful digestive aid.

4. Never drink cold liquids as they freeze the stomach glands and inhibit digestion (body is not capable of producing HCl).

5. Have smaller meals more often. 5 meals a day is ideal–smaller frequent meals keep metabolism at a good pace. The more anyone eats, the more enzymes you need and the more the digestive system is taxed. If children are taught to eat smaller amounts more often at a young age, they'll continue into adulthood. A portion size is only the size of your child's palm.

5. Stop eating by 7 pm each day.

6. Properly food combine if your child has a number of digestive issues (i.e. sensitivities or allergies). Digestion is so poor these days that many of us are turning to proper food combining but this wasn't required years ago. It was the increase of yeast–related problems brought about by antibiotics and refined carbohydrates, such as white sugar and white flour, that created this need in some individuals. Proper food combining involves having fruit on its own with at least an hour separation from other food. It also involves never mixing animal proteins and starches together.

7. As always, ensure your child has adequate levels of good bacteria to assist with digestion. Avoid or limit the factors that contribute to bad bacteria or toxic load (listed in Chapter #1).

90% of food allergies and sensitivities could be eliminated if we chewed well. Completely digested food is actually non–allergic. Also, fruits and vegetables have cellulose membranes, which must be broken down by chewing before they can be properly digested. Many adverse reactions to fresh produce result simply from not chewing enough. By eating raw foods and chewing them well, a large amount of digestion will take place in the mouth before the stomach does any work.

A Rotational Diet
Your child needs to eat whole, simple foods and diversify his or her diet. One of the cornerstones of a healthy diet is variety. The modern world offers a wide variety of different foods from various climates and cultures. There are lots of Japanese, Indian and Thai foods at most health food stores. Try them. Some parents have never tried a mango or papaya or avocado. Open your mind and your child will benefit.

If your child consistently eats a lot of the same food and you are not doing other things to improve their good bacteria and digestion, they will most likely become sensitive to those foods. When I discovered that Taylor could not eat wheat or sugar, I used spelt, honey and maple syrup instead. And can you guess what happened? She became sensitive to spelt, honey and maple syrup. You always hear "Everything in moderation"; the saying is right on.

If you have a hard time feeding your family a variety of foods, there is something called the four–day rotational diet that you can use to introduce variety into your meals. I would recommend you read about the diet even if you do not plan to follow it. The information I'm going to share with you is important to building your knowledge about food sensitivities and allergies.

The Rotation Diet serves four purposes:
1. It is a diagnostic tool, which can unmask food sensitivities or allergies (the elimination diet is better for this though, please read about it further on)
2. It minimizes the development of new sensitivities or allergies
3. It helps children continue to tolerate foods that he or she is already able to eat
4. It allows a child to eat the foods to which they are mildly sensitive on an occasional basis.

This diet was first called the Rotary Diversified Diet. It was developed by Dr. Herbert J. Rinkel in 1934. He believed that by rotating a variety of foods, the probability of adverse reactions occurring could be minimized. Today the rotation diet is taught in Nutrition schools across North America. If a child eats peas at one meal, he or she would have to refrain from eating peas again, in any form, for 3 more days. This is a healthy way to ensure that your child receives a variety of nutrients in their diet. Any nutritionist can help you put the diet in place for your child so that your mind is put at ease, in terms of meeting your child's nutrition needs.

The other purpose for this way of eating is to aid the reintroduction of previously reactionary foods. If your child stays away from a food that once caused a reaction for a period of time, and then that food is reintroduced into his diet, the food will continue to "work" for your child as long as it is used in rotation. We now know that if you have made the improvements to your child's digestion and/or intestinal wall, this way of eating is not necessary but variety is always a good thing.

In case your child reacts to a number of foods, all you need to begin a seven-day food cycle are twenty-one foods to which your child is not reactive. Otherwise, it would be advisable for your child to eat a greater variety of foods.

The whole point of the rotation diet is to let the body recover from the effects of a food before eating the food again. In general, it takes up to 3 days for a meal to pass through the human digestive system. To be safe, allow four days between ingestions of a particular food.

How do you detect your child's food sensitivities and allergies?

Detecting food sensitivities and allergies in a child

You already know that food sensitivities are tricky to detect. Most allergies are easier to detect but there are some that are not. No matter what, the earlier you can detect your child's specific problematic foods, the better! You want to prevent your child's reactions and subsequent health from becoming worse.

As you are learning, some children simply feel unwell while others are unable to learn or behave appropriately because of reactions to food. A child's early years and entire future can be adversely affected by delays in recognizing the many faces and forms of food sensitivities. You must discover the foods and substances that are causing your child's symptoms, conditions or disease; they are different for everyone and everyone's reactions to offending foods are different.

Scratch tests or skin testing performed in doctor's offices, only measure immediate hypersensitivity reactions i.e. allergies. They do not measure digestive problems i.e. sensitivities to foods, chemicals or the environment nor do they measure delayed reactions. In addition, these tests can be invasive and are not 100% accurate.

In detecting food allergies, a scratch test may not produce a positive result. This is because the IgE antibody that is present when there is a true allergy may be localized to some other tissue such as the intestine or nose. In this case, the IgE antibody has not entered the general circulation (blood stream) and therefore would not be present in the skin. The test works best in detecting inhalant allergies.

> Dr. Skye Weintraub states, "The most dependable skin tests for food allergies give accurate results only 30–40% of the time...some people never learn whether they have allergies or sensitivities to foods."[8]

There are a number of methods currently employed for detecting food sensitivities i.e. blood tests, enzyme testing, Interro or electro–dermal screening. Naturopaths or nutritionists perform most of these tests. None of these tests are 100% accurate however they have helped many people narrow down the foods that need to be removed from a child's diet.

The only reliable means for detecting symptoms caused by food is to learn how to read your child's body. It is vital that you discover which foods will help your individual child reach optimal health. I wish I could give you a blueprint of children's bodies but I cannot; every child is different. Become the expert on your child. Wheat can energize one child but make another one want to lie down and take a nap. Eggs can improve one child's concentration but cause another to break into itchy and distracting hives.

HEALTH FACT

It is vital that you discover which foods will help your individual child reach optimal health

How do you read your child's body? We, as parents, often need to be taught how to do this. In our busy lives, many of us don't automatically pay attention to which food makes our child energetic or tired, happy or sad or excited or anxious. We sometimes don't look at which foods bring about bowel movements and which ones constipate. Some nights your daughter can't sleep. Could she have eaten a certain food that caused her insomnia? You might think that playing soccer brings on bouts of asthma in your son. Have you looked into which foods are mucus forming to begin with and taken steps to avoid them?

From reading Chapter #1, you now know some symptoms and foods to watch out for, particularly the foods to which your child is addicted, and that it can take a few days from consumption for your child to react to a food. "How am I going to remember what my child ate four days ago" you ask? That's going to be pretty tricky without the use of a food and symptom journal. It is only through recording the foods that your child is eating and any reactions you observe, over a period of time, that you can clearly see the patterns. You might say, *"Wow, every time my son has cheese, he gets sore legs two days later. I thought it was the hockey that was making his legs hurt!"*

Keeping a food and symptom diary

Keeping a diary, depending on how many details you include, is the only method for determining your child's food reactions with 100% accuracy. Your diary can also be used to check or back up the results you received from any of the tests that you now know are not entirely accurate. It can also be a useful tool for diagnosis and treatment if you decide to solicit the help of a health professional.

The way to keep a food and symptom diary is to record:

1. The date on the top of your page.
2. A list of the foods, drinks, vitamins, spices, gum, toothpaste, drugs or anything that has entered your child's system that day. Don't forget about bath water, pool water, second hand cigarette smoke or fumes from cleaning supplies.
3. The activities your child engaged in that day or any extenuating circumstances; a different family member or a babysitter might have cared for him or her. When your child is left with someone else, they might be fed foods that you are unaware of or your child might be reacting to something in that person's home such as a pet. A food diary will show the symptoms if that is indeed what is going on. Every time my daughter, Taylor, had a swimming class, she caught a cold, which is what alerted me to the potential for an allergy to chlorine.
4. Physical or emotional symptoms that your child experiences, if any. Please refer to the list of symptoms, conditions and diseases that can be caused by food in Chapter #1. Examples include the energy levels of your child each day and the quality of sleep your child has each night. You may want to mention the duration and severity of your child's symptom as well.

Keeping this log makes it easier, over time, to see the patterns. Until you know your child's culprit foods, you'll need to write down everything your child consumes. Once you've eliminated the culprits, you only need to write down the new foods you're trying on your child.

Many of you are busy parents. You may have other children or a full-time job and you're saying to yourself "I don't have time to do this! Forget it. I guess I'll never know the foods to which my child reacts." Don't give up before you've even started! All you need to do is grab a sticky note and scribble down a few details. For example:

Wed May 26th–Tried yogurt
Thurs–Runny nose.

I recommend keeping a food and symptom diary for a minimum of two weeks in order to establish the culprit foods. You need not be overly concerned about trying to determine whether your child's reaction to a culprit food is an allergy or sensitivity. You want to stay away from the foods that cause reactions, period!

Detecting food sensitivities and allergies in a baby that is exclusively breastfed

A baby can be exposed to allergenic foods through breast milk. Many medical doctors, lactation consultants, midwives etc challenge this statement in itself. You'll hear these experts say that babies cannot react to breast milk; it is the perfect food. They are right; babies are not reacting to the breast milk itself but to the food or chemicals that their mothers have consumed, which enter and remain in the milk! Many experts will tell you that the food a mother consumes becomes broken down and pre-digested in the mother's milk prior to her baby consuming the milk. If this is the case, why did my daughter, Paige, react so badly when I ate ribs, the only food I cheated with in the whole six months I breastfed her? I have countless other examples of my eldest reacting to my breast milk, one of which you read about in the "Our story" section.

When an exclusively breastfed child has an adverse reaction or symptom, the first thing that should be examined is his or her mother's diet. Once food as a culprit has been ruled out, *then* other areas should be examined. In most cases, symptoms such as colic, excessive gas, eczema, diaper rash, diarrhea, constipation, and others are as a result of food sensitivities.

If your baby or child has any adverse reactions and he or she is exclusively breastfed, a food and symptom diary can also be of great benefit. By recording what mother eats and what baby's symptoms are, you will be better able to determine the offending foods over time.

It bears repeating, the foods that are most likely to cause problems for yourself and your child are those that you eat often and in large quantities or "binged" on during pregnancy, those you crave and those that you dislike but eat because you think they are healthy. Anything with a drug-like action, such as coffee, tea, wine (especially red wine), beer and spirits, are other suspects, particularly for babies with colic.

Once you think you have determined the foods causing your child's symptoms, you may want to follow an elimination diet to turn "culprit" foods into "safe" foods.

An elimination diet

Food allergy pioneers, Dr. William Crook and Dr. Doris Rapp, first described the elimination diet or elimination-provocation technique. Some of the most well known experts in food allergies and sensitivities rely on this technique for determining problematic foods although it seems that every expert working in this field has a slightly different approach to implementing the diet.

An elimination diet can help you detect your child's problematic foods and, at the same time, help your child's body heal as those foods are eliminated from his or her diet. If your whole family can follow an elimination diet together, this will make the process easier for your child. As an added bonus, each of you will benefit from eating healthier food! (Please refer to Chapter #6 for ideas)

One mother told me that she could not eliminate all sugar from her daughter's diet. She felt that it was so cruel, not to mention the fact that she didn't know what her child would eat that didn't contain sugar. **When it is so hard to wrench a food from your child's diet, it is probably a culprit.** We all know that sugar doesn't do a stitch of good for anyone. It is important to understand that there are many wonderful, healthier alternatives to sugar, which you will read about later. I'm not going to tell you that you *have* to do anything when it comes to feeding your child. Your child's symptoms will tell you how badly he or she needs your help; I am simply telling you how you can help your child when you decide it's needed.

Here is the approach that I have found works most effectively with children:

1. Have your child abstain from eating several foods (See common foods causing symptoms, conditions and disease, listed in Chapter #1) for approximately one week. Your child will just eat non–allergenic foods (See Chapter #6) and then you will add each commonly allergenic food back into the diet, one at a time, carefully watching for symptoms over the next 4 days. However, an elimination diet can also be executed the following way:

2. Have your child abstain from eating one suspect food for a period of time and then reintroduce it. If the child's symptoms reappear, it is evidence that your child is sensitive to the food.

The idea here is that when a problem food is out of your child's diet for a period of time and then reintroduced, reactions are provoked and symptoms that you would otherwise be unable to notice, become obvious. The elimination diet allows your child's body to speak and be heard. The objective is to create a period of "silence" where there are no symptoms coming about from food at all. Then, when a problematic food is reintroduced, the symptoms can be heard. This is why it is better to follow the first approach to the elimination diet, excluding all foods that are likely to be causing problems.

Whichever method you choose, you need to be very diligent ensuring your child does not even have a small amount of a potentially problematic food. Remember to check ingredients in any packaged foods and try to stay away from restaurants that week. You don't want all your hard work to become worthless! If your child has a condition, it would be wise to enlist the help of a nutritionist or naturopath (See Chapter #8) to help you manage an elimination diet and any resulting reactions.

When a child follows an elimination diet correctly, he or she will experience improvements in his or her overall wellbeing. Some specific examples of what you will observe include improvements in:

- Any symptom or condition
- Attitude
- Behaviour
- Cognitive performance
- Energy levels
- Mood
- Reading ability
- Writing ability

Withdrawal symptoms
An adult usually experiences withdrawal symptoms from having a food removed from his or her diet, sometimes for up to three weeks after the food has been removed. A food cannot be reintroduced until those symptoms dissipate. Luckily for you, most children feel much better very quickly after removing problematic foods and you can start reintroducing one food at a time back into their diets once they have felt good for two or three days.

Occasionally, some children do feel worse in the first few days of an elimination diet. Sometimes, the diet may need to be continued for ten, fourteen or even twenty-one days before you'll notice a significant improvement.

Some of the common temporary withdrawal symptoms from food are:

- Aching in all parts of the body i.e. flu-like illness
- Behavioural abnormalities
- Fatigue
- Headaches (mild to severe)
- Heart palpitations
- High temperature or fever
- Pains in parts of the body that have not been affected before
- Temper tantrums

Withdrawal reactions to foods can be eased by giving your child Vitamin C (Please see Chapter #6 for more information).

Reintroduction of foods

Remember that when you reintroduce each food, you are watching for symptoms to appear *over the next 4 days*. And when you reintroduce a food, it is best to do it in the morning or early afternoon to minimize the impact of the offending food on your child's and your own sleep. So when you reintroduce a food on Monday morning, watch for symptoms on Monday, Tuesday, Wednesday and Thursday. All the while, carefully maintain your food and symptom journal.

What I've found with my children is that when they were babies, their reactions to foods occurred within 24 hours of consumption and once they hit one-year-old, reactions started to take longer, up to three days from consumption. On the fourth day, their bodies return to normal so that I can be reminded of what normal is before introducing another new or suspect food.

When deciding what food to reintroduce into your child's diet, you might want to take into account the following:

1. Is the food nutritious?
2. Is the food low in sugar and chemicals?
3. If you want to test poultry on your child but the chicken you have has additives, do you have access to organic chicken?
4. Do you have plans over the next few days that you do not want thwarted by your child's adverse reaction to a food?

Keep in mind that when you are adding a food back into your child's diet, ensure that you test the food in its purest form. For example, use a pure dark chocolate bar from the health food store in order to test chocolate rather than a regular chocolate bar containing dairy, wheat, corn, chemicals and other ingredients.

Once you detect your child's sensitivities or allergies, set priorities as to the changes you want to make. It is really important to pace yourself and your child as you undergo dietary changes. You may decide you want to try a new food on your son every week or every other week or once a month. Some of you may be so worn out from living with the reactions to foods that you will want to just enjoy peace within your family now that you've discovered the culprits and try nothing new!

Whatever you do, the less said to your child the better. This is always the rule of thumb. You don't need to tell your child what you are doing. When you are ready, simply feed your son or daughter a new food and watch for a reaction. If your child does react and he or she wants to know what caused the reaction, let them know what it was and then refrain from saying anything more. The last thing you want is for your child to be anxious about a food they are about to eat; a reaction can become a self-fulfilling prophecy. It will be tricky for some to prevent over-focussing on food and reactions but if you can stay calm and approach dietary changes with balance, your whole family will benefit.

It's very important to remember to replace foods that trigger symptoms with foods or groups of foods that have a similiar nutrient content. For example, if you drop wheat, you must ensure that your child has another source of good-quality unrefined carbohydrates such as spelt. You'll find that the food alternatives that are recommended in Chapter #6 are healthier for your child and less likely to incite reactions. Further journaling helps organize your plan of action.

Other journaling

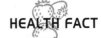

HEALTH FACT

Once you determine the foods to which your child reacts, it will be helpful for you to record separate lists of:

> It's very important to remember to replace foods that trigger symptoms with foods or groups of foods that have a similiar nutrient content.

1. New foods for your child to try and, possibly, the date you're aiming to try each one
2. Foods that your child responds well to
3. Foods that your child does not respond well to
4. The various meals and snacks that you feed your child on a regular basis
5. The various alternative therapies or supplements that you try on your child and your thoughts on how they are working.

Many parents want to know how long to leave a food out of their child's diet once they determine it to be an offender. The answer is extremely subjective. A good rule of thumb is to leave a food that caused a minor symptom in your child out of his or her diet for two to three months and simultaneously work on improving your child's levels of good bacteria and digestion. If you don't work on your child's digestive process, the culprit food may remain a problem and he or she might eventually start reacting to other foods.

If the food caused a more severe reaction, potentially an allergic reaction, a good rule of thumb is to leave that food out of your child's diet for one year and simultaneously work on your child's digestion and healing his or her intestine. These time frames give your child's body an opportunity for the inflammation to diminish and for healing to occur.

In summary: Once you've determined which foods cause reactions in your child, it is extremely important that those foods be completely eliminated from your child's diet, at least initially. In terms of the foods that your child is all right with, try to make sure that you do not offer your child the same food more than once in a 4-day period. You do not want your child to develop more sensitivity. Simultaneously, work on improving your child's digestive and intestinal tracts with the ideas in this chapter. Later, depending on how severely your child reacted to an offending food, that food can be reintroduced slowly, closely watching for any reactions.

Eliminating reactions to foods

When you know for certain that your child has food sensitivities or allergies, what do you do?

What do you do to eliminate your child's food sensitivities?

1. Detect and remove your child's problematic foods from his or her diet.
2. Improve your child's digestion through the use of diet, supplements (Learn how to replenish good bacteria and enzyme activity in Chapter #6) and the "steps for optimal digestion".

What can you do to eliminate your child's food allergies?

1. Detect and remove your child's problematic foods from his or her diet.
2. Eliminate anything causing your child's gut to be leaky i.e. stress, candida, parasites, drugs, sugar, caffeine, viruses, and bacteria (Refer to list in Chapter #1 of the causes of bad bacteria or toxins).
3. Heal your child's gut lining through the use of diet (See Chapter #6), supplements and the "steps for optimal digestion".

Some children avoid a culprit food for years and their allergy never goes away. That's how you know more is involved. As you know, it took me two years to heal Taylor's leaky gut and eliminate her allergies and sensitivities. *I removed all of the common allergens from her diet, replacing them with healthier alternatives and gave her the necessary supplements (acidophilus, essential fatty acids and Vitamin C).* I then fed a culprit food to her after a year and then every few months or so, until the food worked on her. The Canadian School of Natural Nutrition teaches that it takes approximately two years to heal the leaky gut of an adult.

You've just read how I healed my daughter, Taylor, but don't panic! Her situation was extreme. Why did I remove *all* the common allergens? Why did it take two years? Taylor had problems with all the common allergens. This is extremely rare! You may only need to substitute one of the common allergens from your child's diet, replace it with a healthier alternative and give them some supplements–that's it! You can relax. It took two years for me to heal Taylor's gut because she was severely lacking in good bacteria and as a result, had some major challenges! To this day, I have not personally met any child with as many allergies or sensitivities as Taylor had. She had to be our teacher though, didn't she?

Paige had no allergies until the age of five, at which time she started at a new school and decided she wanted to drink from the water fountains alongside her friends. I had warned her about the dangers of chlorine and other contaminants in tap water, but she decided to sneak water from the fountain at this time and she did so for many weeks. It caused her all sorts of health challenges, such as constipation, tantrums, and fatigue. Most noticeably, her body reached its toxic load and her sensitivity to dairy became an allergy. Her allergy was so bad that even if she had a small amount of dairy, she would experience joint pains that were out of control. So, she avoided all forms of dairy for a year, replacing them with healthier alternatives, took the necessary supplements and avoided the items on the list in Chapter #1 that deplete good bacteria. Her dairy allergy is gone.

The next chapter explains more thoroughly how you too can accomplish this seemingly monumental task.

Ten smart strategies for avoiding symptoms, conditions and disease

I. Breastfeed your baby

Breastfeed your baby, if you can, for the following reasons:

- Colostrum alone is high in protein and antibodies. It gives nursing babies natural immunity and protects their gastrointestinal tract, which is not yet mature enough to handle more complex foods. Passing antibodies onto infants helps prevent bacterial and viral infections.
- Breast milk is in its raw state; it contains loads of natural enzymes to aid in its digestion. Infant formulas and cow's milk have been heat-treated through pasteurization at temperatures high enough to kill all the enzymes. If an infant's immature digestive tract cannot supply all the needed enzymes, incomplete digestion takes place. Partially digested protein particles can pass through the naturally permeable intestinal lining and enter into the general circulation more easily, causing an allergic response i.e. colic. Infant formulas are also much higher in protein content than breast milk and are based on the allergenic milks, cow's milk and soymilk, putting an additional strain on a baby's digestive tract. This is why feeding infant formula to babies increases the frequency of sensitivities and allergies.
- The fat contained in human milk, compared with cow's milk (which most infant formulas are based on), is more digestible for babies and allows for greater absorption of fat-soluble vitamins into the bloodstream.
- Human milk, and only human milk, contains an enzyme that breaks down the fat in the milk to form individual free fatty acids, which inhibits the growth of bad bacteria and parasites in the intestine.
- Iron, zinc, other minerals, and essential fatty acids in breast milk are more easily absorbed than those found in formula. Food sensitivities and allergies are linked to deficiencies in a number of key nutrients.

- If you cannot breastfeed exclusively, don't give up; the protective factors in just one ounce of breast milk prevent the onset and minimize reactions to infant formulas.
- Breastfeeding provides your child with skin-to-skin touch or physical contact, helping children to thrive.
- Breastfeeding contains natural pain relief agents which is why a child recovers so much easier from an injury causing pain once he or she is put to the breast.
- Breastfeeding your baby sets the stage for your child's lifelong connection to food as nourishment (See Chapter #10 for more information on nourishing your child with food).

2. Introduce solids slowly (see all of the information written earlier in the chapter)

How you introduce solids to your child will greatly impact the strength of their intestinal wall and digestion capabilities, determining whether or not your child will react to food.

3. Feed yourself and your child foods for maximum nutritional benefit

Feed your child and your other family members more of the foods that our ancestors ate a hundred or more years ago—**natural, alive, good quality foods**. If your child reacts to food, we know his digestion is compromised so it is extremely important that the foods he does eat are filled with nutrients, thereby contributing to his health and growth.

> "It is easier to become addicted to a refined, processed food than to a whole food in its natural state. A refined food has lost its normal protective ratios of synergistic vitamins, minerals and enzymes either by removal or destruction. This alters the way the refined food is metabolized in the body."[9]

Try to reduce, or even remove, any food from your child's diet that contains chemicals, in the form of additives, preservatives, flavours and anything else. All of these put a strain on your child's body, particularly the liver, which is so crucial for detoxification and healthy digestion. These chemicals will raise your child's toxic load and, in turn, weaken his or her whole system.

Feed your children **foods that are high in fibre**. This speeds the elimination of waste and bad bacteria before it can do any harm. In addition to preventing constipation, fibre also cuts down on reactions to food and on fluctuations in blood sugar levels. Fibre is the "broom" that sweeps the colon. Remember, you read about the importance of fibre to diabetics.

Consuming **raw foods** provides the body with live disease–fighting phyto-chemicals and fibre. Cooking depletes vitamins and phytochemicals, destroys enzymes necessary for easy digestion and damages fats and protein. Raw food provides the natural balance of fibre, enzymes, nutrients and the water that we need. If natural enzymes are present in a food, a child's body will need to secrete fewer of its own enzymes to finish the job. Kids often prefer raw foods anyway. Try to incorporate a raw fruit or vegetable into each meal you feed your child. For those that have a hard time digesting raw vegetables because of the cellulose, all you need to do is lightly steam them and digestion will be improved.

Juices made from fresh fruits and vegetables help the body eliminate waste while at the same time speeding up the healing process of the body. When you extract juice from fruits and vegetables, leaving behind the pulp, fibre is lost. How-ever, when you are juicing, this is actually a good thing. Without the fibre, all the nutrients, enzymes and phytochemicals extracted from fresh, raw produce can be quickly digested and absorbed by the body. This is the quickest way to nourish and regenerate cells, tissues, glands and organs. Some diseases or disorders can even be arrested or healed using live juice therapy!

Green drinks, containing spirulina, chlorella, and blue–green algae are referred to by scientists as nature's most perfect foods. These drinks are excellent for reduc-ing inflammation in the body, helping the body eliminate toxins and recurrent infections, as well as energizing the body. Adding a few drops of chlorella to your child's water adds a nice mint taste, which many enjoy.

It is always best to eat a **variety of foods**. Repeated consumption of a specific food stresses the enzyme systems in handling that particular food. If the food is also an allergenic food, the body's capacity to deal with it is greatly diminished. Variety also ensures that your child will be getting a wide cross section of neces-sary nutrients. Lastly, foods work synergistically with one another to create max-imum healing potential. If you introduce a wide variety of different foods and fresh foods, you can start educating your child's taste buds at a young age. Chil-dren have no preconceived ideas about food; it is up to us to help them enjoy the huge spectrum of foods available. Most children older than about 8 months instinctively seek variety unless they have had some bad food experiences.

Feed yourself and your child organic foods.
There are hundreds of studies showing the link between a mother's eating habits and environmental factors on the health of an unborn child.

> ".... A lack of key nutrients and a preponderance of toxins can have an effect on everything from birth weight, IQ, immunity, future fertility and susceptibility to allergies, to cancers, hyperactivity, sleep disorders and normal growth patterns. Choosing organic means

ensuring a good intake of key nutrients while reducing exposure to harmful toxins."[10]

Prior to the Second World War, there was no need for organic food because of the care taken with the soil and the purity that was maintained with the fruits and vegetables being grown in that soil. In fact, fruits and vegetables were organic without being labelled as such. However, in nature, "perfect" fruit has always been rare. One of the reasons that chemicals started being added to fruits and vegetables was to improve their appearance. The organic apple is smaller, has a duller sheen, and the skin is a subtle blend of colours and imperfections; no two apples on a tree look exactly alike. Please do not let the look of organic fruits and vegetables deter you from their purchase.

As well, please don't let the media or others deter you from believing that organic food is truly organic. If a food has a "certified organic" label, it means that each ingredient and every process qualifies it as organic and chemical free.

Organic foods contain no:
- Preservatives, pesticides, artificial fertilizers or food colouring; these chemicals affect digestion and immunity, causing food sensitivities and allergies.
- Genetically modified ingredients, which result in new proteins being formed. Remember, adverse reactions to foods often occur because the body cannot break down proteins.
- Heavy or unnecessary antibiotics; only antibiotics that are necessary for individual animal treatment are used.

Also, organic food is grown in nutrient-rich soil. An organic apple has ten times more nutrients than non-organic. As a result, organic foods taste better than non-organic foods! When children become accustomed to eating nutritious organic food, good eating habits are formed which will help them stay healthy for a lifetime.

I have a fabulous example demonstrating the authenticity of certified organic foods. Our family had a hamster, which was Paige's very best friend for a long time. I fed it different kinds of organic lettuce and nuts and seeds. It came time for us to take a vacation and our neighbours agreed to look after our hamster for us. Now I am past worrying about what others think, but back then, I didn't want my neighbours to know that we were feeding our hamster expensive organic lettuce! So I bought the regular lettuce, which they fed our hamster for one week. I told them that they didn't need to clean the cage in our absence. When we returned after one week, our hamster's cage was filthy and smelled really bad. When I had been feeding the hamster organic lettuce, the cage hadn't needed to be cleaned for at least two weeks! I experimented with this again a few months later and sure enough, the non-organic lettuce required a cage cleaning twice a week versus every 2 weeks with organic lettuce! I should also mention that what I fed the hamsters that we owned over the years, created wonderful, fluffy, soft and relaxed little creatures! All I fed them was organic lettuce, nuts and seeds.

So how much needs to be organic? The answer is to choose organic whenever possible. Buy as much as you can afford. You've probably noticed that the cost of organic products has reduced and the availability has increased over the years as the demand has increased. There is no doubt that organic products do still cost more than non-organic. By cutting out all the convenience and junk food and focusing on quality foods such as fruits and vegetables, you may find you're actually able to spend less on groceries in the long run. Just think of the improved health that organic food brings and you may start viewing the cost of organic food differently too!

> "It is no coincidence that an increased number of miscarriages, stillbirths, childhood cancers, birth defects, heart disease, allergies and auto-immune conditions in children has coincided with the expansion of the processed, convenience food market, based on intensively farmed foods. Children need good, nutritious, fresh, healthy food and they need an environment that is as free from chemicals as possible. From the moment a parent makes the decision to have a baby, the emphasis has to be on reducing the load of toxins in food and in the products used in the home. The best and safest way to do this is to go organic."[11]

Please refer to Chapter #6 for specific foods to feed your child and the Appendix for recipe ideas.

4. Eliminate the foods to which your child reacts

Sensitivities or allergies do not cause every disease but they can be involved in almost any disease. They can weaken the body so that other life threatening diseases can gain a foothold. This is because allergies weaken the immune system over time so that the body cannot defend itself from foreign invaders and tissue degeneration. The most common way allergy kills is not by anaphylactic shock reaction but by the slow multiple symptom syndrome. It is so prevalent that if you have not been told the cause of your child's health problems or symptoms, you should consider sensitivities or allergies first.

5. Ensure proper elimination of toxins (See Chapter #4 for more information)

If this doesn't happen, your child's whole digestive system cripples and their immune system weakens. If a child is constipated, it is not possible for his or her body to absorb the vitamins and minerals that it needs. We already read about foods that help create elimination of toxins. Feed them to your child in large quantities.

6. Pay attention to probiotics, vitamins, and minerals (See Chapter #6 for more information)

Food contains vitamins and minerals, particularly if it is organic and is eaten raw. However, most of the food that we eat today is neither organic nor raw, and it doesn't contain the vitamins or minerals of foods grown in nutrient rich soil. It is absolutely necessary that we supplement our children's diets with probiotics, vitamins, and minerals if we want to increase their good bacteria and truly support their immune systems.

7. Give your child filtered water

Water is the most important substance needed by the body, after air. Increasing your child's water consumption might be the first step you take in improving your child's health, particularly your child's digestion.

> The *Tao of Detox* explains the importance of water in this way, "Water is also the element that extracts nutrients from food, transports them into the bloodstream and delivers them in solution into the cells for metabolism. 90 percent of the blood and 85 percent of the brain are water; even the bones contain 30 percent water. Water is thus required for nourishment and the replenishment of vital fluids, as well as for detoxifying the blood and tissues and eliminating wastes (including candida!). "[12]

Winning the Food Fight by Dr. Joey Shulman explains that water helps the body maintain a normal temperature and an acid/alkaline environment. It also discusses water's ability to relieve fatigue, asthma, allergies, crohn's, colitis, irritable bowel syndrome, skin conditions and help with weight loss. Water also provides necessary minerals.

> "The water used by most people throughout the world today carries more toxic elements into their bodies than it washes out."[13]

Tap water contains bad bacteria from chlorine, fluoride, up to 100 other chemicals and heavy metals i.e. aluminum, cadmium, lead, copper. The quality of bottled water can be difficult to determine. You'll need to do some research to obtain a pure, clean source of filtered water for your children.

Children need to develop a taste for water; that is difficult to do if the only drinks your child consumes are juice, milk or pop. Ensure that children are given water in a container they enjoy drinking from. If a kitchen has a water dispenser that the children can access easily, there will be far more water consumption. Sipping water throughout the day rather than gulping down a cup at a time is preferable.

If a child is adequately hydrated, they may react to certain foods less. *The Tao of Detox* says, "Dehydration produces a state of chronic toxemia and is one of the primary causes of daytime fatigue, sluggish metabolism, depression and inability to concentrate. It is also a major contributing factor to cancer. Several studies have demonstrated that by drinking only 5 glasses of pure water per day, the average person may reduce his or her risk of colon cancer by 45%, breast cancer by 80% and bladder cancer by 50%."[14]

Dehydration is often the hidden cause in cases of chronic pain, including headaches and chronic fatigue. Dehydration dries the blood and other bodily fluids, causing cells to shrink and retain their toxic wastes. When cells are properly hydrated, they expand and become active, spontaneously cleansing themselves of toxic wastes. People take billions of dollars worth of chemical drugs to control pain, yet most of this pain can usually be relieved simply by drinking sufficient quantities of pure alkaline water each day.

HEALTH FACT

Children are more prone to dehydration than adults because of their size and higher activity levels.

Children are more prone to dehydration than adults because of their size and higher activity levels. By the time a child is thirsty, he or she is already dehydrated. Children sometimes go through stages where they lose the urge to drink or say they are not thirsty; this causes the body to eventually stop signalling that it needs water. It is important to stay on top of this.

A formula for calculating how much filtered water your child should consume in a day is:

$$\frac{Weight}{2} = x \qquad\qquad e.g.\ \frac{70\ lbs.}{2} = 35$$

$$\frac{x}{8} = \text{number of 8 ounce glasses a person needs per day} \qquad\qquad \frac{35}{8} = 4\ \text{cups approximately}$$

Water helps children exercise longer and more efficiently. It reduces stress on the cardiovascular system and improves athletic performance. Your child will also need to drink more after exercising to avoid dehydration. If you see poor concentration, constipation, diarrhea, urinary tract infections, fever, chills, headaches, dry mouth, dry skin or poor skin elasticity (returns to normal slowly if pinched), rashes, muscle aches, nausea, crankiness, lack of tears when crying, sunken eyes, lethargy or apathy, then your child needs more water. *If their urine is darker than a very pale straw yellow or is strong smelling, your child needs more water.*

One last point that needs to be made is that drinking water helps fill the stomach and decrease hunger. Why would you want that, you might ask? There needs to be a balance between water and food consumption. When I see one of my daughters making a beeline for snacks over and over within a short time frame, I know she is dehydrated. We have already talked about the problems that result when a child overeats. Your child should be able to eat one snack and feel satisfied. For more information on amounts of foods that children need to stay healthy, please refer to Chapter #6.

8. Provide your child with the regular opportunity to relax and sleep

The rhythm of a child's day should be like breathing; in and out, activity, then rest. The rest provides the body with an opportunity to fight sickness.

Stress

More and more adults are starting to see the real stress that children of all ages are under today. Children certainly feel stress and anxiety. Many children today are actually more sensitive to things being out of balance than are adults. Over-scheduling, working parents, and peer pressure, combined with a general lack of exercise are only some of the causes of this stress. High consumption of white sugar, white flour products and other refined foods also stress the body. If your child is eating foods to which they are sensitive, this also increases the stress levels in their body. Witness the domino effect. High stress = weakened adrenal glands = increased cortisol levels = high inflammation in the body = increased reactions to food, all of which result in harm to the intestinal lining. In high-stress situations, it may only take a few foods to create a symptom.

Older children with multiple food sensitivities or allergies (over 30) often have weakened adrenal glands. The adrenal glands produce hormones such as cortisone and epinephrine, which help to prevent or decrease the intensity of reactions to food.

Stress shuts down the digestive system in order to prepare the body for fight or flight. If this happens enough, it can lead to a decrease in stomach acid and digestive enzymes. Subsequently, the digestive system begins to receive less blood, oxygen, and nutrition, which then weakens the immune system. This results in an increased risk of infection and illness.

If your child is irritable, impatient, wakes up in the night and can't fall back asleep or craves salt, he or she may not be handling stress very well. Kids can also have depression, difficulty concentrating, behaviour problems, lack of motivation, recurring fatigue or total exhaustion, anemia, hypothyroidism, hypoglycemia, indigestion, irritable bowel syndrome, malabsorption, blue circles under eyes (not bags so much), food cravings (i.e. salt), or a low body temperature as a result of stress or being born to stressed out parents!

Inadequate adrenal gland function *can* be inherited from a child's parents, especially if it was the mother that was over stressed or had a poor diet.

The Tao of Detox puts it best when it states "Only when the nervous system is at rest in the restorative parasympathetic (relaxed) mode can the body neutralize and eliminate toxins, process and excrete digestive wastes, regenerate its cellular structure, and restore itself to a balanced state of health and vitality."[15]

The best two approaches for fixing the adrenals (stress glands) in children involve sleep and food:

- Put your child to bed the same time every night and let him or her awake the same time each morning.
- Stress depletes our bodies of vitamins and minerals and often when any of us are stressed out, we don't want to accept the nourishment from food. The way we eat our food and often our food choices themselves, create indigestion. Foods rich in vitamins and minerals or supplements are key in battling stress. Vitamin C directly supports the production of stress hormones (adrenal glands have higher content of vitamin C than any other organ). Vitamin B is referred to as the "stress" vitamin as it makes such a difference to a child undergoing stress. The need for protein also increases during stress.

Of course, communication between child and parent is crucial. Time alone with a parent on a regular basis builds the trust between a parent and child so that the child will feel comfortable opening up to Mom or Dad. Strong negative emotions create inner stress; those feelings need to get out (i.e. journaling, arts and crafts, exercise, and deep breathing) in order for the body to stay healthy.

If you implement or help your child to implement some of these ideas, you will lower the stress that each of you feels:

- "Be more spontaneous and live fully in the moment
- Embrace joy and enthusiasm in everyday life
- Learn to ask for what you need
- Meet your needs while being sensitive to others
- Be more openhearted, willing and able to love, and be loved
- Let go of fear
- Let go of control
- Surrender your self–guilt, self–pity, grudges, and depression
- Let go of the past
- Live life from the inside out, rather than from the outside in
- Love yourself"[16]

"Often, the difference between the non-allergic person and the allergic one is the difference between strong, responsive adrenal glands that can direct the body's defences quickly, and weak, sluggish glands that do not have the capacity to do the necessary work."[17]

Inadequate Sleep

When a child is tired, nothing is easy. In addition to the problem of feeling tired, lack of sleep can compromise a child's immune system, increasing susceptibility to food sensitivities or sickness. It can diminish a child's mental function; and increase their risk of harmful accidents. If a child goes a while without adequate sleep, she can find herself focussing more on the negatives than the positives. Fatigue can also mess with your child's appetite, making them eat more to gain more energy or eat less because they are too tired.

Most children between the ages of five and twelve sleep 8–12 hours a night. If a child wakes and feels rested 5-10 minutes after waking up, they are getting enough sleep.

Sleeping patterns can also be affected by the timing of meals, reactions to foods and the quality and quantity of food eaten. Certainly, a regular routine of waking up, eating, going to bed and refraining from feeding your child just before bed, will help your child fall asleep faster and sleep more soundly.

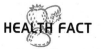

HEALTH FACT

It is up to you, the parent, to ensure that your child is given ample OPPORTUNITY to sleep.

Here's the most important thing to know. It is up to you, the parent, to ensure that your child is given ample *opportunity* to sleep. That opportunity is lost if you are constantly allowing your child to go to bed late and then waking them up to go to school or if you or your spouse is being noisy enough that your child awakens early on a Saturday morning.

9. Ensure your child exercises regularly

Children today are entertained by sedentary pursuits–television, video games, and computers. Nearly two thirds of American children exercise less than two hours a week. Couch-potato kids fatigue more easily than active ones and are more apt to develop diabetes, high cholesterol and obesity as adults. In a study published in the Journal of the American Medical Association, participants with low fitness were 3 to 6 times more likely to develop diabetes, hypertension and metabolic syndrome than the participants with high fitness. Clearly, lack of fitness and good health during youth is likely to translate into increased risk of health concerns when older. Poor health conditions don't have to be a normal part of aging.

Family First by Dr. Phil lists the following benefits of physical activity in children. It:

- "Promotes clear thinking
- Boosts creativity
- Stimulates the brain and learning
- Increases energy and mental concentration
- Produces positive changes in the body that enhance self–esteem (which in turn supports better cognitive learning)
- Helps develop motor skills and coordination
- Helps manage stress and anxiety
- Reduces depression by increasing levels of important brain chemicals i.e. seratonin and other feel good neurotransmitters that are often depleted in depression."[18]

Two other huge benefits of exercise are that it helps improve sleep and *digestion of food!!!*

Your child needs to get out and play, move, exercise, and have fun physically! The American Heart Association recommends that all children age two or older should engage in fun physical activity at least thirty minutes every day, plus thirty minutes or more of vigorous exercise at least 3–4 days a week to build and maintain a healthy heart and lungs.

One of the most valuable contributions you could give your children is to exercise yourself.

Brain Gym is a form of exercise that activates the brain and helps children grow physically, mentally and emotionally. By performing 26 simple and fun movements, children are better able to focus, organize, comprehend and communicate. Grade levels, confidence and attitude improve dramatically with the use of Brain Gym.

According to Jill Hewlett, Educational Kinesiologist and cofounder of Brain Works Global Inc. "The brain's alertness is the result of cognitive fitness–a state of optimized ability to reason, remember, learn, plan, and adapt."[19]

For more information please go to **www.brainworksglobal.com**

10. Help to make sure your child is happy!

You are ultimately responsible for your child's health and well being. Infections, eczema, constipation, autism, obesity and diabetes are common symptoms and conditions found in children today but that doesn't mean we, as parents, should just sit back and watch our children suffer, waiting to outgrow them. If we do that, more and more symptoms will appear. Please see Chapters #7 and #10 for further assistance with your child's emotional well being.

Even if you adopt just a few of these smart strategies for health, your child will benefit immensely.

How to make the best use of this chapter's information

1. Read about preventing and minimizing food reactions—whether you are thinking about conceiving, already pregnant, breastfeeding, introducing solids or feeding your older child. Don't forget to read about the ways to decrease the reactions your child is having to his or her formula!

2. By reading the prior chapters, you linked symptoms to food. In this chapter, you can read about keeping a food and symptom journal and following an elimination diet, in order to detect the specific foods to which your newborn (exclusively breastfed or bottle fed) or child is reacting.

3. Then, if your child is reacting to food, read about the ways to eliminate food sensitivities and allergies.

4. I invite every parent to read the ten smart strategies for avoiding symptoms, conditions and disease.

CHAPTER 6

EAT THIS!

How to Feed Your Child

"No race in history has ever attempted to live in the diet that North Americans are now eating. There is no scientific proof that we can healthfully live on it. There is now appearing considerable evidence that we cannot. More and more authorities are becoming aware that adequate diet is an absolutely necessary pre-condition to a healthy life."[1]

Some of you are seeing the link between food and symptoms, conditions and disease and you want to feed your child in the best possible way in order to prevent health challenges of any sort. Some of you understand that your child is reacting to food. You see the problem feeding your child their particular culprit foods. The question is, what are you going to feed your child until their levels of good bacteria improve?

Finding that answer was a daunting task for us, let me tell you. I used to scour the shelves at three different health food stores on a regular basis in order to find Taylor good-tasting foods and provide her with options. Nowadays, there is a great selection of healthy foods, even at the local grocery stores! Then I had to wrap my head around paying an arm and a leg for a product that, once opened, we couldn't even stand the smell of, never mind the taste. Through lots of trial and error, I eventually found lots of good-tasting options. I remember hearing my husband say more than once, "Here's your $10 homemade sandwich, Taylor"…because her sandwich consisted of organic poultry, specialty bread and supplements. Oh, the frustration of it all…

Then there was the issue of recipes. I cannot tell you the number of times that Taylor and I both got so excited about trying out a new recipe only to find that the treat was no treat–it tasted ghastly! So many times, the challenge of feeding Taylor seemed insurmountable but again, I persevered. The slogan "Where there is a will, there is a way" comes to mind.

The idea of trying to put one meal on the table, for the whole family to enjoy, became a noble one. Before learning of Taylor's sensitivities, we all ate the same meal. Then Taylor started having her own meals and Craig and I had our own thing. Then, needing to be Taylor's ally and knowing that she was eating the healthiest of foods, I joined Taylor and ate the same meal as her. That left Dad eating the unhealthy food all by himself.

Each time I prepared Craig's meal, I knew it wasn't right that he continue to eat unhealthy foods when I knew better but I decided to let time take its course. Craig had to want to eat healthier and I had to find recipes that he could stomach! I found that once I found good tasting recipes, he ate healthier. Before I found those tasty meal ideas, even though Craig was a really good sport, there were some dinners I know he just wanted to throw out and have me start all over again, but he never told me so. I felt enormous guilt. Here was this good man, working hard to provide for his family every day, coming home to one lacklustre meal after another.

For the past few years, I have served one meal to our whole family. We've also reached a balance where most nights we all eat the same meal and some nights Craig eats out. At least three times a month, we all enjoy a "Treat Day" (You'll read about those later in the chapter) where we eat regular food together. In fact, once Craig ate and enjoyed enough of our healthy meals, he started to see the problems he encountered whenever he did eat out but he won't want me to share his symptoms with you!

I had another challenge. Once I found store bought-foods that Taylor could eat and actually liked, I never wanted to be without them. Whenever I went shopping, I would pile up my cart even though there was still plenty at home. The health food was expensive and I would purchase greater quantities than I needed. Later, I became conscious of the fact that I was coming from a place of fear and deprivation; I was afraid that I would not be able to feed or satisfy my daughter.

It wasn't until 2 years after Taylor's constipation bouts ended, that I finally graduated from survivor mode to actually becoming concerned with the health of the foods Taylor was eating. I knew it was more important for me to eliminate the foods that were "bad" for my child than it was to feed my child the "good" foods. She had been fine with plain potato chips so I let her have them more often than other parents might have. You see, they were something she could eat so I didn't care about the health of them! I figured she was already healthier than the average child because she couldn't have sugar or chemicals or other nasties. This was definitely true but the more I researched food and its impact on the developing child, the more I realized that now was the time to pay attention to health, as well.

It is a huge challenge for parents of food-reactive children to ensure that their children's diets are both balanced and nutritious, as well as being appealing, tempting, delicious and child-friendly. Children need a multitude of different nutrients to ensure that they grow and develop properly. What's more, they need to learn the enjoyment of good food and recognize that it does not need to pose a threat to their lifestyles. They need to have treats along with nourishing meals, instilling healthy eating habits that will remain with them for the rest of their lives. This chapter and the Appendix are specifically designed to help you meet this challenge.

Feeding Your Child for Lifelong Health describes the "Five major areas where you can expect food to have an especially big impact:
- Promoting healthy weight gain and preventing obesity
- Avoiding allergies
- Optimizing bone strength and height
- Boosting intelligence
- Preventing childhood cancers"[2]

Foods to limit or keep away from your child
- Refined sugar and sugar products
- White flour products
- Packaged or processed foods (foods that have been altered from their original state)
- Foods that have been fried in hydrogenated oils
- Dairy products, especially cheese and cow's milk
- Red meat
- Foods to which your child reacts
- Juice, tea, or soft drinks with added corn syrup, sugar, glucose, or colourings.

Foods to feed your child (also referred to throughout the book as "healthier alternatives")
Let's take a look at what was eaten before the 1940s. All fruits and vegetables were "organic". Wheat and oats were not altered and bread was purchased fresh, one loaf at a time. Refrigerators were rare and if you were lucky enough to have one, they had little freezer space so there were no readily available tubs of ice cream, Freezies or Drumsticks! Store-bought ice cream was considered a big treat. There was no television, therefore no t.v. dinners or pre-packaged meals. No fast food restaurants existed. No preservatives, colours, flavours, or marshmallows were added to food. It was a whole different world…a world where the majority of children were healthy, a world where everything was simpler, a world that we can learn from today.

When my daughter couldn't eat any of the common allergens, I learned that the way she was eating was the way to prevent and treat all symptoms, conditions and disease. ***The same 'best principles of eating' apply to all symptoms, conditions and disease.***

All your child needs to eat is:

- Fresh vegetables and fruit (An apple a day really does keep the doctor away as long as your child eats different varieties of apples, preferably organic). Apples are "live foods", there is large variety of them to choose from and they a superior source of fibre. They contain essential fatty acids, vitamins, minerals and antioxidant compounds.
- Whole grains i.e. rice, amaranth, buckwheat, spelt, kamut, quinoa and yeast–free breads. All are complex carbohydrates, required for sharp mental per-formance.
- Legumes (complex carbohydrates) i.e. navy beans, black beans, lentils, split peas, chick peas, lima beans, black eyed peas and soy (twice per week). These are loaded with protein, complex carbohydrates, fibre, vitamins and minerals.
- Nuts and seeds, which are high in vitamins, minerals and good fats. Stay away from peanuts, soy nuts and cashew nuts.
- Fresh, lean poultry (chicken or turkey); poultry is high in iron.
- Cold water fish (twice per week) containing loads of brain–building fats.
- Eggs, (high in choline) which help build memory.
- Kefir or other yogurt from the health food store, if tolerated.
- Oils such as olive, sesame, flax, hemp or coconut oil (the most stable oil for cooking). Ghee, the clarified butter, is another good fat.
- Herbs, spices, raw unpasteurized honey, pure organic maple syrup (free of formaldehyde) and vanilla extract, Himalayan or sea salts, baking powder (free of aluminium), baking soda, carob chips or powder.
- Fortifiers such as brewer's yeast, blackstrap molasses, hemp protein powder or hemp hearts, and spirulina.
- Beverages: water being the best. All fruit juice, except orange juice (citrus, high in natural sugars and inflammatory) diluted half and half with water with a maximum of one cup per day.

These foods provide:

- Good quality protein, which is the building material for all brain cells and enzymes and vital for growth and repair of body tissues.
- A good source of fat to help a child's brain relay messages efficiently.
- Carbohydrates to provide energy, brain power and build body tissues.

Fruits and vegetables

Fruits and vegetables are packed with vitamins, minerals, antioxidants, fibre for bowel health, water and sugars, which the body metabolises slowly for a steady energy supply. The fructose in fruit has a steadying effect on blood sugar and does not have the jarring effect on the body that table sugar (sucrose) does.

Vegetables are probably even more important than fruit. Encouraging a taste for vegetables is extremely important for overall health. Vegetables are of vital importance in preventing all the major degenerative diseases such as cancer, heart disease and stroke. Vegetables are also important for bone health as they contain magnesium, which is needed to balance out calcium.

The goal for children is to have three portions of fruits and five or six portions of vegetables a day minimum. Four ounces of organic juice (sugar and chemical free), combined with four ounces of water, counts as a portion but only one eight ounce cup of juice is recommended a day. Make vegetables the centrepiece of your child's meal, with smaller amounts of protein and grain. Your child's body will benefit.

We also need slower-burning types of energy from good fats, proteins, and other carbohydrates to function throughout the day.

Good Fats
Good fats or essential fatty acids are discussed in detail further on in this chapter. Your child needs one to two sources of good fat per day.

Protein
Protein, derived from amino acids, is important for the building and rebuilding of body cells. It is also a vital nutrient for the brain.

> *Is Your Child's Brain Starving?* states, "Protein acts as a "blood sugar buffer", helping to slow the absorption of sugars into the bloodstream after meals. Meals that are low in protein and high in carbohydrates (starches and sugars) have a tendency to drive blood sugar levels upward initially and can result in rapidly dropping blood sugar levels later on. Studies have indicated that children with behavioural problems commonly have difficulties with blood sugar regulation. Kids can become restless or hyperactive after starchy or sugary meals as their blood sugar rapidly rises, then, as their blood sugar drops, they can become very distracted, moody or aggressive. Eating a good breakfast, high in protein, high in fibre, with moderate carbohydrates (sugar or starch), and moderate amounts of fat, helps keep blood sugar levels from going up and down like a roller coaster. This is one of the main reasons why studies show that eating a good breakfast improves mood, behaviour and academic performance."[3]

Protein also produces enzymes that assist with digestion and detoxification. Don't forget that protein comes from many sources, not just animals. All vegetables and fruit contain protein e.g. one cup of broccoli contains almost 5 grams of protein. Protein-rich foods also contain fats and carbohydrates. Your child needs 4 sources of protein a day, paying attention to portion size.

Carbohydrates

Carbohydrates provide the body with energy and are also vital nutrients for the brain. The no-carbohydrate diets are not in any way healthy for the body. Children's bodies need two portions of slow-releasing complex carbohydrates a day. Let me explain.

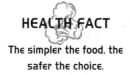

HEALTH FACT

The simpler the food, the safer the choice.

Carbohydrates are made of starches and sugars. The main difference between the carbohydrates is how easily they are converted to blood sugar and the length of time this takes. The slower the better, as it gives more sustained energy over time. Slow releasing carbohydrates are found in whole grains (brown rice), porridge, barley, pulses and beans, and vegetables. Potatoes, sweet potatoes, parsnips and fruit are other good sources of carbohydrates because they are all rich in vitamins and minerals needed for optimum health. Fast releasing simple carbohydrates are found in refined grains, corn, sugar and drinks. After digestion, all useable carbohydrates from starches are turned into blood sugar. Starches also provide fibre, which is needed for healthy bowels and to regulate blood sugar levels.

The simpler the food, the safer the choice. For example, single food dishes instead of casseroles enable you to avoid combinations of foods, which might contain a problematic food. With homemade pasta sauce and other sauces, you eliminate the problem of the sugar and chemicals that are found in store-bought sauces. Lucky for us, most children like their food plain.

As the awareness of food reactions grows, so has the variety of allergen-free products. The following foods contain no dairy, wheat or chemicals and have few, if any, of the common allergens. They can be found at health food stores or health aisles in large grocery stores. I've underlined the brand names that my family and clients find the tastiest. Having this list should save you a lot of time in purchasing health food that, otherwise, might end up tasting horrible! Don't forget that homemade is always preferable to store bought.

Children's Breakfast Ideas
(Choose at least one idea from this list each day)

"Children who skip breakfast, or who consistently eat cereals high in sugar, do not perform as well in aptitude tests, both verbal and non-verbal, when compared to children who eat slow releasing complex carbohydrates and protein."[4]

"Sugary cereals, donuts or pancakes with syrup are too high in processed carbs and sugar, which will accelerate the production of the brain chemical called seratonin. High levels of this chemical can induce sleep and mental grogginess—exactly what a child does not need for alert, effective performance in school or prior to taking a test."[5]

A healthy breakfast includes a piece of fruit or vegetable, some complex carbohydrates (whole grains) and protein. If protein is included, it makes for more morning brainpower than carbohydrates alone.

Below, you will find a list of options to feed your child. I have underlined the most popular and best-tasting brand names of the healthiest packaged foods. I apologize in advance for the fact that some of these brand names will not be around in years to come, when you are reading this book, however, by then, there will be even more options! Now, you parents that don't like to spend hours in your kitchen will have lots of snack and meal ideas.

Whole Grains
Stephano's Bakery Granola cereal
Gogo Quinoa puffs
Envirokids cereals
Barbara's Bakery Brown Rice Crisps cereal
Quinoa/Buckwheat/Millet/Oat hot cereal
Spelt/Kamut Flakes
Kamut puffs
Shasha & Co. Spelt Raisin Bread
Sticklings Organic Spelt Bagels and Buns
Van's wheat-free waffles
Oat, rice, spelt or kamut cakes
Brown rice wraps
Spelt filo pastry (frozen section of health store)
Don't forget, you can add fruit i.e. banana or berries, raisins, coconut, dried berries or apricots, chopped dates or carob chips to your child's cold or hot cereals.

Spreads and Syrups
St. Dalfour jams (many flavours)
Nut or seed butters
Unpasteurized honey
Apple butter
Maple syrup spread
Maple syrup (organic)
Fruit syrups
Agave nectar

Safest dairy alternatives (protein source)

Enriched rice, almond (sugar-free one) or hemp milk

Goat cheese–soft herb or plain–hard cheddar/mozzarella/marble on vegetables or crackers

Sheep cheese–lemon, rosemary and other flavours

Kefir, sheep, goat or soy yogurt

Saugeen County low lactose 'live culture' yogurt

Other Breakfast Protein Sources (not already mentioned)

Egg whites/whole eggs (boiled, scrambled, fried or omelette)

Turkey bacon

Turkey breakfast sausage·

Chicken or turkey sausage

Fish or hemp oil/powder

Fruit and vegetables

Recipes (See Appendix)

Flip-flapping Pancakes

Funky French Toast

Banana Mama Muffins

All Star Zucchini Muffins

Marvelous Muffins

Oaty Granoly Bars

Nutty Banana Bread

Fruit Smoothie

Shriek Shake (green drink)

Breakfast Combinations

Grilled tomato and turkey bacon sandwich on spelt bread with a bowl of berries

Grilled tomato and mushrooms with melted goat cheese on kamut toast

Bowl of oatmeal with grated apple, sunflower seeds and almond milk

Toasted cinnamon and raisin spelt bread with coconut butter and a boiled egg with a glass of mango juice

Oatcakes spread with almond butter and jam, with sliced orange on the side

Soy yogurt with toast spread with hummus and grapefruit slices

A slice of turkey or goat cheese wrapped in a slice of rice bread or added to a rice cracker with a chunk of cucumber

Scrambled egg with sliced turkey breakfast sausage and avocado in brown rice wrap

Children's Snack Ideas

We already talked about feeding your child a minimum of three portions of fruits and five to six portions of vegetables a day. Choose two ideas from the other snack ideas listed each day.

Fruits, Vegetables and Legumes

Organic fruits and vegetables (These are your first line of defence!)
Celery with a nut or seed butter (see below)
Vegetables with hummus/baba ganoush (*Fontaine Sante & Sunflower Kitchen*, both make a delicious tasting garlic hummus and other dips that children adore)
Sun-rype fruit to go squiggles
Fruit Source mini bites
Gourmet Fresh avocado dip with vegetables/crackers/rice cakes
Eden Organic applesauce
My Organic Toddler organic fruit friends (freeze dried fruits)
Organic dried fruits or legumes (chickpeas, peas)

Grains

Glutino gluten free cracker flax
Elco Rice Crackers–onion and garlic/sesame/plain
Vitaspelt pretzels
Veggie Chips
CheeCha Potato Puffs
Plain baked potato chips or *Kettle Chips* Honey Dijon flavour
Suzie's kamut spelt or rice cakes (plain or with a nut butter and/or jam)
Lundberg Rice chips–Sante Fe barbecue flavour
Envirokids organic crispy rice bars
Glenny's brown rice marshmallow treats–original/vanilla
Mr. Krispers baked rice krisps

Nuts and Seeds (protein source)

Raw or sprouted nuts and seeds
Nut and seed bars (*Honeybar, Taste of Nature, Bumblebar*)
Garlic and herb almonds
Tamari flavoured almonds
Pumpkin seed, cashew, almond, sunflower or tahini butter
Ground flax seed

Cookies and Treats (for occasional use)

Barbara's Wheat-free Fig Newtons

Shasha & Co. spelt cinnamon heart cookies

El Peto Products Ltd gluten free birds nest/carob chip cookies

Mi-del gluten-free ginger snaps/arrowroot cookies

Healthy Times cookies (oat)

Whole Alternatives certified organic microwave popcorn

Carob chips or *Cocoa Camino* organic chocolate chips, plain or melted, with maple syrup and drizzled over an apple on a stick, a bowl of strawberries or ice cream!

Glutino chocolate bars

Glutino vanilla dream bites

Pamelas Products ginger snapz, chocolate chip cookies or brownies

Rice Dream ice cream

It's Soy Delicious ice cream

Cool Hemp ice cream

Barkat gluten free ice cream cones

Efruiti gummy candies

Recipes (See Appendix)

Crunchy Chocolate Chippers

Must Eat Carrot Cake

Huggable Honey Cake

Clap Your Hands Carob Cake

Awesome Icing

Delectable Carob Fudge

Sticky Caramel Popcorn

So Tasty Carob Almond Spread

Golden Gingerbread Cookies

Humble Hemp Cookies

No-No Bake Cookies

Crazy Craisin Baked Apples

Meringue Kisses

Chocolate Bottom Cups

Quick as a Bunny Crisp

Doublicious Chocolate Pudding

Healthy Rice Crispy Squares

Simple treats to make

Baked apples with cinnamon

Dark chocolate chips on home-made puddings or ice cream

Bananas baked in their skin or peeled bananas dipped in melted carob and
   frozen

Poached pears with vanilla, cinnamon or melted chocolate

Popsicles (watermelon, melon, mango, strawberry and banana) or blend a
   banana, almond/rice/hemp milk and carob powder and freeze.

Children's Lunch/Dinner Ideas
(Choose two ideas from this list each day)

Falafels using rice wraps/bagels, hummus and vegetables

Hummus/bean spread/nut butter/pesto/baba ganoush/salsa and crackers

Brown/basmati rice and chickpeas/lentils/beans

Homemade pizza using **Shasha & Co** spelt pizza crust or rice crust, tomato
   sauce and vegetables and/or tofu

Tinkyada rice pastas or Artesan Acres kamut pastas (penne, spirals, spaghetti)
   or **Hockley Valley** spelt pasta and **Mediterranean Kitchen** tomato sauce/
   Cdn Herb & Spice Co sun dried tomato spice combo/pesto/**Lumiere de Sel**
   Himalayan salt (wild garlic flavour)

Sunflower Kitchen soup

Ursula's Catering split green pea soup

Sol vegetable/grain patties

Eden Organic baked beans

Molly B's gluten free perogies

Ian's gluten free crunchy chicken cutlets or fish sticks

Casa Fiesta tacos

Fajitas made with **Food for Life** brown rice wraps (freezer section)

Buncha Farmers chicken/turkey/beef gluten and sugar free potpies

Scrambled tofu/tofu fingers/slices with spices/honey, mustard & soy sauce

Sushi

Herbed, grilled or plain vegetables

Vegetable stews

Organic pre-made **Cascadian Farm** french or home fries

Fish, Poultry and Meat (protein source)

Canned wild salmon or **Raincoast Company** tuna

Rainbow Trout with mustard, honey and vegetables

Breaded organic turkey or chicken breasts

Organic turkey or chicken dogs/sausages

Organic ground turkey or chicken burgers/meatballs

Wild salmon burgers

Turkey kielbasa

Sliced turkey or chicken

Shish kabobs

Sandwiches (on sliced kamut/spelt/rice-bread/bagels/buns/wraps)

Hummus/baba ganoush/avocado dip
Tuna or salmon
Nut/seed butter & jam/honey/banana
Organic turkey or chicken slices
Turkey bacon
Egg
Grilled vegetable
Mashed avocado
Apple butter
Goat cheese & tomato

Recipes (See Appendix)

Healthy Shake N' Bake
Salmon Bits
Tangy Tuna Casserole
Chock Full O' Chicken Noodle Soup
Satisfying Shepherd's Pie
Maple Tofu Fingers
Scrumptious Bean Spread
Homerun Chickpea Balls
Tasty Burgers
Vege Chili
Vege Filled Lasagne
Yeast-free Pizza
Four Ingredient Mac and Cheese
Oh-So-Sweet Potato Hummus

Lunch or Dinner Combinations

Vegetables, shrimp or chicken strips, slivered almonds and rice stir-fry
Three-bean salad using canned beans and vinaigrette in a brown rice wrap
Baked chicken with rosemary, lemon, olive oil and toasted sesame seeds served
    with roasted baby potatoes or a steamed green bean and tomato salad
Quinoa with some flaked fish, peas, small pieces of cooked onion and red
    peppers
Vegetable samosas using ready-rolled spelt filo pastry and a filling of your
    choice (goat cheese, curried cooked veggies, sun dried tomatoes, hummus)
Spelt pasta with tuna, mayonnaise and diced sun-dried tomatoes
Mushroom and asparagus risotto
Chicken meatballs, tomato sauce and brown rice spaghetti

Easy drinks to make

Smoothies made with fresh soft fruit such as bananas, strawberries or blueberries, melon, papaya, or peaches and water, orange or apple juice, or milk and crushed ice

Any juice mixed with sparkling mineral water makes a fizzy drink

Old fashioned lemonade using lemon juice, water, a dash of maple syrup and ice cubes

Hot chocolate using warmed rice milk and a good quality chocolate powder such as Green and Blacks

Certainly those of us in York Region are blessed to be so close to **Nature's Emporium Wholistic Market** *www.naturesemporium.ca*, a gigantic health food store, which carries all of the aforementioned foods and much more. They are located at 16655 Yonge Street in Newmarket. Their phone number is 905–898–1844.

We are fortunate that bakeries exist today that make breads and foods from alternative flours. I encourage you to find a bakery of this kind in your neighbourhood. Every month, one of my friends drives 1.5 hours round trip to visit the bakery in my neighbourhood and freezes her purchases. It is called **Bagel Flame Bakery**, located in Aurora. Their phone number is 905–841–8766. In my opinion, it sells the best tasting foods of their kind. Here a listing of their alternative products:

Spelt muffins–different flavours

Cinnamon buns made with rice flour

Spelt gingerbread and other cookies

Rice cookies

Spelt apple pie

Kamut/spelt sliced bread/bagels/buns

Rice sliced bread/bagels/buns/hotdog buns

Rice pizza crust

Calderone's Produce is my store of choice for organic fruits and vegetables but they sell all sorts of healthy foods. They supply to the restaurants in the area so need to have the freshest produce available. They are located at 255 Industrial Parkway South in Aurora. They can be reached at 905–841–4452.

El Peto Products are located in Cambridge and offer pages of gluten–free great tasting products. They can be reached at 1–800–387–4064.

Judy's Magic Mixes are the most amazing gluten–free mixes that I have tried. She makes mixes for pies, cakes, cookies, muffins, breads, pancakes, and waffles. You can order from 1–866–598–9968 or **www.health–trends.ca.**

There are many other healthy food options for children; these will certainly get you started. Remember to remain conscious of how many pre–packaged foods you are feeding your children, as opposed to alive or "homemade with love" options.

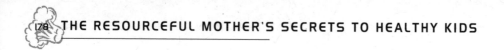

Children's one week menu plan

Sometime during each day:

- Smoothie with rice/ almond milk and fish/hemp oil/ground flax seeds, fruit, and ice or Kid's green drink
- Filtered water or herbal tea (warm or cold), drink separate from meals

Monday

Breakfast: Almond butter on a spelt bagel
Snack: Bowl of berries
Lunch: Baked salmon with vegetables and rice
Snack: Rice crackers and sliced turkey
Dinner: Breaded (spelt) chicken with steamed peas and carrots

Tuesday

Breakfast: Rice crisp cereal with almond milk
Snack: Garlic hummus with rice crackers
Lunch: Baked turkey breast with steamed broccoli and cauliflower
Snack: Fruit platter (sliced apples, cherries and watermelon)
Dinner: Rice pasta with tomato sauce containing herbs and finely chopped almonds, with cooked vegetables (onion, carrots, and snap peas)

Wednesday

Breakfast: Spelt cereal with hemp hearts, sliced fruit and enriched rice milk
Snack: Granola mix
Lunch: Boiled egg with kamut bagel and cut up red peppers and celery
Snack: Cashew butter on a spelt bun
Dinner: Chock Full O' Chicken noodle soup (See Appendix)

Thursday

Breakfast: Van's wheat free waffles toasted with nut butter
Snack: Carrots and celery with hummus
Lunch: Sliced chicken or turkey sandwich on kamut bagel with sliced cucumber and lettuce
Snack: Granola with raisins and dates
Dinner: Rainbow trout, brown basmati rice, sesame seeds and green beans

Friday

Breakfast: French toast using kamut or spelt bread, bananas, enriched rice milk and maple syrup
Snack: Baba ganoush on spelt bun
Lunch: Homemade vegetable soup with a slice of bread with hummus

Snack: Vegetables and La Fontaine Sante tofu spread
Dinner: Rice spaghetti with tomato sauce, peas, avocado and hemp hearts

I would recommend that all foods consumed be organic, if possible.

The need for treats

After what you have read so far in this book, you might be thinking, hasn't this mother ever taken her children to McDonald's? I have (once). My children have also tried many of the junk foods available to mankind. However, these splurges are occasional treats, not the staples of our diet. Over the years, I have modelled the valuable concept of moderation for my children.

The term "treats" can be summarized as any food that your child does not eat on a regular basis. There are three kinds of treats for the food–reactive child:

1. The safe treats–the kind they can safely have without any repercussions e.g. homemade honey cookies, carob bars (healthy chocolate bars) and Soy Delicious ice cream on a cone
2. The unsafe but generally healthy treats–single foods to which your child reacts (e.g. eggs, corn) that will cause repercussions if eaten
3. The unsafe and completely unhealthy treats–the kind that will cause repercussions for any child (e.g. candy floss, marshmallows)

I believe the first category of treats can be given to your child every few days. The second and third categories of treats should be eaten with far more discrimination. For some, these kinds of treats are completely out of the question, until they have stayed away from their problem foods long enough that their bodies are able to handle small amounts.

Some "health nuts" would say, "Your child should not eat any treats. The body only needs and should only be fed healthy food". That is, of course, entirely true! Certainly there is no need to expose a pre-school child, without older siblings, to category three treats. However, when it comes to older children, ask yourself these three questions:

1. Do you want your child living in a bubble? Imagine never being able to order eggs and toast at a restaurant or never having a regular ice cream cone or simply buying a treat from any store they go into (rather than just a health food store). The confidence and joy that a food–reactive child gains from going to a Baskin Robbins store and ordering whatever he or she wants is tremendous. To have no fear of major repercussions is huge for a child's emotional growth. When your child sees their friends enjoying treats, your child itches to do the same. This is simply a fact of life.

2. Do you want your child to have the experience of tasting something that is totally delicious? It's an interesting question because if you always feed your child healthily, many times they will try a category 2 or 3 "treat" and say, "I don't like it" or "It's too sweet". However, that won't happen every time. There will always be something they'll try that will fill their body with ecstasy. For my girls, that treat is ice cream (third category).

3. Do you want your child to grow up without treats then leave home and proceed to gorge themselves with junk food? Deprivation will do that. So that is exactly what will happen if they never have treats as a child. Human beings, by nature, are curious. They also want to experience what others experience. Why? Well, that's human nature too.

So, if you agree with this philosophy, how do you handle treats? How much do you give, how often? This is, of course, entirely up to you but I'll just give you some ideas as to how I handle this.

"Treat Day"

I give my step-mom full credit for this one. In our family, she invented the almighty "Treat Day".

It had been two years since my eldest had been in any pain from constipation. Taylor forgot what the pain felt like, so she was no longer afraid to experience it. At the age of four, she started sneaking food. She began with babysitters, telling them she could eat certain foods when she couldn't. It proceeded to her having a small piece of cake at a birthday party that I had not accompanied her to. I was astounded because Taylor had always been completely on side with me when it came to taking care of her body. It didn't take me long to think it through. This was a child, a child who craved treats, real treats but never was able to have them. Could I blame her for being dishonest? No. Once she started experiencing minor repercussions from these treats, she stopped sneaking as often but she didn't stop all together. In addition, almost every day, she asked me for treats. No mother wants to always tell their child "No".

In comes the concept of "Treat Day". This means having a "Treat Day" once in a while so that your child can experience other foods but ensure that his or her body doesn't go into overload. **You see, it is better for your child's body to have one day of eating some unhealthy choices as opposed to eating one or two treats every day.** Important: Do not use this day to feed your child a food to which they react (e.g. eggs), if you want your child to be able to handle the food one day. Strictly avoid any foods to which you want your child to overcome their sensitivity or allergy.

These days, I use "Treat Day" for all three categories of treats. The concept can only be put into play if your child:

- Is able to handle unhealthy treats without major repercussions
- Knows what he or she is missing. The way your child will learn what they are missing is by being around older children who eat "normal" food on a regular basis or if an older sibling is having the occasional treat. Younger siblings always want what older siblings have, no matter what it is! I certainly could not allow my eldest to have "Treat Day" and deny my youngest that pleasure. Mind you, my youngest didn't have the major repercussions from having food that her sister experienced.

Here's how the concept of "Treat Days" works for a child two years old and up…

You explain the concept of "Treat Day" to your child. An example of what you might say is "I know how much you love treats and I want you to have them. It's great that your body can handle treats of this kind now; remember when you couldn't have these things? Here's the thing, if you have too many treats, your body will start telling you that it can't handle them again. Also, you are asking for treats wherever we go, bugging me all the time. So here's my idea. You can have treats every once in a while on what's called "a treat day". We can make a calendar and mark all the days on it that you can have treats."

Both of my children loved this idea. I said "Okay, let's look at our calendar to see when we have birthday parties or special occasions coming up." We found that over the next month, we had one to three special occasions a week. I felt that we could have a treat day once a week for that first month and we would see how things went. On the weeks where there was more than one special occasion, I asked the girls to choose the event at which they wanted to enjoy treats. They wanted to have treats at friends' birthday parties but didn't feel the need to at family events. In this way, we were able to put stickers on the calendar marking four allotted Treat Days over the next month.

The build-up in excitement as the treat day fast approached was quite tremendous. Initially, they continued to ask for treats whenever they saw them. I would always respond, "It's not Treat Day" or "Wait for Treat Day". I never gave in and because of this, Treat Days remained sacred. Eventually, they stopped asking for treats in between those days, as they knew I would never waver.

When Treat Days arrived, my older daughter would awaken, immediately remember, and come flying into our room, yelling "It's Treat Day today!" The younger one (three years old, at the time) would slowly awaken, as she always does. The first thing she'd say was "Is it Treat Day today?" and her arms would go up and down in a silent cheer once I told her it was.

At first, the girls would only have what the others around them were having on those days. Then they got smart and started asking for other treats on those days…things they had never had before but wanted to try. Nobody would be eating gummy worms at a birthday party but one of my girls would bring it up out of the blue and ask if they could try some that day. I felt that they were having enough at the birthday party and told them so. I found that my daughters knew they were getting carried away and dropped the subject. Eventually, if they were given candy by someone else on a non-treat day, they would say, "Can I have this on Treat Day?" I would say "Yes" and put it in a special spot for them to have on the next Treat Day. Children never forget that you have a treat waiting for them, by the way. So, don't even think about eating that treat yourself, supposing they'll forget all about it by Treat Day because they won't! Sometimes we would go grocery shopping together and they would see something they wanted to try on the next treat day. Sometimes I would allow this and sometimes I would not, depending on how I saw their bodies reacting to the current treat load.

It is up to you to decide how many treats to give your child on a treat day. If you give them too much or allow too many treats just prior to bedtime, your child might take hours to fall asleep and then have frequent wakings throughout the night. You need to look at your child's symptoms as the determinant. If their symptoms are bad for their health, such as diarrhea or your lives are being 'ruined' by poor behaviour or constant tears, you know you need to either cut back on the treats or do away with Treat Day all together. You might decide that only one treat is allowed on a treat Day. You have to determine how much you will allow yourself and your child to suffer. If your child's body has healed to such as extent that he or she can withstand numerous category 3 treats on Treat day, you will, no doubt, be very excited by this development. However, you may want to think about how your child's overall health will be affected by consuming these types of treats on a regular basis. It is easy to say, "My child is healed" and allow frequent Treat Days until your child is, once again, eating poorly all the time, which might have been exactly where you were when you picked up this book.

Speaking to your child before Treat Day is upon you is the very best thing you can do to ensure the day goes smoothly. You can discuss the number of treats they can have and/or decide upon the actual treats they will have. Feel free to put in a caveat such as "We don't know how your body will handle this, so we're going to take each Treat Day as it comes. Next Treat Day may be different".

I explained earlier the importance of feeding your children as similarly as possible. The same holds for Treat Day. If one child is suffering more from the treats than the other, then Treat Day needs to be scaled back to meet the needs of that child. The other child will be happy to have any treat; they don't need to know their allocation of treats is being scaled back. Treat Days are something with which you can play; nothing need be set in stone.

One word of caution. If your child is looking forward to treat day for any length of time, you cannot then say "No Treat Day" as a punishment for misbehaviour. Pick another consequence for their actions, not the sacred, long awaited Treat Day. I fully believe food should never be used as a bribe or punishment.

There are also better times in the day to give your child treats when it is Treat Day. Breakfast and late evening are not the optimal times. ***Right after a meal is ideal; sweets cause fewer blood sugar fluctuations if they are consumed following a meal of whole foods than if they are taken between meals.***

For those of you that are single parents, with your child visiting their other parent, you may be faced with a challenge if the other parent doesn't feed your child healthy foods. This scenario is very common. Use the Treat Day concept to your advantage. Your child may have Treat Days for the weekend they are with their other parent and eat healthy the rest of the time with you. Why should your ex have all the fun, you ask? There are many other ways to have fun. Remember, you care too much about setting the foundation for your child's lifetime of health to feed your child badly. If your child is visiting their other parent more often than just two days a week, suggest to your ex that he or she pick the Treat Days in which your child be fed treats but that it can't be every day of each visit. Let your child's symptoms explain your reasoning for this approach.

HEALTH FACT

Remember, you care too much about setting the foundation for your child's lifetime of health to feed your child badly.

Supplements to feed your child

Avoiding the foods to which your child reacts is the most important step you can take to helping your son or daughter overcome food sensitivities and allergies. It is not, however, the only step. You also need to heal your child's gut, whether it has a lack of good bacteria (food sensitivities) or is actually leaky (food allergies). This is done with supplements i.e. vitamins and minerals. Supplements are aptly named; these vitamins and minerals are supplemental to a healthy diet.

Gas, bloating, abdominal pain, indigestion, constipation, diarrhea, fuzzy thinking, difficulty concentrating, fatigue, mood swings, hypoglycemia, itchiness, sinus problems are some of the early symptoms you can look at to determine if your child's gut needs healing. Chapter #1 provides you with a more complete list of symptoms, conditions and diseases that indicate the need for intestinal healing.

"Can't my daughter get all the vitamins and minerals she needs from the foods she eats?"

> *Empty Harvest* states, "When the European settlers began arriving in the sixteenth century, Planet Earth was still in pristine condition after thousands of years of use. The water was absolutely pure. You could stop anywhere and drink it, as long as it was flowing. The land, no matter where you went, was fertile. If a seed fell out of your pocket, it would grow."[6]

It was only during the 20th century's Industrial Revolution with man's grasp on technology, that humans began weakening the Earth, the source of our entire livelihood. The immune systems of both the earth and its inhabitants, intricately connected to the soil, water and air, have suffered immeasurably.

Food grown in depleted soil makes malnourished bodies on which disease preys. Modern farming methods have wasted, poisoned, sterilised and eroded the soil without regard for the very planet we live on, all in the name of the mighty dollar. As a result, our food is naturally lower in vitamins and minerals than it should be.

Along with the demineralisation of our soil, there has been another assault to our food supply. Just after World War One, science began showing man how to bleach, refine, chemically preserve, pasteurise, sterilise, homogenise, hydrogenate, artificially colour, de–fibre, increase sugar and salt, synthetically fortify (enrich), and can the food supply.

Do not forget that vitamin and mineral imbalances can pass from mother to child during pregnancy. You can see how each generation can become unhealthier if the nutritional imbalances are not corrected somewhere down the line. Remember, nutritional imbalances are not in your child's inherited genes, but are in their body chemistry. Therefore, they are usually easy to correct with nutritional therapy.

In summary: Ideally a balanced, healthy diet contains all the nutrients we need. Unfortunately, today, even a balanced diet is lacking in essential minerals or trace elements because of the soil in which our food is grown. Cooking, canning, processing, and refining are further destroying vitamins and minerals.

Therefore, the more nutrient–rich, raw, certified organic fruits and vegetables your child can eat, the better. If he or she is eating these foods frequently and you are not noticing any of the symptoms discussed in this section, your child may not require supplementation. **The body digests vitamins and minerals from foods better than from supplements.** Knowing this probably helps you understand why it is best to give your child vitamins and minerals with meals. Certainly 'whole food' supplements are superior to any other kind of vitamins and minerals as they are made from whole foods as opposed to being synthetic.

> "More than 50% of American children under the age of three years do not get the recommended amounts of several essential nutrients without a daily multivitamin/mineral supplement."[7]

Raising Psychic Children refers to a researcher, named Stephen Schoenthaler, who studied inmate, juvenile delinquent and school populations, found that children's IQs increase and their delinquent behaviour significantly decreases after they take vitamin and mineral supplements.

The book also refers to another researcher, Dr. Richard Carlton, who found that vitamin and mineral supplements lead to significant improvements in academics and behaviour. Carlton reported "some children gained three to five years in reading comprehension within the first year of treatment, and all children in special education classes became mainstreamed, and their grades rose significantly."[8] Carlton also noted that the students taking vitamin and mineral supplements became more sociable and exhibited better moods.

What do vitamins and minerals do generally?

Vitamins and minerals are necessary for every human being to function properly.

Certain vitamins act as antioxidants–substances that protect the body's cells from the damage caused by air pollution, chemicals, alcohol, etc that trigger food sensitivities and allergies. Minerals are essential to both structure and function within the body. We have to get more of these in our diets–one way or another.

Supplements also balance some of the unhealthy aspects of our children's diets and correct some of the damage caused by poor eating habits.

Lastly, our modern, overscheduled lives place demands on our bodies causing them to require extra nutrients. Pollution, noise, stress, food additives and many other factors combine to put stress on the body. Stress of any kind–whether it is emotional or physical–increases our need, and our children's need, for nutrients.

Every child, past the stage of breast-feeding needs a good multi-vitamin and mineral complex. Unfortunately, the more a supplement costs, the better quality it is. You will need to determine what you can afford. Don't be afraid to ask a knowledgeable employee at the health food store for the best brand of Vitamin C, for example, for your child and then ask for the one that is second best, once you see the price of the first brand and so on! Please stay away from any supplements that you find in a drugstore; these are generally not high quality supplements.

Symptoms of food sensitivities or allergies can be similiar to those caused by nutritional deficiencies so you will need to address both areas, when raising the healthiest child possible.

Probiotics/Good Bacteria

As I've clearly stated many times, good bacteria is crucial to healing the digestive tract and intestine. Probiotics are good bacteria. They are the opposite of antibiotics. They replenish the healthy bacterial flora in the intestinal tract that is destroyed by prescribed antibiotics or antibiotics that are fed to the animals we eat. Probiotics discourage the growth of yeast, harmful bacteria and parasites in the intestinal tract and prevent bacteria from getting into the bloodstream (See Chapter #1 for a reminder of the factors that contribute to bad bacteria or poor intestinal flora).

Restoring the balance of healthy bacteria in the gut helps nutrients be better digested and absorbed, improves bowel health and ensures proper elimination. Probiotics are also responsible for making certain vitamins and enzymes and we know that lack of certain enzymes creates reactions to foods. Lisa Petty in her book, *Living Beauty* explains that probiotics help return our intestines to a balanced state, maintain hormone balance, promote mineral absorption and bone formation and boost the immune system.

For all of these reasons, it is strongly recommended that your child be given probiotics every single day. As the Acidophilus, the most common probiotic, makes your child's intestine healthier, you will notice that they begin to have more frequent and larger bowel movements, aiding waste elimination.

> *Coping with Food Intolerances* tells a story: "A seven–week–old baby was brought to the office because of severe colic and bloody diarrhea. The baby cried or nursed and slept for no longer than two hours at a time. Mom was extremely exhausted because of the lack of sleep in almost two months. Her paediatrician had recommended stopping breast milk feeding and using formula. Mom was determined not to give up and with a radical diet change, the addition of the probiotic HMF, she was finally able to see changes in her son and she got adequate sleep as the colic and bloody diarrhea improved."[9]

Breast milk already contains acidophilus but some children need more, as you can see from this example. Acidophilus has very little taste. You can feed your baby acidophilus powder using your fingertip or off of a spoon. I strongly recommend that acidophilus be added directly to every baby's bottles. An older child can have acidophilus powder in his or sandwich, soup, applesauce, chili or anything you can slip it into without your child noticing! Genestra makes excellent acidophilus supplements. When I started using their acidophilus on my girls, their health improved immeasurably. Chewables are also available. Renew Life makes Flora bear chewables, which my girls used to refer to as "bear candy" as each tablet has a bear on it. I mention these two but there are numerous makes of acidophilus. Purchase one from the health food store, designed for babies or children, depending on the age of your child. While you're there, you might want to consider purchasing acidophilus yourself. It is highly beneficial for everyone.

When researchers tested acidophilus on twenty children in 2007, they found that the frequency of their bowel movements doubled. The children also experienced a 20% decrease in abdominal pain after four weeks of supplementing with probiotics.

What other supplements or foods are great for healing the intestine?

- Vitamin C (You can read more on this further on).

- Aloe vera gel is excellent unless your child has diarrhea (it is a natural laxative)—you can add it to your child's food or drink
- Slippery elm, if your child has diarrhea (good for crohn's and colitis).
- L' Glutamine is an amino acid that helps heal the cells lining the small intestine and stomach; it is the main energy source for those cells. It is probably more effective than any other single nutrient. You can open a capsule of powder and sprinkle it in your child's food or drink.
- Oil of Oregano, but it has a very strong taste so it needs to be hidden in food or put into an empty capsule supplied by a health food store and swallowed by your child.
- Green supplements (chlorella, spirulina and blue-green algae) contribute to the healing of the digestive tract.
- Essential Fatty Acids (please read on)

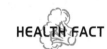

HEALTH FACT

Some children simply need a daily dose of good quality acidophilus to heal the gut.

Some children simply need a daily dose of good quality acidophilus to heal the gut. Many others need more. You can decide which one of these supplements you want to feed your child. Each supplement should be taken on a daily basis for a minimum of 2 months in order for healing to be complete unless your child's diet warrants regular usage of the supplement.

Essential Fatty Acids (EFA)

EFAs boost metabolism, energy levels, improve digestion and promote cellular healing. **The #1 nutritional deficiency in children is a lack of Essential Fatty Acids.** It is most important that your child be given EFAs, as our bodies cannot manufacture them. We need to obtain them from breast milk, foods or supplements. Low EFA consumption is the least recognized nutritional deficiency. This deficiency leads to immune system breakdown, setting the stage for allergy.

> Dr. Leo Galland states, "My research shows that people who have allergies need more essential fatty acids (EFAs) than people who don't. The reason seems to be that in people with allergies, one of the enzymes involved in EFA metabolism is weakened or doesn't function properly."[10] He cites further research to substantiate his claim.

From the time your baby is conceived until the age of two, the brain and nervous system are forming new tissue and creating neural pathways, which pave the way for learning. **Children are particularly dependent on EFAs for brain development; without them their brains cannot grow to their full potential; EFAs are literally that important.**

Cells and organs will degenerate if EFAs are not consumed. EFAs also inhibit inflammation, which is what occurs with every adverse reaction to food. In addition, Essential Fatty Acids help heal the intestinal wall, lubricate the intestine and soften stools.

Just giving your child EFAs, alone, can reverse his or her reactions to food. When my daughter Paige decided one day to eat a capful of strawberry flavoured EFAs, she had her largest formed bowel movement ever! Prior to that, she missed bowel movements after eating certain foods. Suffice it to say, we upped the EFAs after that!

"Every child will benefit from EFAs, now dangerously deficient in our diets. EFAs are converted into substances that keep our blood thin, lower blood pressure, decrease inflammation, improve the function of our nervous and immune systems, help insulin to work, encourage healthy metabolism, maintain the balance of water in our bodies and affect our vision, co-ordination and mood. There is also exciting new research showing that it can have a positive effect on children's behaviour and ability to learn."[11]

Well Being Journal wrote about Alex Richardson, a psychologist at Oxford University, who conducted a study at 12 primary schools. He researched 117 children, ages 5 to 12, with average academic ability but who were underachieving at school. The children that were given Omega 3 for 3 months did substantially better at school than those in the control group. In spelling, these children performed twice as well as expected, whereas the control group continued to fall behind.

Symptoms of EFA deficiency

Attention Deficit Disorder
Bad temperament
Bleeding gums
Bumpy skin on face or back of arms
Clumsiness
Cold hands and feet
Constipation
Dandruff
Depression
Dry, rough, cracked, or peeling skin
Dry, brittle or oily hair
Dry eyes
Eczema
Excess earwax
Excessive thirst

Fatigue
Food or environmental sensitivities
Frequent urination
Hair thinning
Hyperactivity
Lowered resistance to infection
Lack luster hair
Sinus problems
Sleeping problems
Poor concentration
Weak, brittle or split nails

EFA Depletors

It is important to note that high sugar (refined) and saturated fat intake, drugs/antibiotics and second-hand smoke interfere with EFA metabolism.

Food sources of EFA

There are three EFAs that are essential to health, Omega 6s, Omega 3s and Omega 9s. They are found in flaxseed, hemp seed (I don't believe it is available in the United States), other raw, unsalted nuts and seeds (especially pumpkin, sunflower, and sesame), cold-water fatty fish (salmon, sardines, cod, trout, and mackerel), fish oils, avocado, beans, green leafy vegetables and organic eggs.

Omega 3 is anti-inflammatory. Omega 6 is inflammatory. Make a guess which one we need more of. Omega 3, of course. Flax is 60% omega 3 and 40% omega 6. Hemp seed has three times more Omega 6 than Omega 3. Fish oils have no Omega 6 so you can imagine how good they are at reducing the inflammation caused by food! Fish oils are the optimal choice for ensuring your child is receiving the necessary essential fatty acids. You simply need to purchase a high quality fish oil (devoid of mercury) in a liquid or soft gel chewable. They come in flavours such as strawberry, orange, lemon and others. Most naturopaths rely on fish oils, particularly for brain-related symptoms.

I give my children fish oils *and* ground flax. Flaxseeds have the highest proportion of Omega 3 and also contain Omega 6. Flaxseeds are easier to slip into your child's foods, from a vegetable source, less costly and do not contain the toxins often found in fish. I refer to flaxseeds rather than flax oil, as the seeds do not go rancid as quickly as flax oil (however flax oil would be the best form of EFA to add to formula). Flaxseed oxygenates the cells and acts as a barrier to bacteria and viruses. Flaxseed also contains essential amino acids i.e. protein. It supplies many vitamins and trace minerals and is an excellent source of fibre. It has historically been used to heal digestive ailments such as inflammation of the stomach, intestines and colon and significantly helps with constipation.

The body better absorbs ground flaxseeds than whole flaxseeds. You may grind flaxseed using a coffee grinder (that has not been used for coffee) or buy it already ground in the refrigerated section at the health stores or in the health aisles. You can keep some in a container in your fridge for immediate use and then freeze the rest of the ground seeds. Ground flaxseeds can be used on cereals and salads and added to sauces and soups. I even put them on my girl's sandwiches, mixed in with the hummus, almond butter or jam etc. My girls are little detectives, like most children and would certainly revolt if they noticed or were bothered by the seeds in their food.

HEALTH FACT

80% of the brain is made up of DHA, which is why it is so important that it be consumed.

Flaxseed and fish oil contains Docahexaenoic Acid (DHA), which is needed for proper brain function and a healthy heart, especially in children. 80% of the brain is made up of DHA, which is why it is so important that it be consumed.

DHA

- Increases cognitive function
- Fetal and brain development
- Increases activity in children
- Enhances learning and achievement
- Decreases behavioural problems and hyperactivity
- Decreases aggression and hostility
- Decreases eczema and acne
- Helps with slow growth

Daily required amount of EFAs

One tablespoon of EFAs is required each day.

Minerals

"(The) mineral content of soil used to grow today's (crops) is one sixth of what it was fifty years ago, due to commercial farming methods…"[12]

Without minerals, the body cannot make enzymes. Enzymes are made of minerals. Enzymes are necessary for overall health because they help to ensure that food is properly digested. When food is properly digested, the body can obtain the vitamins and minerals it needs. Because of this, many believe that minerals are more important to health than vitamins!

We obtain minerals from vegetables, spring water, nuts and seeds, and natural ocean products (plant, sea vegetables). According to The Canadian School of Nutrition (CSNN), sea vegetables contain more than 60 minerals whereas organic vegetables have only 20 minerals! Sea vegetables are definitely not considered favourites amongst children. However, you can cook pasta, soups, rice and sauces with a piece of seaweed in the pot at the same time and then remove the seaweed when the food is ready to be served. The minerals from the seaweed are absorbed by the food being cooked. The other option is that you buy seaweed shakers (e.g. Nori seaweed) and shake them into your child's food, just like pepper. You'll be amazed to hear that the food will not taste fishy!

Himalayan salt is also rich in minerals and can be purchased in different flavours in a shaker format. The roasted garlic flavour tastes amazing on pasta with some olive oil.

Minerals can also be purchased in a liquid format and a few drops can be added to your child's drinks or food.

These sources provide all the minerals your child needs if they have no deficiencies. However, most children today have certain mineral deficiencies and need to also supplement with individual minerals but only for a period of time, until levels return to normal or symptoms of the particular deficiency disappear. Remember: Low stomach acid (See Chapter #3 for more information on this) is one of the main causes of poor absorption of minerals!

Blood tests at a doctor's office may show mineral levels in your child as normal but it is important that you check the symptoms of each mineral deficiency to ensure that the medical test is correct. Medical tests have a very large range for what is "normal".

Magnesium

The #2 deficiency in children (and adults) is Magnesium. It is estimated that 80 percent of the population is deficient in magnesium.

Magnesium is vital to the production of over 300 enzymes, particularly those involved in energy production. It is required in more than 500 biochemical processes within the body. It also assists in the absorption of calcium and potassium. Magnesium helps our body rid itself of the toxins we consume and face daily. A deficiency of magnesium causes our bodies to release more histamine, which increases severity of allergic symptoms i.e. coughing, congestion, irritability, fatigue, and muscle spasms. The more dairy your child consumes, the more magnesium they need. A deficiency in magnesium interferes with the transmission of nerve and muscle impulses, causing irritability and nervousness. Magnesium is a sedative, meaning it calms the nerves and muscles and is helpful with hyperactivity and insomnia.

In a study described in *Raising Psychic Children*, children who received magnesium supplements showed a significant decrease in hyperactivity. One study found that 95% of ADHD children were deficient in magnesium.

"A child that is ticklish, sensitive, impulsive, and excitable can be low in calcium and magnesium, especially magnesium. Rhythmical activities like thumb sucking, bed rocking, hair twisting, and foot jiggling usually indicate low levels of calcium and magnesium. More stress increases these activities. These children are restless, squirmy, disturb others, and fail to finish tasks. They tend to be more restless in a crowd or the classroom, but less trouble on a one-to-one basis."[13]

Other symptoms of Magnesium/Calcium deficiency include:

- Abdominal pain
- Anxiety
- Asthma
- Chronic fatigue
- Chronic pain
- Constipation
- Cramping in calves
- Depression
- Dizziness
- Grinding teeth
- Headaches
- Hyperactivity
- Insomnia
- Irritability
- Muscle weakness and twitching
- Poor digestion
- Poor sleeping
- Rapid heartbeat

Magnesium depletors

Stress, too much exercise, or a diet high in salt, sugar, refined chocolate or fats can deplete magnesium stores in your child's body. The process of bleaching grains from foods like brown rice or whole wheat actually strips the grains of most of their magnesium; another advantage to feeding your child whole grains.

Food sources of magnesium

Magnesium is found in apples, apricots, avocados, bananas, peaches, cantaloupe, grapefruit, blackstrap molasses, oats, whole grains i.e. brown rice, raisins, figs, garlic, green leafy vegetables, nuts, sesame and sunflower seeds, beans, black-eyed peas, carrots, fish (i.e. halibut and seaweed such as kelp and dulse–you can buy shakers of these at the health food store), dark good quality chocolate and others.

Supplemental sources of magnesium

Nature's Calm drink powder and Dr. Reckowig's magnesium tissue salts are two favourites of children.

Daily required amount of magnesium

3 mg of magnesium per one pound of body weight is the daily requirement. If you buy magnesium supplements, be sure to buy Magnesium Citrate, as it is the most easily absorbed by the body. Adding a cup of Epsom salts to your child's bath is a great way to get magnesium into his or her body.

Zinc

Zinc is the #3 deficiency in children. Prescription for Dietary Wellness states that approximately half of all children are deficient in zinc. Zinc is probably the most important immune mineral. Studies show how low zinc levels reduce the number of T-cells and slow the healing of wounds. Zinc is important in healing the intestinal wall. It is also helpful with skin problems and can actually heal eczema; the body needs zinc to absorb vitamin A. Recent research has uncovered the fact that zinc actually converts some of the EFAs to their active form. Zinc rich foods help the nervous system and are amazing for the growth and development of the brain. Too much calcium or protein or stress depletes the body of zinc. Zinc is also responsible for taste and smell capabilities. If your child is a picky eater, there is a chance that he or she may be deficient in zinc and therefore unable to really taste their food.

In summary, zinc is crucial for children with sensitivities or allergies. It is needed for cell repair, efficient digestion, immune function and emotional health.

Other symptoms of Zinc Deficiency include:

- Fatigue
- Impaired growth
- Hair loss
- Recurrent colds and flu
- Recurrent infections
- Skin conditions
- Thin fingernails that peel
- White spots on nails

Zinc depletors

Strenuous exercise, high protein diets and allergies increase the loss of zinc from the body.

A zinc deficiency is often found in a young child who gets most of their nutrition from milk and cheese.

Food sources of Zinc

Foods high in zinc include fish, poultry (particularly the dark meat), egg yolks, legumes, pecans, all types of nuts and seeds, beans, lentils, sea vegetables and whole grains.

Supplemental sources of Zinc

Metagenics liquid zinc and Dr. Reckowig's zinc tissue salts are two favourites of children.

Daily required amount of Zinc

Children need around 10–15 mg of zinc per day.

Supplements for the digestive system

Even if a child eats a wide variety of healthy, organic foods, a girl or boy can be malnourished because of an inability to digest and absorb foods properly. A properly working digestive system makes a healthy immune system, which protects the body against bad bacteria and allergens. Digestive problems can result from the body being exposed to problematic foods and chemicals.

> Dr. Elson Haas writes in *Staying Healthy with Nutrition*, "I have come to believe that the digestive tract and its function may be the single most important body component determining health and disease. Maintaining normal digestion, assimilation, and elimination is a necessity, and when these functions are faulty, we may not be aware that these dysfunctions are contributing to so many other problems. Another key digestive factor is that hydrochloric acid (Hcl) is a stimulus to pancreatic secretions, containing the majority of enzymes that actively break down foods. The poor digestion of proteins, fats, and carbohydrates then further contributes to poor assimilation and nutritional problems. Thus, when they are needed, supplemental support of digestive enzymes may be even more important than Hcl."[14]

Excessive gas, belching, burning, diarrhea, constipation, cramps, undigested food in your child's stool, and poor tolerance to starches and legumes are all symptoms signalling that the digestive process is not working properly. These symptoms should not be ignored.

Digestive enzymes

Enzymes are needed for every chemical reaction that takes place in the human body. No mineral, vitamin or hormone can work without enzymes. Enzymes digest food, help the immune system work and build minerals into bone.

Remember: Minerals make up enzymes and enzymes are needed for the proper digestion of food. If food cannot be digested, its nutrients cannot be absorbed and used.

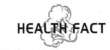

I already detailed the importance of feeding your child foods that are easy to digest and the Steps to Optimal Digestion. Of particular importance to the production of enzymes is ensuring that your child chews his or her food well. When food is chewed well, it becomes thoroughly mixed with enzymes from the saliva. Enzymes work on the surfaces of food so that the more the food is chewed, the more exposed surfaces there are for enzymes to work on.

Eating less food in general and more raw food are other ways to increase enzyme content in your child's body. Raw honey is an enzyme dense product and so are beans, grains, nuts and seeds. Nuts and seeds have up to twenty times their original enzyme content after being soaked in water for 12 to 24 hours. Grains and beans are more easily digested (less gas producing!) when they have been soaked for 24 hours prior to cooking.

If you have tried all these methods and your child is still reacting to food, your child may need digestive enzymes.

The usual treatment for an enzyme deficiency is to exclude the foods that a child cannot deal with from their diet. For example, a child may have a shortage of enzyme lactase, which breaks down the sugar in milk. (In fact, most children stop making this enzyme between early childhood and adolescence. 70% of the world population is lactase deficient!). Instead of a child avoiding eating dairy, they can take digestive enzymes to help have a milder or non–existent reaction to lactase and prevent further reactions to food. Digestive enzymes ensure food is properly broken down and digested, as well as help the digestive organs rest. Digestive enzymes also decrease inflammation and heal the intestine.

Many food–sensitive people find that taking intestinal digestive enzymes helps control their reactions to food. Dr. Michael McCann found that 25 to 50,000 units of protease, before eating allergenic foods, prevented or reduced a food reaction in more than 90% of adult patients. These enzymes are responsible for breaking down the proteins into their non–allergic components (amino acids).

If enzymes are taken with a meal, they help digest the food (certain ones help digest protein and others help digest starch). If taken between meals, they get into the bloodstream where they 'clean house'.

Sources of digestive enzymes

Genestra makes an excellent peppermint flavoured chewable digestive enzyme that many children seem to enjoy with meals. There are many other options that can be found at your local health food store.

To learn more about the power of digestive enzymes, I would highly recommend reading *Allergies, Disease in Disguise* by Carolee Bateson-Koch DC ND.

Vitamins

Vitamin C

Approximately half of all children are deficient in Vitamin C. Vitamin C is the cornerstone of health and one of the basic vitamins. For children with food sensitivities or allergies, Vitamin C is a must. The bioflavonoids within Vitamin C make the gut less leaky. This is the supplement I chose to heal Taylor's gut. Vitamin C is one of nature's best anti-histamines as it has anti-inflammatory properties. And it is also a natural laxative.

If your child has recurrent infections (colds, coughs, ear infections), make sure that he or she has extra Vitamin C, which helps to boost the immune system. Constant, low-grade infections are a sign that the immune system is not functioning at optimum level. Many experts recommend extra vitamin C as a matter of course, to help ward off illness. Vitamin C also improves memory and performance.

> Dr. Rona says that, "Vitamin C is important for the following reasons. It:
> - Aids in formation of collagen and the health of bones, teeth, gums, nails, muscles, ligaments, and all other connective tissue;
> - Strengthens blood vessels and prevents bleeding and plaque formation in the arteries;
> - Promotes healing of all body cells;
> - Increases resistance to infection;
> - Aids iron absorption and utilization;
> - Is an antioxidant that helps prevent cancer and heart disease;
> - Is a natural antihistamine in high doses."[15]

If your child is reacting to food, has hay fever, bleeding gums, stiff joints or joint pain, slow wound healing, recurrent nosebleeds for no obvious reason or bruises easily, he or she might be deficient in Vitamin C.

Food Sources of Vitamin C

Vitamin C is found in all green vegetables, sweet peppers, sweet potatoes, summer squash, watermelon, honeydew, berries, citrus fruits, avocados, cantaloupe, pineapple, blackberries, kiwi, and tomatoes.

Supplemental sources of Vitamin C

Camu C is the best form of Vitamin C for maximum absorption. Ester C is second. Capsules opened up into juice or swallowed with water work best as opposed to the chewables. I do not recommend time-released Vitamin C, as the body eliminates this too quickly.

Daily required amount of Vitamin C
Between 100 and 1000 mg of Vitamin C is appropriate, depending on your child's age.

In Conclusion
All the supplements discussed in this chapter are better absorbed by the body if consumed with food.

With all supplements, you need to be careful that you don't overdo it when feeding them to your child. The most common side effects of too many supplements are headache, nausea, and diarrhea.

Just like introducing new foods, when you introduce supplements into your child's diet, it is important that you test each supplement on them for at least 4 days to ensure there is no reaction before introducing another new supplement.

Integrating improved nutrition into your child's life
I've talked a little about integrating improved nutrition into your child's life, stressing the importance of making gradual changes. Following, you will find a specific example of how to implement a major change gradually.

Say you decided to follow the elimination diet and you discovered the foods to which your child reacts. Your first priority is keeping culprit foods out of their diet for an extended period of time. Discussing the changes with your child or others will be covered in the next chapter.

The second priority is replacing the food with a healthier alternative. If you eliminate all problematic foods at once, you can gradually introduce the healthier alternatives one at a time, ensuring you try only one new food in a four-day period. Alternatively, you can remove one food group at a time, testing the healthier alternatives for that food group, one at a time.

An issue many parents face is how to get their child to live without their much coveted glasses of cow's milk each day. All you need to do is:

1. Decide which healthier alternative with which you would like to replace his or her "regular" milk
2. Pour one quarter or one fifth of the glass up with the alternative milk i.e. enriched rice milk, and then fill the rest of the glass with cow's milk
3. Gradually increase the amount of rice milk in the glass until your child is only drinking rice milk from the glass. This could take days, weeks or months depending on how sensitive your child's taste buds are.

You could use this plan of action with other foods such as replacing unhealthy juices with healthy juices or unhealthy flours i.e. white unbleached flour with healthier flours i.e. spelt flour.

Certain foods are direct substitutions, such as replacing beef hotdogs with turkey hotdogs. You will simply need to see if your child likes the turkey dog or not. Certainly, Hockley Valley spelt pasta is white and tastes like white pasta so this makes healthier substitution easier.

There will be times when you might not want your child to try new foods or supplements in case of a reaction because you wouldn't want a special occasion, trip or visit from a family member to be jeopardized. Certainly, whenever you introduce new foods or supplements to your child, choosing a time when your child is feeling good and there is not much else going on in your household is ideal. When does that happen, you ask? My response has become my mantra: where there is a will, there is a way!

In time, you can devote more time improving the overall health of your child by increasing the number of vegetables or fruits you offer, increasing the amount of filtered water your child drinks, serving more smoothies, introducing a green drink, cooking with sea vegetables or simply serving more live foods. This takes place over the many years that your child lives at home with you. Please know that any improvement you make will directly improve the health of your child but if you integrate improved nutrition into your child's life too quickly, the stress of doing so could lead to the opposite effect. Besides, we all know what happens when humans make changes cold turkey; it's very hard for us to stick to those changes!

Setting up your kitchen

Here are some ideas for helping others navigate their way around your kitchen when they are preparing a meal for your child:

1. You can post the list of foods to which your child reacts on the fridge for all to see.
2. Create a cupboard that only contains "safe" snacks and meals for your child. That way, everyone in your family and any caregivers always know where to find foods that your child is able to eat.
3. Fill one or two shelves in your fridge with only your child's "safe" foods.
4. Create space in a cupboard for the baking ingredients that are "safe" for your child.
5. In another cupboard, set aside some space to put foods that you want your child to try.
6. In another cupboard, hide treats for your child that can only be brought out for special occasions i.e. for when a grandparent or babysitter is caring for your child.

7. Cookbooks with healthly recipes for children can be kept together in one spot.

8. Supplements for your child need their own home and should be out of reach of your child.

9. Your food and symptom journal needs to have a special spot in your home so that is easily accessible to make notes in throughout the day.

10. Your "props" for making your child's meals interesting (See Chapter #10) need some cupboard or drawer space.

The cost of feeding your child healthy foods and supplements

I touched on this subject briefly when discussing organic foods and supplements. You will find that food packed with nutrients will fill your child up more, so that they don't need to eat as much as when regular foods are consumed. I notice that when my girls go to a birthday party and eat lunch there, they are hungry very soon after the party ends because their bodies are searching for the nutrients they didn't receive from the pizza and cake.

Another point to consider is that very often when children are perpetually sick, their parents need to take time off work. Once these parents are absent for a certain number of days, their pay starts getting cut, workloads increase and their relationship with their employer might become strained. These parents will find that healthy eating keeps their children healthy and in school, which is obviously the best of both worlds.

The bottom line is: If our children do not have their health, they suffer and then, we all suffer. Isn't it worth making sacrifices in order for our children to have their health? As a loving parent who cares, your answer will always be a resounding "Yes!"

Dr. Dick Thom says, "I am often told that healthy food is too expensive. Health does not cost; it pays. Studies have shown that if you spend wisely, consumers could reduce their annual food budget. Use the following suggestions:

- Eat out less often as it is twice as expensive to eat out as healthful cooking at home. Bring your lunch to work or school.
- When you do eat out, make wise choices with less expensive items.
- Buy fewer packaged foods.
- Buy less meat.
- Buy more beans, whole grains, vegetables, and fruit.
- Store food properly so it doesn't spoil.
- Don't waste money on junk foods, such as soda pop, hot dogs, candy, potato chips, etc.
- Grow some of your own food in your own organic garden."[16]

The amount of work involved in feeding your child differently

Here's your most likely scenario. You have read everything you need to do to integrate nutrition into our fast–food world and you are starting to get rather worked up, to say the least. Does following my suggestions require advanced planning and more time spent on execution? Yes! You are thinking about all the changes your family is going to undergo and all the work you now have just to feed your child, never mind all the other responsibilities that come along with raising them! Back in the Introduction of this book, I discussed the fact that many parents' jobs are harder than ever before and now I'm suggesting that you do even more work? The truth is that it is *more work short term but less work long term*; I promise you! Your life as a parent will become easier.

HEALTH FACT

The truth is that in this day and age we have to earn health.

Initially, grocery shopping, cooking and baking were arduous tasks for me. I needed to scour ingredient lists, learn about alternatives to the common allergens, find those alternatives and experiment with different recipes. I had to learn a whole new language of food. I can assure you that now I spend no more time in the grocery store or kitchen than you do; I simply work with different foods. Now that we can implement the concept of "Treat Day", I no longer have to plan the meals for each outing. You will need to go through the same learning curve as I did, but your learning curve will be much shorter because you have the benefit of being guided.

If you look back through your life, you will realize that many of your greatest accomplishments were achieved with hard work. The truth is that in this day and age we have to earn health. It doesn't just happen; we have to work for it. Children need to be taught the all–important concepts of hard work and perseverance; the best way for them to learn is by your example. When you put in the hard work in the short term and you see the benefits for your child, you realize how worthwhile your efforts can be.

If your child is small, returning to a natural, healthy environment is easier. You will have less to undo. If your child is older, reintroducing healthier foods and cleaning up your child's body will probably be harder but you will have the advantage of having your child's help and their reasoning abilities. They can more easily understand why certain foods are unhealthy and the reasons for making positive changes. The next chapter will further assist you in accomplishing this very task.

How to make the best use of this chapter's information

1. This chapter tells you everything you need to know about feeding your child in order to prevent, minimize or eliminate symptoms and sickness and help your child become the healthiest possible! Good tasting brand names and a meal plan are even included.

2. Once you begin feeding your child these healthier options, you can look into the supplements your child needs (healthy food is always first priority!). Acidophilus and essential oils are mandatory for every child (and adult, for that matter!). Then, if your child has allergies or a condition, review the list of supplements to choose from, in order to heal their intestine.

3. The last sections of this chapter explain how to integrate improved nutrition into your family's lifestyle—slowly and simply.

CHAPTER 7

LET'S TALK ABOUT IT

Recommendations for Effectively Communicating About Feeding Your Child Differently

---

This chapter is my personal favourite. It contains ideas for cultivating the best relationship possible with your child. It also makes recommendations for talking to your child and others, when your child is eating differently than the majority.

In order for you to be your child's ally and effectively communicate about eating the foods that are right for them, *you* first need to understand food and reactions and everything that goes along with them. You should be starting to feel that you understand these matters now that you have read the preceding chapters.

I would like to share with you some of the feelings I had, before I truly understood the information I impart in this book. For a long time, I felt as though my child was disadvantaged because she couldn't eat the foods that all her friends were eating. Taylor sometimes felt left out or, even worse, that something was wrong with her. Right off the bat she was different, before personality even came into play. People couldn't give her treats; storekeepers, friends and relatives accustomed to showing their love by giving children treats, believed that I wasn't allowing them to love my child. Some babysitters were scared to look after Taylor for fear they might give her the wrong food.

For an even longer time, I was afraid for my child's present and future. I was afraid she would become constipated, be in pain, or she might become even sicker down the road and that I might be the person responsible for letting this happen. I worried that I was the cause of her health challenges, in the first place.

I wondered what she would have to look forward to at special occasions like Halloween, Christmas and Easter. What would she do at birthdays when all the others were having candies and cake? As Taylor got older and started spending time each day away from me, I worried that someone would feed her the wrong food. I wondered who could care for her if I went on holidays. At the time, no one, except for me, took her food sensitivities seriously. I feared that she would live a life in constant pain if I were not there for her. When I was with Taylor, I was uncomfortable having the responsibility of feeding her. Is there really any worse fear than not knowing how to feed your own child? If that weren't enough, I worried that I would need to check her bowel movements every day for as long as she lived at home.

Initially, I felt sorry for myself, as well. Why did I have to deal with all these extra worries and have to learn more about these matters than other parents? Simply raising a child was difficult enough, in itself. I also felt very alone, knowing that it was all up to me whether my child would heal or not. There was no one else to lean on; no one else to shoulder the load. Oh, there were people that worried and some that tried to help but no one spent day in and day out with Taylor and me. No one really saw what was going on, experienced the gravity of our challenge or felt the depth of our emotions.

Like all parents, I wanted everything for my child. I really believed her food sensitivities and allergies would seriously hamper my desires from being fulfilled. Luckily, I was wrong.

Communicating with your child

> "Parents feelings about their children's (adverse reactions to food) are likely to be profound, complex and influential. Your feelings are bound to affect your child's feelings and vice versa... You have the power to make your child anxious, scared or resentful about their (sensitivities or allergies) or accepting and positive."[1]

Once you understand the following important aspects of helping your child, you will have the confidence to talk to them in the most effective way. ***These ways of communicating will also benefit the parents who are simply trying to feed their children healthy foods.***

Step #1 Education—Become educated about your child's food sensitivities and/or allergies:

- Understand which foods present a problem for your child
- Get to know what happens to your child's body when they eat problematic foods
- Learn how to avoid the problematic foods, find the alternatives and improve your child's overall health
- Develop tools to handle situations when your child does end up eating a problematic food
- Determine how to minimize, if not eliminate, your child's symptoms

Step #2 Trust—Ensure that your child trusts you implicitly:

A child that is being fed differently from the majority needs to trust their parents for the following reasons. He or she:

- Needs to believe you when you tell your child to stay away from a food
- Needs to trust that you will help if they react to a food
- Needs to understand that you are doing your best to take care of them and not just trying to control them

Trust is the foundation of any successful relationship. Your child *must* trust you. If you always speak the truth to your child even when it comes to the smallest thing, your child will trust you implicitly. Another way to build your child's trust in you is to tell your child ahead of time, whenever possible, what is going to happen. So, tell your child the schedule for the next couple of days and prepare them for what is going to happen when, say, they visit the dentist. Then, let him or her see it unfold the way you described. Remember to explain why something did not go as planned, if this occurs. Just as you like to know what is ahead for yourself, your child wants to know what lies ahead. ***More importantly, every time you tell your child something will happen and it does, you build your child's belief in you.***

Now, say you have given your child reason not to trust you, maybe multiple reasons. You need to turn that around, especially now that your child is staying away from certain foods. No matter what you did, all you need to do is apologize to your child. It sounds so easy but it can be one of the hardest things to do, which is why so many parents end up dying before apologizing to their children. It can be something as simple as keeping your child waiting, while you talk to a neighbour, when your child was expecting to go to the park. It could be yelling at your child. It could be lying to your child. It could be years of not being present for your child if you are a workaholic. Whatever it is that you did to make your child not trust you, apologize. Ask for a new start or tell your child that things will be different now, because you have learned from your mistake. All a child wants is to feel loved and understood. By apologizing, you show your child that they are loved, respected and understood. Then, watch your child's trust in you grow.

Step #3 Communication—Learn how to communicate most effectively with your child:

Communicating with your child in the right way is paramount. You will need to talk with your child to help them understand that having food challenges is a positive, not a negative. Here's why:

- **Having certain food sensitivities or allergies promotes health**

Just as adults say, "Why me?" some children feel food sensitivities or allergies are an unfair burden. Dwelling on life's injustices is unproductive and incorrect. If you determine that your child has only one or two food sensitivities, (say, to sesame seeds) well, that's just a hassle. However, if you determine that your child has a problem with one of the top three common allergens or has numerous food sensitivities, well, that's tremendous! You will find your child healthier alternatives and he or she will benefit, overall. If your child reacts to other common allergens such as soy, caffeine or chemicals, even better (Please refer to Chapter #2 for the reasons behind this).

Society is the least healthy that it has ever been; yes, some people are living longer but their quality of life leaves a lot to be desired. The main contributing factor to our poor health is diet. If your children doesn't eat the staples of the North American diet, there is no reason to feel sorry for them. They are better off. There's no question about it. Teach your child about doing things differently from the majority, that it's a positive thing to be different, not a negative. You can say to your child, "I will feed you differently because I will not let you be less than who you truly are. I want you to be the best person you can be." Help your child to understand this as early on in life as possible, so that they always know that eating differently is a positive thing.

If your child reacts to major food groups and you turn the challenge into an opportunity to clean up your child's digestive and intestinal systems, in addition to feeding your child healthier alternatives, it will result in even more improvements to your child's current and potential health!

- **Having food reactions decreases the chances of your child having weight issues**

Removing foods that a child is reacting to can knock 10 pounds off of a child right away, in addition to the power of eating healthier alternatives. As early as 5 years old, a child begins to notice and think about weight. Remember, weight is not just an issue of vanity but also an issue of health. Not to mention the fact that an overweight child has a difficult time responding to tasks with energy, optimism, and enthusiasm. Another reason to applaud food sensitivities and allergies! When my children were sensitive to all the common allergens, it was next to impossible for them to have weight issues. They couldn't eat refined white flour or sugar, the two biggest culprits for weight gain. It was still possible, if they ate too many natural sugars or were overeating in general, but they were not going to acquire the sweet tooth that refined flour, candy, pop and chemicals create in children who eat "regular" food.

- **Having food or drug sensitivities promotes the use of natural remedies**

(Please see Chapters #3 and 9). Because Taylor reacted to every drug her body came into contact with, I had to learn natural means of helping her when she was sick or in pain. I found that the natural remedies worked faster and more effectively than the medications. The natural remedies did not deplete her body of the good bacteria or cause side effects. I've already told you that once I changed Taylor's diet, I found that she rarely became sick. Paige had a healthy diet right from the start and, I don't mind repeating, has never had a drug enter her body. The fewer drugs that enter your child's body, the stronger their intestinal wall will become and the healthier they will be.

Encourage your child to observe the lack of health in the world around them

This is risky business. They should be able to see the failings of the typical diet without becoming judgmental of their friends and family. You want your child to notice the health of those around them and see the link between their friends eating chocolate every day and their subsequent poor concentration in class.

If you do not encourage your child to look around at his or her classmates, you will not be able to fully instill the importance of a healthy diet in your child's mind. Ask them, "Have you ever noticed how the other children in your class miss school because they are sick?" They will undoubtedly respond, "Yes". "Well, have you ever wondered why your friends are sick so often, sometimes really sick but you don't get that sick or miss as much school?" "You do not get really sick because you eat healthy food!" "Each time your teacher checks your ears with the scope (this happened at two schools), know that she will probably never find anything because you have never had an infection in your life and you probably won't, as long as you keep taking care of yourself". You cannot stop the discussion here, however.

Explain to your child that most other children do not understand how foods affect them. Food puts them in bad moods, gives them rashes or makes them have diarrhea but they don't know they are reacting to food and neither do their parents.

Now, you can see there is a fine line between helping your child to understand the power of food and making them feel superior to others. I feel that it is extremely important for children to understand the link between food and sickness. Looking at others in order to see the connection is very effective for children. If you concur, remember to explain to your child that other people do not understand the connection but they probably will one day. It is not their job to school their friends. I tell my girls that everyone learns at their own pace, depending on the life circumstances brought before them.

- **Having reactions to foods promotes respect for one's body and taking responsibility for self**

Health conscious parents or parents of food-reactive children sometimes walk a tightrope. On the one hand, they need to warn their child about which foods to avoid but on the other hand, they do not want to instill fear. So, what can you say to prevent them from harming themselves? This is where trust *and* communication come in. The most powerful tool we can give our children is to teach them how to listen to and respect their own bodies. *They* need to connect with their bodies enough to understand which foods make them feel good and which foods make them feel badly. Today, if I tell my daughter that she cannot have a food, she knows I am telling the truth and she doesn't question it. Parents ask me on a regular basis, "I can't believe your child listens to you when you tell her she can't have that food. What's your trick?" My children know what happens to their bodies when they eat certain foods. They trust me when I tell them which foods will make them feel poorly because they've experienced it for themselves. To show you how I reached this point, I will use my daughter, Paige, as an example.

How to teach your child the link between food and symptoms

Paige was only two years old and had recently started school. At my girls' school, snacks were laid out on a table for all the children to indulge in whenever they liked. This is the way some Montessori schools work. Talk about the most challenging situation for a child that cannot eat regular food! For two months, Paige only ate her own snacks that I provided for her. She knew not to eat the other children's foods, however tempting they appeared. Then, she started sneaking cups of fruit juice filled with sugar and chemicals. As well, after school, she and her friend would head off around the side of the school and Paige would share her friend's snack, thinking that the moms couldn't see them. Remember, Paige was young and hadn't as yet experienced any consequences from eating the wrong foods. The second time that I saw Paige sharing her friend's snack, I asked her to stop. Not wanting to listen to me, yet looking right at me, she rammed a cookie into her mouth faster than I believed possible. Then she proceeded to grab her friend's last cookie and stuff it into her mouth just as quickly as the first. The other moms and I stifled our laughs, while at the same time, trying to control the situation. Sure enough, Paige didn't have any bowel movements for days as a result of her forays. She didn't sleep well and became pale and unhappy. Then, one morning, she started hitting the other children at school and her teacher raised it as an issue with me. That day, while driving home from school, I asked Paige if she was hitting the other children and then "Do you feel good inside when you hit other children?" Her reply, of course, was " No." I asked her if she noticed she was-n't going to the bathroom or sleeping well, either. I pointed out to her that when she doesn't feel well or hits other children, it is because she is eating foods that are bad for her. I then asked her if she would try to eat only her own foods for the next

> **HEALTH FACT**
>
> The most powerful tool we can give our children is to teach them how to listen to and respect their own bodies.

couple of days, just to see if she felt better. She agreed.

The rest of the day, I fed her organic vegetables and put supplements in her drinks and food to get her bowels moving and the unhealthy foods out of her system. She had two large bowel movements by the time she was back at school the next day. That day, Paige ate her own food and drinks and was well behaved in the classroom and at home. She continued to eliminate, started to sleep more soundly and the colour returned to her cheeks. My words to her were "Good girl! You see, you're eating your own food and you're going to the bathroom again; you're feeling happy again!" At the age of two, I was teaching my child to be conscious of her own body, to listen to its messages and know that if she didn't, there would be consequences. That is how we teach our children to understand the relationship between food and the body. It is also another way to help our children come to trust us. Most importantly, it is how we teach our children to be responsible for their own health.

You may need to teach this lesson a few times, in this way, before your child reaches a point of total trust, listening when you say, "No, you cannot have that food". Children will give you the necessary guidance on how much detail they need by their questions. Answer their many questions with short and simple statements. Sometimes your child will ask the same question over and over until they fully understand the answer. It is important to avoid overwhelming your child with words or information.

HEALTH FACT

We teach our children to be responsible for their own health.

Once that incident was over with Paige, I never spoke to her about it again. We carried on with our lives, did fun things, and talked about all sorts of other matters. If you constantly speak to your child about food and the body, or your child often hears you talking about it, you will incite anxiety in your child around the issue. Always keep this fact in mind.

Helping your child make the connection between food and symptoms *is* something you need to communicate whenever you observe a new symptom. If you are not certain, you can discuss the possibilities with your child. Maybe your child has sore knees every time he or she eats dairy or has nightmares after swimming in chlorine. Whenever Paige had sore knees, at the young age of two, she would say, "That's because I ate ice cream". I, being most impressed, would be extremely complimentary of her cleverness. This, in turn, encouraged her to put two and two together whenever she had a symptom. "I threw up because of the corn, right Mommy?" "That's right, Paige." I would respond, my voice brimming with pride!

One day, my eldest daughter said, "Is today treat day?" I said, "No, the next one isn't until Saturday". She replied "Oh good, I didn't want another treat day for a while." She knew she didn't feel well, having had all those treats, and she didn't like feeling that way!

For children who are unclear as to how problem foods affect them, they can keep their own food and symptom journal, from age five or six onwards. This is a very effective way to teach your child how their body reacts to foods.

Teach your child about proper elimination

When teaching your child to be conscious of their body, it is also important to teach what to look for in the elimination of waste or toxins. If your child's urine is a pale yellow or straw colour, he or she is drinking enough fluids. If your child's bowel movements are from his or her wrist to the elbow in length, soft and light brown and there is at least one a day, all is fine. If your child is not seeing the ideal results in that toilet bowl, they will know themselves that something is not right. It is no longer a question of believing you, the parent.

Will these lessons stay with your child when they are all grown up and living their own life?

One afternoon, I started to ask Taylor, "When you grow up and you don't live with me anymore…"; she jumped in, saying, "I'm always going to live with you Mommy". I replied, "Well, say you decided to move out. Do you think you'll eat treats every day because I'm not around?" Taylor replied "That would be crazy, Mom. I don't want to feel yucky every day. I would only have them once in while, just like now."

Now, of course, not every child responds this way but I'd be willing to bet that if your child is taught properly about their body and how it works, your son or daughter will respond similarly! That, coupled with the fact that most adults live their lives very closely to the way they were raised, creates a good probability of success. It's usually only when you're not conscious of something that you allow it to continue. Once we are aware of the repercussions of doing anything, we often stop the behaviour.

▪ Having reactions to foods promotes a healthy enthusiasm for life

It's difficult to feel upbeat, have good relationships with others, and accomplish our goals when our bodies are busy reacting to food. I can tell you that there is no way that I would be writing a book if it weren't for my positive attitude derived from eating the foods that are right for my body and subsequently, feeling good inside.

▪ Having reactions to foods promotes good appearance

It seems minor to bring this up after you've just read the biggest advantages to having food sensitivities or allergies, but I wouldn't be honest if I didn't talk about appearance having some significance. Interestingly enough, having good appearance promotes respect for oneself, which is of great importance. Staying away from common allergens can keep our skin clear, our hair thick and shiny, our nails strong and shiny, our eyes bright and alive, and our bodies slim. Just being healthy inside can improve our outer appearance immeasurably. When we look good, it's a proven fact that others respond more favourably towards us; it's simply human nature.

You will need to describe your child's food, supplements or natural remedies using positive words

I recommend occasionally using words to describe your child's food such as "healthy", "special", "delicious". Some parents might say, "My child hears a food described as healthy and stays clear of it". There are two reasons why your child might feel this way:

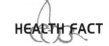

HEALTH FACT

Staying away from common allergens can keep our skin clear, our hair thick and shiny, our nails strong and shiny, our eyes bright and alive, and our bodies slim.

- Your child has not been fed healthy foods for the better part of his or her life.
- Your child's experience with healthy food has not been a good one. He or she tasted a healthy food and didn't like it.

Give your child great tasting healthy treats and you'll see the attitude shift. Ensuring that other family members are eating healthy foods further solidifies the change in attitude.

In case your young child is not listening to you about the importance of healthy eating, children are also taught about health in school in the early years. So, if you, every once in a while, remind your child that their food is healthy, when they start hearing it in school, they make the connection. Then, they are pleased that they are following what they learned about in class.

If your child loves a particular sport, you might mention to them that these foods/supplements provide more stamina and energy, enabling your child to participate at a higher level. If they are struggling in school, you can tell them that these foods/supplements will make completing schoolwork easier, whether concentrating, reading or writing. If your child is chronically ill, you can tell them that these foods/supplements will turn their situation around in time.

If you give your child supplements or remedies and your child questions you, mention that the powder, for example, will make them healthier and that is why you are doing it. I recommend using positive words like that, instead of saying, "It will fix you", making it seem as though there is a problem. When Paige was 5 years old she knew that when she took vitamin C, it kept her healthy and prevented her from catching colds. When she did get a cold, she asked me for the vitamin C.

Listen to your child's worries, turn his worries into challenges and arrive at solutions together

- **Your child is worried about being food-reactive**

Children love food. *Your Child—Allergies* states, "Food is comfort and pleasure, sustenance and reward, fun and sharing. And food – when prepared by their parents – is a symbol of love. To be excluded from certain kinds of foods, as many allergic children are, can feel deep down like an unfair punishment."[2]

Reactions to food complicate a child's life. There's no disputing that. Every child wants to be part of the group. They worry about rejection. Their self-esteem has not yet been built up through life experience. Then, when they are doing something so obviously different from the rest of their peers and the world in general, their self-esteem can suffer immeasurably. If your child has obvious symptoms, he or she might look different, as well. A child may not want to play sports for fear of having an asthma attack. Others continually have watery eyes or mucus running down their faces. We all know how much children tease one another, particularly for being different, which, of course, makes matters far worse than they need to be. Your child might also be suffering, while at the same time, being teased or even bullied. They might be really itchy and trying to focus on not scratching or having frequent tummy aches or be running back and forth to the bathroom with diarrhea. This adds stress to the mix, as well. Stress weakens the immune system, which in turn can cause symptoms to worsen.

Children in these circumstances might hate the world, depending on their age, or feel sorry for themselves. There is no end to the emotions that a child with food or chemical sensitivities might feel. We do know that children are full sensory beings. A traumatic event for them might be inconsequential to an adult.

If your child is negative or has bad feelings about their food sensitivities or allergies, it's important to let them speak their mind and then, for you to acknowledge those feelings; they are very real. ***Many times, parents have a hard time letting their children "own" their feelings.*** We tell them that their emotions are wrong or inappropriate or we try to convince them that they don't feel that way. When we respond this way, our children do not feel safe. Their feelings do not go away, they become buried and sometimes, children end up ashamed to have those feelings. This creates "emotional blocks" in children. *Your Child's Self-Esteem* states that children's tested IQs have jumped from 60 to 100 points when emotional blocks are removed. Children cannot absorb new information at school or in the world when their focus is turned inward. Children that "own" their feelings know it is all right to be themselves, even if their feelings are different from Mom and Dad's. What a great impact this realization has on their self-esteem!

Many children think they've done something bad or wrong to cause their food sensitivities or allergies. These kids may act out or become self-destructive. Parents must let them know they did nothing to bring on their food sensitivities or allergies and that they will do everything they can to minimize or eliminate their reactions, reminding them of the positives of reacting to certain foods.

It is important to remember that if you do not provide your child with the time or atmosphere to speak freely to you, he or she often won't. Ensure that your child has pockets of time every day to talk to you about whatever their heart desires. That time for my family is at night, before my daughters go to sleep. Once your child does share their feelings and you support them by telling them that it is okay to feel the way they do, remember to speak in simple language. Let your child know that *most* people want to eat unhealthy food because it looks and smells good. It's everywhere, it's cheap and usually doesn't take long to prepare. Let them know that most people do pick unhealthy choices because it is all they know. Point out the fact that these choices often cause them to suffer from many symptoms and illness or that they probably will eventually. There is literally no way that sensitivities or allergies to many of the common allergens can ever be viewed as a negative if you really understand them. Food sensitivities and allergies are a wake-up call to improve the health of the body before sickness or disease sets in!

Here is an example of the simplicity of a conversation that you could have with your child. One day I told my 6-year old that her body was her best friend. About a week later, she told *me* that her body was her best friend and proceeded to say, "If I feed it properly, it will be happy and I'll feel good inside".

▪ Your child is being teased for eating differently

Children will tease. Children need to know that those who tease are often not happy with themselves, so they take those feelings out on others. By doing so, they end up feeling worse about themselves. Having said that, we must let our own children know that teasing is unacceptable; it only serves to hurt the feelings of others. Thankfully, that is a teachable skill. The more we can do to help our child's self-image, the better he or she will interpret and respond to life's unpleasant moments (Please read on for further assistance in this area).

When my daughter was 5, she told me that another child in her class was teasing her about what she ate for lunch. She said, "Ew" or "That looks yucky". Taylor asked me if she could just take a sandwich to school every day to avoid this situation. Now, I could have complied with this or I could have turned this into an amazing lesson for Taylor to learn about how great it is to be different. I guess you can gather that I chose to do the latter. "Taylor, why don't you ask Melissa if she has ever tried falafels (chickpea burgers)?" I have never heard of anyone not liking falafels and this is what Melissa was teasing her about on this particular day. "If Melissa says "no", then why don't you say "Well, if you've never tried them, how do you know if you like falafels or not?" I know that at some schools, there is a "No sharing" policy. I haven't heard of a "No sniffing" policy yet, except for children with peanut allergies. I suggested Taylor ask her classmate if she would like to taste or smell her food, telling her that she would probably see the situation turn around once Melissa did this. If this girl didn't like the food in question, it would generally be because she was not used to the food. Taylor's response could be "Well, I love it and you know what? Having a sandwich every day is not very exciting, so I'm going to bring different things to school for lunch each day. You know what else? Tomorrow I'll be bringing pancakes (her own version) with maple syrup for lunch!" Now a simpler response that I could have taught Taylor is this: "My food may look yucky to you but you know what? I actually love it and it's really healthy." You can offer your child a variety of responses.

If another child continues to tease your child, it is important to encourage them to explain to the teasing child how the teasing makes her feel inside. Often, young children do not realize that they are hurting another child when they tease. Occasionally, another child will continue teasing your child no matter what measures your child takes to put an end to it. This is when you will need to teach your child the art of ignoring. Often, once a child is ignored for a period of time and no longer gets a rise out of another, the teasing ends.

▪ Turning negative thought patterns into positive thought patterns

Your child says: "I can't eat candy, chocolate bars, or Oreo cookies."
Your positive parental response:
- "You can eat healthy versions of all of those foods."
- "You can eat some of those foods on "treat day" but the rest of the time, your body wants healthy foods."
- And, if they still persist..."Those foods make you have a sore tummy or make you have eczema etc, but one day you'll be able to have those foods every once in a while."

Your child says: "The other kids bring hotdogs to school for lunch."
Your positive parental response:
"Oh, would you like to do the same? You can take your hotdogs to school too!" Sometimes young children start to think that they cannot do what the other children are doing with food just because they eat different foods.

Your child says: "It was Luke's birthday today and all the children got to eat treats except for me."
Your positive parental response: "Why didn't you have one of your special treats?" If you've properly communicated with teachers, they will give your child their treat reserved for special occasions, at the same time the other children are having theirs.

Your child says: "Today Suzie's mom brought in Halloween treats for all the kids."

Your positive parental response: "Well, I hope you got one too to keep for treat day/when you're bigger/to give to Daddy/to give to Grandma." Children want treats to be eaten and enjoyed. If they know they can eat the treat eventually or that they can feel pleasure giving the treat to a family member that will enjoy it, they will be satisfied.

▪ Your older child is worried about making any dietary changes

Many of you will make necessary changes to your older (age six onwards) child's diet gradually and without comment. If your efforts are detected and unappreciated, you can explain to your child that you would like to try making some changes to how your family eats and see if there is a difference in everyone's symptoms, conditions or disease. Notice, I am not suggesting alienating your child.

Set a time limit on the changes, say, 2 weeks. You might say, "For the next two weeks, we are eliminating dairy, just to see if our health improves. If we see no difference, we will go back to the way we were eating before." For children, two weeks is usually an achievable goal and long enough to see improvement. If your child says "no way", suggest one week. If your child or teen still says "No way" then maybe, they have been given their own way far too much in life. If this is the case, the severity of your child's symptoms will determine what they will be willing to do in terms of making the necessary dietary changes. If your daughter has pains in her stomach, on a regular basis, which prevents her from going out with her friends, she will give the changes a try. If your son has eczema all over his back and dreads the changing rooms at school, he will try the new way of eating.

You cannot force your child to eat healthy foods. All you can do is work towards integrating healthy choices into your whole family's daily lifestyle. Maybe eventually, your obstinate child or children will follow suit. "Children learn what they live. "

Step #4 Confidence—Instill confidence in your child

Outside of feeding your child healthily, I believe the very most important thing you can do to raise a happy child is to build your child's self-esteem. Yes, it will develop over time, but there are steps you can take to build your child's self-esteem faster, so that eventually they are the strongest possible.

We already know that the everyday challenges of childhood–feeling different, being teased, feeling left out–aren't any different for health conscious children than those who are not, but they can be magnified. In fact, food sensitivities or allergies tend to put everything under a microscope.

It's important to be your child's greatest advocate. All of the good you are trying to do can be undone if your child perceives there is something wrong or unlovable about them, making these changes necessary. Living a healthy life benefits everyone; dietary changes should not be portrayed as punishment for being unhealthy or overweight.

If your child feels different or is being teased, you may want to implement techniques to increasing your child's self-esteem. There are numerous books available that can help do this.

If your child has high self-esteem, they know their value. Your child's feelings of self-worth form the core of their personality and determine how they live all parts of their life.

Your Child's Self-Esteem says, "In fact, self-esteem is the mainspring that slates every child for success or failure as a human being."[3]

HEALTH FACT

It is up to you to show your child that they matter just because they exist.

Self-esteem comes from the quality of the relationships that exist between a child and those who play a significant role in their life. It is up to you to show your child that they matter just because they exist.

Here are a few ideas for increasing your child's self confidence, no matter the age:

- Spend time with your child, as much time one-on-one as possible, showing that you enjoy being with them. Ask your child questions about matters that interest them.
- Play with your child, even it's just for 10 minutes a day. For some, it is one of the hardest things to do, dropping all of your responsibilities and thoughts and just being in the moment with your child.
- Offer your child plenty of love and support. Explain to your child that you love them regardless of how they behave or the mistakes made; you can even tell your child that there is a name for what you share and it is "unconditional love".
- Consistently show respect for your child's rights and opinions.
- Compliment your child on specific good things he or she does or says and minimize the importance of your child's mistakes. If *you* focus on your child's mistakes, that is what they will focus on.
- Children believe what they are told–they have no other reference points.
- Organize fun places to go and unique things to do. Your child might not be eating what others do, but they are doing activities that others are doing.
- Clearly define limits on your child's behaviour–a child needs and wants discipline and limits; rules help your son or daughter feel that they matter.
- When it comes to healing a rift in your relationship, nothing beats loving touch and children are particularly sensitive to this. Even when one of my daughters and I are having a disagreement, it will take all my strength but I will reach for her, fold her in my arms, hold her on my lap and all is well. Loving touch should be a part of each and every day.

Education brings confidence in your decision-making and reduces worry. Your child also will have more confidence by being better informed, so the more you share with your child about what you learn about food, the better. Of course, be cognizant of the fact that you cannot talk about food incessantly!

The mind has a very powerful influence on health. If your children know that you love them and you are doing your best to make them feel better, feel better they will.

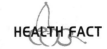

HEALTH FACT

Your job is to help your child make positive food choices, whether you are present or not.

Step #5 Encouragement—Encourage your child to make the right choices for themselves

Your job is to help your child make positive food choices, whether you are present or not. As you continually provide them with healthy food choices, you help create a palate in your child that appreciates healthy food and is more able to withstand the constant temptation of unhealthy choices.

As well, if you give your child a firm belief in their own self-worth and their ability to make good decisions, life will be that much easier for your child.

Elementary school years

By this point, children have been taking responsibility for a portion of their own care for some time. You can now start to explain what is happening in the body when symptoms of food sensitivities or allergies occur. By third grade, children are able to understand bodily functions e.g. how the lungs work normally.

Your child can begin making some decisions about his or her health. For instance, if your child's school has an ice cream day as a fundraiser, your child can choose to partake in that or eat the food offered at a friend's Christmas party that upcoming Saturday. A child left out of decision-making will not assume responsibility on their own.

Once your child is about five years old, they will start going places without you and another parent may not always know what the children are up to. Consider that your child may no longer have pain or suffering when eating certain foods but still experiences symptoms from some foods. Your child goes to a friend's house and the two of them head off to the kitchen, on their own, to get a snack. At this age, your child will usually know what they can and cannot eat, as long as you have explained this to them. What would you say if your child comes home and tells you, "Suzy ate M&M's but I had yogurt, thinking that was healthier." Your child cannot eat dairy and knows it. If you react with anger, your child might decide to never be honest with you again. It is important that you react calmly, pointing out what your child did that was right. You might say, "You are so good not to eat the M&M's. It's okay that you ate the yogurt, as long as you don't sneak food like that often. We both know what happens to you if you eat problem foods all the time, right?" It is important to tell your child that you are proud of how she handled a certain situation. Keeping things positive is essential for all children finding their own way in this world.

High school years

Many teenagers are capable of taking full responsibility for their health around age thirteen.

Eventually, your role will transition to observing how they are doing and having occasional discussions about their health. Negotiate with your teen how he or she can communicate with you so that you are both comfortable. The last thing your teen wants is you pestering them about what they ate that day or what their bowel movements look like!

Some teens need to be taught that there is another choice they need to make. Teens can feel better or not. They can listen to their bodies and stay away from problem foods or they can ignore their body's signals and feel lousy.

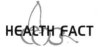

HEALTH FACT

A child left out of decision-making will not assume responsibility on their own.

If you have a teenager that decides to feel lousy, it is your responsibility, as long as your child is under your care, to help them overcome this. It is up to you to find a way to encourage your child to straighten out their diet. Communication is the best means. You may need to share some facts with your child, both verbally and with the use of books or articles, ensuring this is a short conversation not a long lecture. In a calm tone, explain to your teen that if they do not eat properly now, their symptoms will develop into conditions and eventually, possibly, disease. I am telling the truth. It usually takes a lot of work to acquire a disease. As I mentioned earlier, it is very rare to just wake up one day and find out you have cancer; your body gives you plenty of warnings ahead of time, which, unfortunately, most people ignore. You might have colic as a child and then constipation, which might lead to irritable bowel syndrome and then a bleeding ulcer. If you still haven't paid attention to your body's signals, cancer ensues.

We all know how common it is for teens to do the opposite of what parents want in order to win a power struggle. However, if your teen wants to feel lousy most days, you may be dealing with a lack of self-respect or low self-esteem issue, which although very common, takes time to mend. When this is the case, it means that your child needs to feel understood by YOU. This is a whole other subject but it usually involves a conversation wherein your child expresses their feelings about their upbringing, which, if all goes well, incites compassion and understanding in you. When you feel ready, you will apologize for the mistakes you made in raising your child. You probably were never aware that you made these mistakes and truly felt you did the best job possible. However, it is only after this discussion takes place that the two of you can agree to start fresh as a team. Hard work but so good for the soul....

Some parents and children are not at a place in their lives where they are ready to tackle this conversation. Until the time is right, you can simply tell their child, "When your symptoms become worse and they will, I'll be here to help you improve your way of eating." If you can encourage your teen, on their own, to see a naturopath that performs testing, the tests will demonstrate the areas of imbalance and the severity. Your teen will have a professional opinion of their dietary issues and not just have to take your word for it.

Your ultimate success will come when your children no longer need you. Our goal as parents is to raise children so that they are free to fly on their own and do so in good health!

Step #6 Set an example—Set a great example for your child

You know your child better than anyone. You know what is important to his or her wellbeing and you can visualize the end result of implementing positive lifestyle changes. To succeed with implementing any new ideas, you must accept that you will be a role model for the rest of the family. Others are always watching you. If you can embrace the dietary changes yourself, you will show your family, through your actions and not just your words, how dedicated you are to them and how much you love them.

> *Healthy Habits* says, "Your behaviour affects the validity of your words. Say you love him but don't act like it, and your child will doubt your affection. Say it's important to eat healthy but keep all the unhealthy food for your own consumption, and your child will continue to covet those foods. Say its fun to exercise but make no effort to be physically active or always complain when you are and your child will lose motivation."[4]

Your children assign you great power. You are their model of adulthood because you protect and nurture them and spend the greatest amount of time with them. If you explain to your child that it is a good thing they cannot eat unhealthy foods and then you proceed to eat ice cream by the carton or buy candy floss at an amusement park while your child cannot share in the fun, how powerful will your words be? How are you making your child feel? You must ensure you follow your own advice. Be an ally to your child and stay away from the foods to which your child reacts. If you need to be a closet eater every once in a while, that's okay. However, if you really believe in teaching by example, you need to show your child what it means to be a healthy adult so that your child has something to aspire to and that means cheating only on rare occasion.

HEALTH FACT

You are their model of adulthood because you protect and nurture them and spend the greatest amount of time with them.

If your child is offered something, his or her response might be, "I cannot have that" and your response might be, "I can't, either." Or "We're both sensitive to that."

It's vital that your child feels safe in the knowledge that you, the parent, know how to take care of them. If you are knowledgeable about the foods your child can and cannot eat, know the alternatives and remain calm when symptoms appear after trying something new, your child gains confidence and comfort in dealing with their particular challenges and can stay calm too. It all begins with you.

If you had sensitivities as a child or still do, tell your child about how it felt or feels for you and how your life differs as a result. For example, I shared the fact that when I eat chocolate, I get pimples. At my brother's wedding, the girls saw me eating chocolate cake and reminded me that I get pimples from eating chocolate cake. I immediately put the cake down and thanked the girls for helping me as I had forgotten. The girls were happy to help me out and they saw how quickly I put down the offending food, which set a perfect example for them.

HEALTH FACT

It all begins with you.

If you are the picture of health, your children will see that and know that healthy eating is responsible. Guess what they'll want to do next? Emulate you, their shining example.

John and Stasi Eldridge talk about the role of a mother in their book. "She is playing the most irreplaceable, essential, powerful, life-impacting role imaginable."[5]

"If a child lives with tolerance, he learns to be patient.
If a child lives with encouragement, he learns to be confident.
If a child lives with praise, he learns to be appreciative.
If a child lives with acceptance, he learns to love."
–Sinai Sentry[6]

Being afraid to eat and using fear to your advantage

The *Food Allergy Survival Guide* says, "When something as innocent but essential as food causes pain and discomfort, it is a scary situation. When foods that others can eat without ill effect give us a splitting headache, nausea or other distressing symptoms, it is easy to feel apprehensive about eating. Understandably, some people with food sensitivities become afraid to eat almost anything. As a result of avoiding foods for fear of the reaction they may produce, some allergic people become malnourished or develop eating disorders. To a certain extent, fear is necessary and our ally, as it drives us to be careful about what we eat. It can motivate us to find and consume only foods that we can tolerate. However fear may be overwhelming and lead to feelings of loss of control, dread at the thought of going out and terror at the thought of having to eat food prepared by someone else. If our children are the ones with food allergies, we feel a special fear and responsibility for their health, happiness and wellbeing. While these fears are not unfounded, they are also not productive. It is possible to regain control and shed our feelings of helplessness."[7]

It is entirely possible to shed our feelings of helplessness. There is simply no reason why your child should feel the way this author describes. Use the *Food Allergy Survival Guide* as well as this one to ensure that your child always feels safe in this world. Reread steps one to three at the beginning of this chapter so that neither you, nor your child, end up living in fear.

Communicating with other members of your immediate family

A food–reactive child can incite the following feelings in the rest of the family members:

- Stress–the extra time and worry that is involved with having a food–reactive child
- Guilt–the most loving and caring parents and caregivers have food–reactive children
- Fear–that the sibling, son/daughter will not recover from their symptoms
- Resentment–at the attention the food–reactive child receives

Having a food–reactive child becomes "a whole family affair". If one child has sensitivities or allergies and the others do not, sometimes the others resent the attention the sensitive child receives or the special meals prepared for them. Some siblings act out. There's bound to be resentment unless you do something to prevent it.

A marriage can become strained because one or both parents have put too much focus on the food–reactive child and not enough emphasis on good communication with one another. Sometimes this focus becomes so exaggerated that a child eventually carries the responsibility of holding the family together.

Overprotecting can cause psychological problems for the family. Sometimes a mother is so focused on the food–reactive child and so overprotective that the child's life becomes quite restricted. In this case, the whole family suffers. The child feels smothered and other family members do not receive the attention they need and end up feeling resentment towards the other child.

It is easy to become over–focussed on an asthmatic child, for example, because an attack is very frightening. A feeling of helplessness occurs when you see your child gasping for air. The youngster may be anxious because he or she feels as if the air supply is being cut off. Of course, you need to focus fully on your child in the midst of an attack. However, by learning all you can about asthma, you will be able to react calmly. As you learn more, you will find ways to help your child avoid attacks all together.

A few sessions with a family counsellor can help improve communication and rebuild family ties. Maybe some help with housework will allow parents more quality time with siblings. Perhaps a knowledgeable caregiver for a child with asthma will create time for you and your spouse to enjoy each other.

No matter what, a child's main caregiver has a big responsibility raising a food-reactive child. The stage in which you are first figuring everything out is obviously the hardest and most time consuming. I recommend that the main caregiver take the time whenever possible to explain what they are doing and when they might be able to spend time with another family member. For example, "I'm just trying to read this book to determine what the alternatives to wheat are so I can put together the grocery list for tomorrow. I should be done in about twenty minutes and then I'll be free to do something with you, alright?" Or, if you do not know how long it will take you, you might simply say what you are doing, "I'm having a really hard time finding the information though and I'm not sure how long it will take me. What would you like to do in the meantime?" Then, provide any help that is needed to get the other person set up to do that task. Unfortunately, it takes a lot of thought, time and communication to make each family member feel that they are important but it's worth it. Keep in mind, giving each member of the family equal value is the only way to ensure you create peace within your home. Of course, if you can do any tasks when other family members are away from home or asleep, it is ideal.

Remember: It is only if food sensitivities or allergies are singled out as a "problem", that an unhealthy focus can take place.

Communicating with your food-reactive child's siblings

When symptoms are occurring

There was only one time after Paige was born when Taylor was constipated and uncomfortable for days on end. When that occurred, I did not know when I would be free to play with Paige, who was one year old at the time. I explained to her a few times that I was helping Taylor and when it seemed that Paige couldn't possibly look at any more books, I told Paige that I would take her to the indoor playground once Taylor was back at school. Then, I asked her if she wanted me to call a babysitter that was particularly good at playing with Paige to come to our home and help us. The babysitter came and that night I thanked Paige for being so patient and told her what a good girl she was to let me help Taylor for so long. Then, I made sure that I took Paige to that playground as soon as Taylor was back at school.

Preventing symptoms from occurring

You will have one of these two scenarios:

- One child with sensitivities or allergies and the other(s) without
- Both or all children with sensitivities or allergies, usually they'll share some of the same problematic foods and differ in others

Scenario One

No matter what, the food-reactive child needs an ally. If the whole family is eating one way and they are the only one eating different foods, you, the parent, are creating a problem. Preferably, you should eat the same foods your food-reactive child is eating. Second choice, would be for you to eat differently than everyone in your family, so that both of you are eating differently than the others. This gets into making three different meals for one family though, which I don't imagine you want to get into, unless necessary.

"The children without sensitivities" is an interesting concept. Are you sure they don't have any reactions to food? In this world of processed food, it is extremely hard to find a child without sensitivities, of some sort. Now, suppose for a moment that your other child (or children) doesn't have any food sensitivities. Do you want them eating chemicals and loads of sugar, found in so many of the unhealthy foods out there? In my mind, there needs to be restrictions on a child's diet as long as you are living in North America today. Something to think about. If you agree with this way of thinking, then there is only one scenario, which is scenario #2.

Scenario Two

One child is eating eggs, one child cannot. The one who cannot eat eggs, can eat corn but the other cannot. Neither child is eating chemicals or pop. In a case like this, your aim is to feed the children and yourselves, as similarly as possible, most days. Find food ideas that you can all handle and enjoy. As discussed, many of the common allergenic foods are foods none of us should be eating anyway. Feeding one meal to one family makes your job easier and keeps the resentment between the kids down to a minimum. If there are too many discrepancies in what your children can eat, the way to handle this is on the day that the one is having eggs when the other cannot, the other should be having corn when the other cannot. Try never to get into the habit of sneaking food to your less sensitive child as this breeds favouritism, shows your less sensitive child that sneaking around is acceptable. You can only imagine how your more sensitive child would feel if he or she caught you in the act!

Imagine you have one child and are not aware of them having any food sensitivities, and then you have a baby that has major issues with food. You will, first, need to address the issue at hand. Tackle the baby's issues and then, eventually start looking into whether your older child really does need some dietary changes.

The older child will have eaten one way for years and will, no doubt, resent their new sibling, if foods they love end up being taken away. The best way to handle this is to say that the baby helped you understand how to make everyone in the family feel better. Give examples. "Do you notice that your rash on your face is gone? That's because we're staying away from wheat." Or "Don't you feel so much better now that you're having such large bowel movements?" (Or whatever you choose to call the movements?)

It will be easy to feed your baby differently from their older sibling when your youngest is only having pureed foods. Once your baby is a toddler, you will need to find ways to feed your children similarly.

What do you do if your older child sneaks food to your younger child? A strict no tolerance rule applies in this case. Explain to your older child that you know they were trying to be nice by giving that food to their little brother or sister but that specific food will cause their sibling to have symptoms such as... Most older siblings want to protect their younger sibling. You can ask your eldest to help you take care of the littlest one. They will usually be pleased to oblige. If they choose to rebel and continue to feed problematic foods to your youngest, you will need to decide on the consequences for that older child.

Suppose you're at an amusement park and one of your children wants an ice cream cone but the other absolutely cannot handle ice cream cones. You decide that you really want your one child to have an ice cream cone. This will literally cost you! Before purchasing that cone, you need to take the other child to the store at the amusement park and allow them to pick a toy of the same value as the ice cream. It's not that every single move needs to be perfectly fair to each child, but when you are dealing with diet, you are setting a precedent for a long time to come. How you handle one scenario will directly effect how the next scenario will play out, knowing that food sensitivities can last for a long time (but hopefully not!) You may find that the other child, who originally wanted ice cream, changes their mind and picks a toy. If this happens, you might feel happy that neither child is having an unhealthy treat but you would certainly think about the impact on your pocketbook and waste of money on yet more toys. If the child still wants a cone, what do you do with the one child while the other one is eating the ice cream? You need to have someone else with you, to carry out the rest of this plan. You simply cannot make one child painstakingly watch another demolish an ice cream cone right before their eyes! If you have another adult with you, one can be with the child eating ice cream and the other can take the other child on a ride. You can see from this scenario that this can be done, but what do you think is really best for your children? Try to feed your children as similarly as possible. If your one child can have a cone, ask this child to have a cone on another outing, without the watchful, sad eyes of brother or sister.

This brings up another point. I decided that I would like to spend more alone time with my eldest child, once she was in school full time. She was very excited when I suggested an outing for just the two of us. What does a child who has always had so many food sensitivities or allergies want to do once her body no longer goes into pain from eating certain foods? Eat new foods! Taylor really didn't feel she needed more alone time with me; she wanted treats without her sister around! Needless to say, our outings were few and far between until we could agree on a new arrangement!

Communicating with your spouse

When you are the one bearing most of the responsibility for your child

Because one spouse usually ends up taking on more of the responsibility for child rearing than the other, problems can ensue because they take on most of the stress and worry for a child that belongs to both parents. One spouse may feel that since they are the main breadwinner, their number one priority is work. They expect the other to keep everything running smoothly at home, so that they don't need to worry and can maintain focus on providing for the family. This is a very unfortunate situation because everyone loses in this case. A parent misses out spending time with their child. The child misses out on spending time with their parent. The spouse misses out receiving the support and love necessary in order to provide the same for their child. There are always ways that a working parent can make a difference in the lives of those at home without large time commitments.

You may have perfectly justifiable anger at your spouse for not helping out as much as you would like or for resisting change. Talk about it together privately. Tell your spouse how *you* are feeling (lonely, scared, confused, and sad) without putting blame on the other person and ask if he or she has any ideas as to how you could both make things better. It might also help to explain your personal commitment to doing what's necessary to help your child, including being a role model. Talk about the positive future you envision for your family and attempt to engage your spouse's help on the journey. They may benefit from visiting your family naturopath, nutritionist or other expert helping you understand your child better. Your spouse might also increase their comprehension of the situation by reading the books that you have been reading. If you try all of these methods and feel that you are still not feeling supported, you can seek the help of a counsellor and work out a more equitable way of sharing responsibility. If you are unable to obtain your spouse's help, don't let this deter you. Try to settle for a willing passenger on the journey. Maybe over time, as you quietly go about making small improvements to your child's meals and your spouse sees the positives in your child, he or she will end up becoming your co-pilot, after all.

Without the benefit of at least one parent who is willing to accept responsibility for your child's wellbeing, your child will probably feel very vulnerable, alone and afraid. Also, if neither parent accepts responsibility for their child's wellbeing, your child will not learn to take responsibility for himself. When a child's health is on the line, someone needs to show up and be present.

When your spouse is having trouble coping with caring for your child

Suddenly, someone you've counted on to make you feel better no matter what the circumstance may feel overwhelmed just going to the grocery store. He or she may have once reacted calmly no matter what happened, but now cannot seem to handle anything with poise. Keep in mind that time heals. Give it time and patience and your spouse will likely rise to the challenge at hand eventually. Accepting your own or your partner's personal challenges along with a reasonable plan to work around them is one of the best things we can do, not just for our food-reactive child but for all our children. The plan might involve seeking outside help or taking care of yourself so that you can continue to assume most of the responsibility for your child. Read on for more assistance in these areas.

HEALTH FACT

Also, if neither parent accepts responsibility for their child's wellbeing, your child will not learn to take responsibility for himself.

I was in the health food store one day and a little boy asked his father if they could buy watermelon and his father responded matter of factly, but with kindness in his voice, "Watermelon isn't healthy for us". "Us".... It was a glowing example of bearing the burden, being on the same team, ensuring that little child didn't feel alone in this big, sometimes scary, world. Kudos to that father.

When your spouse gives your child a problem food

Your spouse once was trustworthy and efficient, but now seems to be the opposite. They give your child gum or small candies, thinking it won't cause any harm. Your child suffers. No matter how the other is acting, it's safe to assume that parent feels awful about what happened.

Men and women communicate and behave differently, it is important to realize. Women, understand that men will sometimes try to play a situation down in order to calm themselves down. Inside they may be as shaken as you are, if not more. If you start accusing them of not caring, they will withdraw even more. Talk about it. Share your fears, your frustration. There is a price to pay for anger. Anger and blame can ruin your relationship and your family. Sharing information brings people closer together. Look at what the two of you can learn from what happened and discuss steps to take to ensure it doesn't happen again.

"Date nights" are a wonderful way for you and your spouse to get together in the midst of all of the chaos. Pick one night a week or one night every other week to go have fun together, whether you see a movie or go to dinner. Time alone for the two of you is of utmost importance in remaining a team and creating peace within your home. If this tradition is started when your child is young, your child won't ever question your departure because it will have been part of their routine right from the start. If you have no one to look after your child or cannot afford a babysitter, ask a friend, who also has children, if you can take turns looking after each other's children.

When your spouse feels guilt for causing their child to have food sensitivities or allergies

Sometimes a parent feels guilt for creating a child with food sensitivities or allergies, especially once they learn the causes of food sensitivities and allergies. My husband and I attended numerous parties, drinking excessive amounts of alcohol over many years, prior to having children. Did this contribute to Taylor being so sick? Absolutely! Was this the sole reason for her health challenges? Absolutely not. Did we do other things that contributed to Taylor's lack of good bacteria and leaky gut? Absolutely! Did we know the damage we would be causing our unborn child? Absolutely not. Did our child, who was so sick, benefit in the long term? Absolutely. Do those that know and learn from our family's lessons benefit? 100%. Do I feel guilty? What for?

Even if you have, so far, been unable to put an end to your child's suffering, there is no reason to feel guilty. You are trying, you are learning and everyone around you benefits from your lessons. The only reason a parent has to feel guilty is if a mother or father is not taking the time to pay attention to the health of their child.

Taking care of yourself

> "Every woman who becomes a mother enrols herself in the graduate-level course of higher sacrifice. Motherhood teaches a woman how to deny herself. When money is tight, the children are clothed and fed first. When energy is low, nighttime books still get read. Mothers give and give, long past exhaustion and reasonableness."[8]

You, better than anyone, know your child. You are the most suited to identify the foods, chemicals or drugs to which your child reacts and eliminate them from their diet or environment. You have the power to make your child healthy and happy for the rest of their life. What a gigantic responsibility!

The stress of looking after a child, any child, is huge. When you have a child that is eating differently than the majority, you may feel anxious, a little depressed, or even angry at your circumstances. It can be very unsettling knowing that your precious child is vulnerable to harm every time they eat. A certain amount of anxiety serves a purpose; it makes you careful and alert. If you become educated about food sensitivities and allergies, your anxiety will decrease. The job of caring for a food-reactive child is continuous, from the moment your child awakes until bed-time. Food must be uppermost in your mind, many times a day, every single day of your life. If your child is extremely sensitive or allergic, there is little breathing room for mistakes. If an accident happens, whether or not it was your fault, you are the one that bears the repercussions of your child's symptoms. Technically, I should have started this chapter with 'taking care of yourself', because if you do not take care of yourself, you are no good to the rest of your family. If you allow anyone to zap all of your energy, you are the person that suffers. If you are phys-ically drained, have health issues, are not getting time to yourself or are not truly enjoying life, your child or someone else in your life, might be taking too much energy from you. Don't let it happen! If you are lacking energy, it is impossible for you to have fun in life, one of our main functions here on earth.

HEALTH FACT

If you are lacking energy, it is impossible for you to have fun in life, one of our main functions here on earth.

The challenge lies in the fact that there is always something more that we, as parents, could be doing for our family, our work or our home. It is so easy to stay on the treadmill of trying to please everyone else or feeling guilty that you are not doing enough for your family members. It takes courage to jump off the treadmill, stand back from the situation and say, "I don't need to sacrifice or deny myself any longer. I am going to say "no" to my family sometimes and begin taking care of my needs." You don't need to attend each of your child's sporting events or get groceries in between picking children up from their activities or do everything yourself.

> An excellent book on this subject is *Briefcase Moms*, even if you are not working outside the home. The author suggests becoming comfortable asking others for help and says, "Asking for help is not a sign of weakness but rather a demonstration of inner strength and confidence." You might ask your spouse how the two of you could share what has to be done so that both your needs are met, rather than placing blame on your spouse for not helping enough.[9]

If you allow yourself to be free of the burden of being "Super Mom" or "Super Dad", slow down and learn to serve your own interests, you will find that you will ultimately better serve the interests of your family and others in your life. Being selfish, in a positive way, allows you to be physically and emotionally present at all times and free of resentment. You might just surprise yourself and eventually reach a point where you know in your heart that what you do for your family and others *is* enough. Imagine the example you would set for your child. You would be teaching your child to always nurture themselves, no matter what goes on in your child's world.

It was only a couple of years ago that my husband told me, "You have to stop caring about everyone else so much". I had no idea what he was talking about when he said these words to me. Not long after, I went to see an incredible counsellor who invited me to have a love affair with myself. Again, I had no idea what he meant by that statement at the

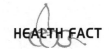

HEALTH FACT

You would be teaching your child to always nurture themselves, no matter what goes on in your child's world.

time but didn't want to admit it! I walked away from the appointment determined to find out what having an affair with myself entailed. I knew that a pedicure would probably be included in part of what I was supposed to do. I had rarely indulged in pedicures, manicures or massages in the past, thinking that the effects of these services were short lasting and therefore, a waste of money. I was so wrong!!!! Pampering and feeling good about yourself is what it is all about! The aesthetician that gave me the pedicure had children and had been grappling with caring for herself, as well! She told me that her counsellor told her to sit on her couch in the middle of the day and read a book for 10 minutes. I pictured myself sitting on my couch and envisioned all the thoughts rushing through my head involving what I "should" be doing. I shared these thoughts with the aesthetician and she laughed, saying that she had the same thoughts. However, I decided to try taking time out for myself and let go of those harmful thoughts. I chose to suntan for 10 minutes on the deck, taking the phone with me in case anyone called. Within two minutes of sitting in the sun, I picked up the phone to call someone and then told myself that I didn't need to make a call at that moment. This conversation went on in my head at least one more time in the ten-minute period. Finally, I managed to make it for 10 minutes. Eventually, I built those 10 minutes up to a whole day of doing only what I wanted to do (once my girls were in school, of course)!!!!! When people would call on those days, sometimes I would answer and they would ask what I was doing. Instead of rhyming off everything I was doing, like I did in the past, I would respond with the words "Absolutely nothing". Many of my friends thought I was joking! I was so enjoying doing absolutely nothing that I was proud to tell others! Some acquaintances tried to make me feel guilty for taking time for myself but I had spent too many years denying myself to care what they thought. If you ask an elderly person what they would have done differently in their youth, so often you'll hear them say they would have slowed down and enjoyed themselves more.

After a few months of spending time doing nothing and having fun, I came to feel really good about myself. I had never afforded myself this luxury in my 40 years of life! You know what else? I came to feel that even though my family is important, I AM IMPORTANT too! To this day, I have never stopped filling a part of every day without doing something for myself that nourishes my soul. Nurturing myself no longer feels like a luxury; I know it is necessary to keep me feeling energized, even-tempered, focused and happy. My family feeds off the positive vibes I exude!

Outside of not realizing our own importance, there is another reason that we don't want to take time out for ourselves when we have food-reactive children. We are afraid of what will happen to our children when under the care of someone else. Most times, however, leaving your child under the care of someone else is a positive experience or can be turned into something positive.

Here's a great illustration. Long after Taylor stopped being in pain with constipation, I went away for a "girls' weekend". Didn't Taylor end up being in pain from constipation that weekend? My husband was in charge. He told me afterward, his voice heavy with emotion, that it was absolutely horrible. Taylor wouldn't move from the couch, she was moaning and groaning from her pain for hours on end. She wasn't hungry. She couldn't sleep. My husband said that he was completely exhausted from tending to her, worrying about her and from not sleeping himself. He said, "We cannot deviate from her special way of eating, not even slightly. I will feed her whatever you tell me is healthy for her." He also talked about how proud he was of Taylor because of how she managed her pain so calmly. These words were music to my ears, coming from a person who never seemed to take what I said about Taylor's health seriously and who was often slipping her foods that she couldn't handle.

By taking care of myself and leaving my husband in charge, he came to understand what I had dealt with for months and, for the first time, began taking responsibility for his daughter's health. As a bonus, Taylor and her father bonded like never before and I came home after the weekend refreshed and ready to take on all my challenges again with a positive outlook because "my cup had been filled."

Weekends away are a great way to get a break and return with renewed appreciation for the miracle of your children and spouse. I invite you to make a list of things that you want to do that would nourish your soul. If you just can't see where you would fit this time in, then you might want to keep a log for a week to see how you allocate the hours of each day and whether the way you spend your time accurately reflects your priorities. When I did this, I found that I was doing far more in a day than I needed. I stopped making lists and began doing only what I needed to do each day. What a difference this made in freeing up hours to enjoy myself!

You can experience joy every day by:
- Dancing in your kitchen
- Meeting a friend for lunch or dinner
- Running or walking in the trees
- Taking a long candle-lit bath
- Sun-tanning on your deck (in moderation)

- Sitting on top of a mountain (yes, a hill will do!) or by a lake
- Attending a class e.g. painting, cooking, dance, whatever interests you
- Attending a spa
- Buying something for yourself
- Having your hair done
- Having your home cleaned
- Decorating a room in your house

Some of you cannot get away without your child so here are some ideas to bring you personal fulfillment while in the presence of your child:

- Talking to a friend on the phone or reading a book while your child plays quietly on their own.
- Meditating while your child watches television (a little time in front of the television never hurt anyone but your lack of sanity could!)
- Holding your child while he or she watches television is relaxing for you and allows your mind to wander.
- Doing crafts alongside your child. Even colouring together can be a short escape for you.
- Having your child read to you, once they no longer need your assistance with the words.
- Listening to music while you cook.
- Going for a hike in the trees together.
- Taking pictures of your child.
- Inviting your friend to join you and your child on an outing.

If you get into the habit of taking care of yourself when your baby is first born, it will be easier for you to keep it up. It is important that you take the time to sleep, shower, eat a nutrient rich balanced diet, exercise, take your vitamins, find time for yourself and experience joy every day. Making your body fit and strong will make you feel better and more confident in yourself, which will improve every aspect of your life.

Exercising literally saved me when I was going through the hardest time with Taylor. She went into babysitting at the gym, met other children who she remains friends with today and learned that her mother would always come back for her. One of the babysitters had been struggling with food sensitivities herself and was a great person to talk to. She even helped me when I said, "I've eliminated all the dairy from Taylor's diet but she's still struggling." She asked whether I'd eliminated yogurt. I followed this suggestion and noticed the increase in Taylor's bowel movements right away. I was also able to converse and become friends with other mothers while we exercised. In addition, the exertion from my workouts released my endorphins, putting me in the best mood and helping me feel energized.

You may need to become creative in finding alternatives so that you can have time to yourself. You might share driving or activity attendance with another parent. You might need your child to go to a daycare or spend a day with a relative or friend for a day a week. You might ask your spouse to be home early from work or ask a friend to come over one night a week so that you can go out, even if it's just to the book store to sit and read in a different but comfortable space. When your child is older, you might ask them to help you accomplish your goals. Tell your child that as soon as you get home from school, the two of you will do something together (i.e. play a game), then you can make and clean up dinner together and after that, it can be your turn to have time to yourself while your child plays alone or reads. This system works really well in our house, especially because my girls receive my attention at the beginning of the evening as opposed to waiting until the end to be with me.

Talking to your friends, a health professional and others with similiar issues will help promote healing within yourself. People always think they are the only ones with a particular issue or going through something. YOU are *never* alone. Think about attending a parents' group for food-reactive children or start your own. In these support groups, you can share some of your difficulties and learn how other parents cope. It is also good to hear from others with the same experiences, that although you try to do everything right, your child still may have challenges.

If you are one who prefers not to talk to others about your difficulties, you will need ways to release your emotions. Keeping all of your emotions bottled up inside is the most harmful thing you can do to yourself. I know. Here are some ideas for releasing your pent up feelings and stress:

- Exercise (in nature ideally)
- Keep a journal (writing about people or moments that you are grateful for really puts things into perspective)
- Play an instrument or listen to music
- Meditate (start by listening to your breathing for 5 minutes)
- Do something creative (i.e. artwork, scrapbooking, woodworking or decorating your house)

Another excellent book that will give you far more ideas than what I've just shared with you is *When you're about to go off the deep end, don't take your kids with you* by Kelly Nault.

> "As mothers, we sometimes struggle with our passions, believing that to deny them is somehow sacrificial and good. God created you and called you with a purpose. To deny your passions is to reject his call on your life."[10]

Communicating with others

Communicating with other family members, friends and acquaintances

How you choose to talk to others about your food-reactive child also shows your child how you truly feel about their reactions to food, so it is extremely important that you think this through carefully.

When it comes to having a child with food sensitivities or allergies and being with other people, there is one thing to keep in mind. The less said the better. Consciously, pick the people with which you want to share your challenges. Good friends, complementary practitioners or maybe some family members are all good choices. The person you just met, the restaurant server or the flight attendant; these are not good choices. Let me tell you why. When you recognize your child's food sensitivities or allergies and choose to feed the healthier alternatives, you are increasing your consciousness and changing your behaviour. You are now doing things differently from the majority. And good for you! What the majority is doing, is not working.

However, just because you are doing things differently, doesn't mean that everyone needs to know. Doing things differently and telling others about it only invites judgement and/or criticism. Often, older children may ask their parents to respect their wish that you not speak about them to others. **What works for you and your child is all that matters.** You don't need other people's approval or their opinions when you already know what works. If you do decide to explain to a stranger what you go through on a daily basis with your child with food sensitivities, you are only using up your precious time and energy trying to explain something to someone who really can't comprehend what you're saying, simply because they haven't gone through it.

It is important to be honest about family challenges, to yourself, to your partner, and to others. Make sure that you never exaggerate some already difficult circumstances when talking to others.

You may find that your friends or family members get tired of listening to you or think you're overreacting, so be wary of the possibility and try to prevent it from occurring to begin with. Certainly, in our own family, word spread quickly amongst the relatives about how ridiculous I had become when it came to Taylor's diet and environment and a number of them turned against me. Thankfully, this was not the case indefinitely, as family members watched Taylor thrive, month after month, year after year. Funnily enough, one said, "Whatever you're doing with her, its working." I thought to myself, "I'd love to tell you exactly what I'm doing" but unfortunately I knew she didn't want to hear what I had to say.

Another thing to keep in mind when you're discussing your child with anyone, if your child has food sensitivities, is the importance of not referring to food 'sensitivities' as 'allergies'. "Allergies" is an overused term and often used erroneously. Because of this, if you tell people your child has food allergies, often people think you're exaggerating the problem or that you are a health freak and are using "allergies" as an excuse to keep your child away from birthday cake or ice cream, for example. My experience is that if you say your child has food sensitivities, others often view you as quite educated and ask, "How did you discover your child has food sensitivities?" (As we know, food sensitivities are much harder to detect than most allergies) Some prefer to simply state the symptom that results if their child consumes a certain food and not even bring up the term "sensitivities". Again, my opinion is to not bring up "food sensitivities" or "symptoms" unless necessary.

Keep in mind, there are always going to be people who will mistake your reasonable efforts to protect your child as efforts to control them or your child. You simply need to know that taking care of your child is your top priority. As your child heals and has fewer and fewer reactions to food, your confidence in doing things differently will increase and the opinions of people, who do not share your circumstances, will not matter.

In many cases, when I had to tell people what was going on, I found them to be very interested in what we were experiencing and it made them count their lucky stars that their children didn't have any challenges with food. Obviously their child's body was not responding to food in any severe way, which was good news for them but I would always wonder what symptoms their child *did* have.

Communicating with older generations

If you explain to grandparents that a certain food is causing a specific symptom in your child, they might remember that their child had those symptoms, as well, but admit that they didn't figure out that food was the problem. If this is the case, your child's grandparents might be very interested to see how removing the problematic food helps their grandchild. Certainly, this would be a positive communication experience!

Unfortunately, if you tell your parents or in-laws what you're up to, many of them might just feel threatened. They raised their children on regular foods and vaccinated them and their children turned out fine. Why isn't their way good enough for you? Well, maybe their children did turn out okay but the way regular food is being made has changed since they were feeding their children and so has the way modern vaccinations are being administered.

They might also think what they did worked okay when, in truth, they were actually unaware of the effects of how they fed their child. For example, you tell your mother-in-law that you're not feeding your child cow's milk because it causes ear infections and she says "Well, Thomas drank lots of milk every day when he was a kid and he had no problems." Meanwhile Thomas is all grown up now and knows he cannot tolerate cow's milk but never mentioned it to his mom. Maybe Thomas did grow up without any obvious health issues but the world is a different place now from when Thomas was being raised. Nothing is as pure as it was back then; not the air, water or food. That is why we are seeing so many symptoms, conditions and disease in our children today. Circumstances now dictate that we do things differently than the way our parents raised us.

The other issue with grandparents in particular, is that many of them rely heavily on giving their grandchildren treats. To them, a treat is their expression of love. If you are not at the point of being able to offer your child treats, you may find that you need a game plan for visits to Grandma and Grandpa's house. Bring healthy treats to their home that your child will be excited to receive from them. You can bring some recipes over for healthy cookies or a cake that your child can make and then enjoy with Grandma and Grandpa. If your child's grandparents refuse to believe the impact that certain foods have on them, bring their grandchild over for a visit after having eaten problematic foods. Be sure to point out the link between the problematic foods and the symptom your child exhibits! Then, be ready to make a quick exit if the symptom is poor behaviour!

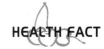

HEALTH FACT

Circumstances now dictate that we do things differently than the way our parents raised us.

Anticipate family members' objections and create positive and optimistic responses. When your child is reacting to food, it isn't the time for arguments or recriminations; it's a time to bring the family together in a shared goal of companionship, mutual respect, and support. However, it is important to know that it is highly unlikely everyone in your family will understand, never mind support, the way you are helping your child.

Communicating with others that are caring for your child
(See Chapter#8 for more information)

Others may not believe that food sensitivities can be dangerous and thus, may not be as careful as necessary. Whether due to denial, lack of understanding or other reasons, clear, effective communication is of utmost importance.

We had a babysitter that continually fed Taylor foods to which she was sensitive. That was what made me reorganize the content of the kitchen cupboards, so that it was clear to whoever looked after Taylor which cupboard contained her "safe" food. However, on subsequent days, the babysitter gave Taylor things from the *fridge* that she could not have. This made me reorganize the fridge. Then one day, the babysitter took Taylor to her house and gave her whole wheat bread from her own kitchen. I asked the babysitter why she did this and she said she thought it was healthy and wouldn't cause Taylor any trouble.

Each time an incident occurred, I calmly explained to the babysitter that Taylor could not eat the particular item she'd been fed and explained that Taylor experienced problems going to the washroom, without getting into a discussion about her pain. Finally, when accidents kept happening, I communicated Taylors' true experiences with certain foods, my voice heavy with emotion. I told the sitter that what she was feeding Taylor was putting her in a lot of pain, which lasted for days and thoroughly explained the consequences of her actions. I then asked her whether she was up to the challenge of simply feeding Taylor the foods I said she could have (ensuring I offered lots of choices) or if she would rather not babysit Taylor anymore. Once she understood the gravity of what she'd been doing, our babysitter apologized profusely and said that she would like to continue to babysit Taylor, making sure she only fed Taylor the foods that I had set out for her. We never did have any more problems with that babysitter. She looked after both our children until she went off to university and we all came to love her.

This scenario shows you that there are times when long explanations *are* needed. I could have simply never asked this babysitter to look after my child again but I only had one other woman to help me at the time and I felt more comfortable having two options. I knew I could find someone else if I had to, but because of effective communication, there was no need.

If an accident occurs while your child is in the care of someone else, find out what went wrong and what all of you, as a team, can do to prevent it from happening again. Give the caregiver the opportunity to tell their side of the story; you may learn something that will prove useful in the future. Ask them to present you with a plan to avoid future accidents. Your forgiveness and trust are key elements. If you treat the other person like a teammate, trying to achieve the same goal of caring for a child that needs extra help, you will have a greater likelihood of success. There may be times when someone you have taken a lot of time talking to, may deliberately dis-regard your instructions, without good reason, and say, "Well, the others were eating cheese (for example)" or "He wanted it so badly that I had to give him a little piece". My suggestion, in this case, is that you find a new caregiver, if at all possible.

Communicating with your child's doctor(s)
(See Chapter #9 for a deeper understanding)

There are millions of people in this world, millions of babies born every day. Babies with colic, constipation, diarrhea, runny or stuffy noses, and eczema and other rashes are everywhere. These symptoms are the norm, not the exception. Why is there so little medical expertise on identifying and managing food sensitivities? I couldn't understand it.

My child was suffering. Our family doctor and doctors at clinics we visited told us her experiences were normal. She would outgrow her constipation. No words can express the anger and pure frustration that I felt, at the time, with each doctor we consulted.

When I asked the doctors whether foods might be causing her problems, they non-committedly replied that foods might have something to do with it, but had no more knowledge on the subject to share with me. As you know, they told me to give my child laxatives, suppositories and enemas. We did try this route and still have the bag filled with drugs to prove it. I wanted to get to and eliminate the root cause of her symptoms!

After I had Interro testing done, I brought the test to my doctor. I wanted to ask her some more detailed questions about its findings. My doctor took one look at the test and said that she did not believe that this form of testing was in any way accurate. Believe me; I wanted her to be right, with every ounce of my being! Yet, I knew that the part of the list showing the major foods to avoid was true. That was the day I learned not to bring up alternative methods with my particular doctor; every doctor is different.

Doctors are revered, the gurus of health. I couldn't help wondering what was preventing them from finding out what is behind so much of the chronic illness in children today. Then I came to understand that doctors are trained more in disease management than in prevention. They are not trained in nutritional medicine; they are trained in prescription medicine. Seek the help of doctors when your child breaks a bone, has a structural challenge or when food or natural medicine is not working. Some medical doctors have done other research and are open to natural methods of achieving health and wellness; feel free to speak openly with those doctors! Otherwise, it is best to recognize that medical doctors will not be doing research on natural methods by listening to you, the patient.

Your child talking to others

I think you'll find that there won't be a lot of this going on. When a child is doing things differently than the majority, they are usually not in a rush to talk about it. What you will run into, is others offering your child regular food.

If your child is offered a candy, for example, here are some ideas of how they can handle it:

- Accept it and say, "Thank you" and then you can encourage your child to save it for "Treat Day" or give it to Daddy or some other person of choice. In my experience, this works wonders because a child takes great pleasure in giving treats to others.
- Say, "No, thank you." If the person insists, your child can say, "I have food sensitivities." That's it, no lengthy explanation, no belabouring the matter. If the person continues to ask questions, you can step in and simply say, "As you can see, the food sensitivities are making him (or her) the healthiest possible."

You may be reading these suggestions and saying, "Yeah, right! My child is going to respond that calmly and maturely…. Sure." If you've already shown your child what happens when an offending food is eaten, your child will have no interest in eating that candy, which is exactly why they can respond maturely.

In Conclusion

Responsibility for health improvement belongs to you, your spouse, your child and your practitioner. If all the team members play their part, there should be no major repercussions and your child should become less reactive and healthier as time goes on. Good communication is essential. Most importantly, know that you have all the answers to your challenges within.

> *"According to Hindu legend, long ago all humans were gods. But they so abused the privilege that Brahma, the god of all gods, decided their wisdom and power should be taken away from them. But he had to hide it where no human would ever find it again.*
>
> *"Let us bury it deep within the earth," suggested one god. Brahma said, "No, they will dig until they find it."*
>
> *"Let us throw it into the deepest part of the biggest ocean," proposed another god.*
>
> *"Humans will learn to dive and someday come across it," insisted Brahma.*
>
> *"Then it can be hidden in the clouds atop the highest mountain of the Himalayas."*
>
> *"They will manage to climb that high someday," Brahma pointed out. "I have a better idea. Let's hide it where they will never think to look: inside themselves."*[11]

How to make the best use of this chapter's information

1. There are sections of this chapter that assist all parents in raising healthy and happy children. They are as follows:
   - Communicating with your child
   - Taking care of yourself
2. In this chapter, some of the things you can learn include:
   - Building your child's trust in you
   - Teaching your child to be responsible for his or her own body, so that they know when things are not right, and stay on track with healthy eating
   - What healthy eating can do for your child and how to talk to your child about implementing it into your family's lifestyle
   - Building your child's self-esteem
   - Setting an example for your child
   - Letting your child "own" their own emotions, which will help keep your relationship with your child strong
3. If your child is also reacting adversely to food, then you will want to read:
   - Communicating with other members of your immediate family
   - Communicating with others

CHAPTER 8

OUTSIDE THE SAFETY ZONE

How to Feed Your Child in the Big Wide World

The last chapter explained methods that you can employ in different settings for talking about feeding your child differently. The goal is to obtain the most understanding and cooperation from your child and others. This chapter shows you a number of ways in which you can manage the task of feeding children differently than the majority when they are surrounded by other children their own age at school, attending social functions, special occasions, or travelling.

Some parents feel that their children cannot partake in regular events because if their child does participate in events where other children are involved, their child will have to eat whatever everyone else is eating. It is not necessary or helpful to a child's development to keep your child away from social events, on a regular basis, for fear of your child eating the 'wrong' foods. Nor is it in the best interest of your child to eat whatever everyone else is eating.

It is my intention to show you ways for your child to take part in all the wonderful adventures of life without sacrificing their health.

Please refer to Chapter #6 and the Appendix for snack and meal ideas to use in the big wide world!

Having friends over

This may still be the comfort of home, but with the addition of friends who ordinarily eat whatever they want, things can get tricky. From the first time a newborn lays eyes on another child, the fascination with other human beings becomes readily apparent. Kids love other kids. Encourage your child to have friends over! The two most important criteria for a successful play date are fun activities and kindness. Food is really at the bottom of the totem pole. However if you serve great-tasting food, as well as meeting the other criteria, the play date will be a raving success! All you need to do is serve snacks that all the kids enjoy. Garlic hummus and rice crackers, all natural fruit Popsicles, Freezies or any flavour of Soy Dream ice cream, even in the middle of the winter, are enjoyed by most children. The majority of children find that spelt pretzels taste like regular

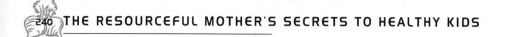

pretzels and they are usually gobbled up quickly. Depending on the children's ages, they can even help you make a fruit smoothie, even helping to choose the fruits. Of course, homemade healthy cookies or cake is always welcomed with open arms by little ones! The originality of the snacks or their presentation (See Chapter #10) goes a long way too.

Leaving your home

Every parent knows that you never want to be out with a hungry child! Whenever you leave the house, always remember to bring "safe" snacks for your child (ren) with you. Even if you think you will only be out for a short while, you can always be delayed. Try to always bring a selection of snacks so that your child can choose a food that they are in the mood to eat. Examples might be freshly cut apples or sweet potatoes (raw sweet potatoes are excellent!), a bowl of mixed berries, or pieces of cut up turkey with rice crackers. Storing a couple of fruit or granola bars in the glove box might come in *very* handy one day if you are stuck in traffic.

Eating out with other families

If you are meeting up with other children, bring some snacks with you that all the children will enjoy. This teaches your children to share and your children will delight in the fact that other children are fond of their "special" food. Maple syrup suckers or candies are good examples of something loved by most children. Some of the packaged foods mentioned in Chapter #6 are hits with other children, as well. If you are in a rush and think you haven't any treats that other children might enjoy, you could pack a bubble-making kit or a little game, something that all the children will like doing together. This, of course, also takes the focus off food.

If you are meeting other children for lunch and both families have agreed to pack their own lunches, you might want to pack your child's version of pizza or some other fun food. The other children will probably have sandwiches or something easier to travel with and will invariably say, "Oh, I wish I could have pizza!" For once, it will be another child wanting what your child is eating, which will definitely make your child feel better about their own food.

When you're out and other children are eating something your child wants, you can tell your child that you will give them something special when you get home. Your child will usually want to know what it is right then and there, so try to have something in mind that you know they love. If you can't think of anything off the top of your head, you can tell them that you are going to give them a new treat. Some children will be content with the prospect of having a treat when they get home and will wait patiently until then. If your child is not one to wait, bring a special treat that you know will excite them but do not display it unless the other children start eating something that your child wants.

Eating in restaurants

I have talked to mothers who will not take their child to a restaurant because they do not believe it is fair for their child to be in a place where they cannot eat the food everyone else is eating. This is a very considerate way of thinking. Unfortunately, by keeping your child away from restaurants, your child misses out on the experience of eating out. Children adore eating out. They love the activity, the atmosphere and being able to watch other people, especially fellow little ones! In addition, you, your spouse, other family members and friends need not be denied the experience of going to a restaurant simply because one or two family members cannot eat certain foods.

So, you've decided to take your child to a restaurant! The first thing to consider is this: are you going to order your child something from the menu or bring food with you? Your answer will depend on the following:

- How many sensitivities or allergies your child has
- How strict you are about your child eating healthier alternatives
- What type of restaurant it is
- The age of your child

HEALTH FACT

Young children's taste buds are sensitive to the subtle flavours in food.

If you start going to restaurants when your child is a newborn, life will be easier for you because they will be breastfeeding or having a bottle, clearly eating differently from the rest of the patrons. Next, your child will eat baby food, until there are enough teeth to start eating non-pureed food. At a young age, your child will become accustomed to doing things differently.

When your child is around one year old, things become a little trickier because they really want to eat what you are eating. For the longest time, the only food in restaurants that my girls were not sensitive to was French Fries (they couldn't even have the ketchup!). Some of you may be dead set against fries but in my mind, having fries the odd time is not a sin. It is a food that kids get excited about and it is something that I can order without having to ask any questions. I must mention that there was one fast-food restaurant where Taylor reacted to the fries. Later, it was discovered that their fries contained dairy and wheat; thankfully, this has been corrected.

The rule of thumb with restaurants and health conscious or food-reactive individuals is to order simple items such as a baked potato, steamed vegetables or poultry or fish without sauce. Young children's taste buds are sensitive to the subtle flavours in food. They do not need butter or other seasonings. If your older child prefers their food seasoned, bring your own "safe" seasonings, sauces and salad dressings from home. Don't forget, you can always bring a whole meal or part of a meal from home and supplement it with restaurant foods. Often young children are simply tickled pink to be with Mom and/or Dad, be at a restaurant and finally, eat off the same "fancy" plates as everyone else.

You may decide to bring a meal from home that needs to be heated up. Without any fanfare or so much as saying, "My child has food sensitivities", all you need to do is politely and quietly ask your server to heat up your child's food and bring it back on a plate like everyone else's. The less said the better.

If you think that telling your server all about your child's food sensitivities or what they can and cannot eat, will ensure you receive a healthier meal, you're likely wrong. Here's why:

- A server may not have studied food or know the ingredients used in foods. For example, a server might think that a vegetable burger is made of vegetables and fried in oil; they might not think that it could contain eggs, sugar, white or wheat flour or chemicals. Do you see how many common allergens can be found in something as simple as a vegetable burger?

- If the server asks the chef for the ingredients of the vegetable burger, quite often the chef does not even know. In all likelihood, they warmed up a pre-cooked vegetable patty that came from a package from a box in the freezer. The majority of mainstream restaurant chefs today do not make their meals from scratch.

- Your server is a very busy individual. He or she wants to take your order, bring your food and get on with the next customer. The faster servers take care of their customers, the more customers they serve and the more tips they receive. When you get into *any* length of discussion with your server, you risk making your server and other customers angry. Remember, your child does not have life-threatening allergies. That is what a restaurant really pays attention to accommodating.

- Most importantly, any time you get into what ingredients are in which foods, or how you could doctor up this dish or that, you are raising your child's angst about food and increasing the chances of your child eating something to which they will react. You are potentially harming your child every time you bring up their situation with a stranger and single your child out. You risk embarrassing your son or daughter and making them feel like the problem.

HEALTH FACT

One study of allergic reactions at restaurants found that half of the reactions were caused by foods "hidden" in dressings, egg rolls and sauces.

You'll want to educate yourself as to what is or can be in foods commonly found in restaurants. One study of allergic reactions at restaurants found that half of the reactions were caused by foods "hidden" in dressings, egg rolls and sauces. There are so many dishes at restaurants that are combinations of food. In the event that there is a risk that a dish will not be prepared to your liking, avoid the hassles and refrain from ordering it.

Freely express your gratitude when you do receive what you asked for and tip your server well, if possible. Each time you successfully negotiate a situation like this, you will gain confidence in your ability to move freely in the big wide world. Just as your friendly, "can do" attitude paves the way for your child's safety, it also helps your child learn how to deal with others. If our children see us approaching new people with warmth, courtesy and ease, that will be their inclination as well. It's extremely important for kids to see parents managing food challenges and making it look simple.

HEALTH FACT

If our children see us approaching new people with warmth, courtesy and ease, that will be their inclination as well.

The day will come when your child asks you why you bring food from home for them. Your response can be, "This way you do not have to wait a long time for your food, like everyone else has to". Also, "If you eat the food here, you will get a tummy ache" (or not be able to go to the bathroom or whatever symptom your child experiences after eating the problematic foods). Remember, as long as your child is aware of what happens to their body when certain foods are eaten, they will be your full partner in ensuring they eat the healthiest foods for their particular body.

Now, maybe you are lucky enough to have a healthy restaurant in your area where you can pretty much order anything they have and know that your child will be all right upon consuming it. We have one such restaurant in our area and they serve foods without dairy, wheat, sugar or chemicals. When they opened, my family was one of their first customers. I came close to crying when I saw their menu for the first time and realized we could not only order something here but that we had choices! My girls were thrilled to be able to choose from a number of non–allergenic foods and loved the experience of eating out, with others around who were eating the same foods! It was pure ecstasy for each of us.

We have remained loyal customers ever since.

Theme Parks

If you're at a theme park and sweet smells are wafting in the air and people are eating treats wherever you venture, it is quite likely your child will want a treat of some sort. Packing one of their really special treats is a good idea or feel free to purchase your child a small souvenir from the park such as a pen or something that can be kept for a longer period of time. Remind them that other children's treats will be gobbled up in no time, whereas your child's treat will be something to treasure always. A meal or a treat at theme parks costs an arm and a leg. Keep in mind that you are saving a lot of money because your child is *not* eating junk food!

Away without you (e.g. friend's house)

We do not and cannot have complete control of our child's environment at all times. That is why it is so important to teach your child to take care of themselves. It will take practice but you'll be surprised at how quickly your child will catch on. From the age of 2 years, you can tell your child which foods they will need to stay away from when visiting friends. If your child reacts to a lot of foods, all you need to do is tell them to only eat their own food, the food you packed for your child. Of course, you will need to tell the friend's parent the same information that you tell your child. Some find it helpful to put a laminated index card, listing the problem foods, in their child's backpack. By talking to your child and the other parent, there shouldn't be any mistakes. If there are mistakes, your child will suffer. When there are mistakes, it is important for you to point out to your child the reason for their suffering, so that the importance of listening to you next time is understood! Encourage your child to share their food with a friend by packing items that you feel will be enjoyed by all.

HEALTH TIP

Encourage your child to share their food with a friend by packing items that you feel will be enjoyed by all.

Off to school
Nursery School

Your child is truly beginning life in the big wide world. You have, no doubt, chosen or will choose your child's school with safety in mind. Today it's rare to find a place that hasn't had to deal with children eating differently than the majority. Communication is the key to keeping your child safe in school. Don't wait until the first day to discuss your child's way of eating or food sensitivities or allergies with the teacher(s). You can start laying the groundwork as early as the April or May prior to school starting.

I would suggest arranging a face-to-face meeting and going about the discussion in the following manner:

1. Tell the teacher that your child reacts to certain foods and that you would like his or her help in ensuring that your child is not fed problematic foods.
2. Describe your child's symptoms or potential symptoms when they eat certain foods, whether it is unruly behaviour, troubles concentrating, nightmares or diarrhea. I feel it is important to describe the symptoms before describing the problem foods so that the first priority is placed on what happens to your child if certain foods are eaten. When you describe the symptoms, you will need to give enough detail so that your child's teacher understands the gravity of the matter yet, at the same time, you don't want to get into a whole long tale of your family's woes. It is important that the teacher does not lose sight of the facts and doesn't get into questioning your beliefs or circumstances.

3. Provide the teacher(s) with a complete written list of the foods to which your child reacts. With my daughters being allergic or sensitive to all of the common allergens, I provided the teacher with a list of foods that my child could eat safely, as that was a shorter list than the former.

4. Develop an action plan together as to how feeding your child will be dealt with under different circumstances. Some of the questions you might ask are: Can you, the parent, supply your child's meals and snacks? If so, where would those foods be kept in the school and how would they get to your child? Is there a "no food sharing" policy? How will you maintain good communication with the teachers regarding treats for special occasions? Does the teacher give you a day's warning before an in-class birthday party? Have you made provisions for field trips? Ask about the different circumstances that might come up during the year; in certain instances, making and eating food may be part of learning about different cultures e.g. latkes.

The easier you make things for the teacher, the better off everyone will be. Suggest providing all of your child's snacks, including ones for special occasions. Ask whether you should bring in the snacks at the beginning of each month, week or day. It would be helpful for you to bring in a selection of snacks that is kept in a cupboard or drawer for your child to choose from at any time. It would be a bonus if your child could bring in fresh snacks i.e. fruit or baked goods every day or every once in a while. You may want to ask whether the teacher would allow you to use the school fridge, microwave or freezer, which would give you even more flexibility.

Teachers may feel apprehensive or stressed about doing things differently for your child. That's okay. It's better to be like that, than carefree. You are on the same team. You might say "I know that people may feel a little nervous with my child at the beginning but that won't last long. I'll ensure that you have everything you need to make things run smoothly and easily and I'll always be available when you need me." Let your child's teacher know how much you appreciate their efforts on your child's behalf.

Some teachers may have ideas as to foods that your child can eat that you did not put on the list of acceptable foods. It is great when a teacher can be this thoughtful; ensure you thank the teacher and then tell them that your child cannot eat anything that you have not read the label for and approved.

You will also need to place some of the responsibility on your child's shoulders for making sure that they do not eat problem foods at school. It is not all up to the teacher to make sure things run smoothly.

Elementary school

Once you get past pre-school, the way things are run become more streamlined, which makes life easier for you. The majority of schools have a no food sharing policy and children bring their own food to school. The only matter you may need to discuss with your child's teacher is what to do on specific food days i.e. pizza days or special occasions (i.e. birthdays, field trips). As soon as my children hit grade one, their teachers knew nothing of their reactions to foods. My girls would bring home any treats they were given and save them until "Treat Day" (Please see Chapter #6). Both girls opted out of pizza days, choosing to indulge on their "Treat Days" instead.

Off to sleepover camp

Having your child that eats differently than the majority go anywhere without you for a week or more is one of the greatest challenges you'll face. As a matter of fact, it can be one of the greatest challenges for families that *don't* have to contend with food issues!

Obviously, you cannot entertain sending your child to camp if your child:
- Is younger than 7 years old
- Reacts to a number of foods
- Has a very adverse reaction to any food, unless they are older

Camps, like most places in North America, are very familiar with coping with children who cannot eat everything on their regular menu. These days, it is common to find camps with dairy–free, vegetarian and other specialty menus. If your child reacts strongly to chemicals, assume that your child is not ready for camp yet. Chemicals are ingredients used in almost everything made in North American kitchens. If your child reacts to a category of food (i.e. dairy) or reacts to a few foods, you may want to follow these steps.

Step 1
Choose your child's camp wisely

Obviously, it is important to choose the appropriate camp beforehand, if possible. When seeking the camp that is most appropriate for your child, it is helpful to look for the following:
- Camp owners, managers or counselors that are very comfortable and familiar with feeding children differently
- Permission to speak to the camp cook within weeks of your child leaving for camp
- The ability to pack a cooler with your child's special food contained therein
- Nutritionists on staff
- Other health conscious families that have frequented the camp

Step 2

Acquire the camp menu plan

You may have the opportunity to meet the camp cook somewhere along the line, in the process of choosing your child's camp. If so, simply introduce yourself and ask if you might be able to call with questions before camp commences. A few weeks prior to your child's departure, call the cook and ask if the menu has been formulated for the time period that your child plans to be at camp. Then, kindly ask if they would mind faxing you the menu once it is ready. Also, ask the cook if they can make substitutions for certain items on the menu, where required. Yes, this is a case where you might need someone else to help your child remain safe. You will then need to ask the cook if you can call back once you've reviewed the menu.

Step 3

Fully understand the foods your child will be eating

Once you receive the menu, determine the obvious problematic foods for your child and check for situations where the problematic foods might be used as ingredients. If you are unsure of what ingredients might be used in certain foods, feel free to call a Nutritionist to assist you. Then, prepare a list (preferably written) of questions to ask the cook. You can only call the cook once with your queries, even twice is pushing it, so planning is paramount. Remember, the cook is talking to you out of courtesy only. He or she does not know you or your child, nor can you assume that the cook has much time or interest in chatting with you. The less you inconvenience the cook, the better their relationship will be with your child.

If your child reacts to dairy or you would like your child to avoid it since you know the harm it can cause, ask the cook what type of milk is used to mash the potatoes or make the pancakes. You may be surprised to learn that " a little bit of cow's milk" is used even in the dairy–free meals and that there are no dairy–free alternatives for the mashed potatoes or pancakes. Can you tell that I am speaking from personal experience? Unfortunately, I am.

Step 4

Teach your child how to make the menu plan work best for them

Once you are aware of all the ingredients in each food, you can teach your child which of the foods are problematic and what the alternative foods could be. For example, if your child is sensitive to dairy, write "dairy" beside the pancakes and the mashed potatoes. Then, record the foods that your child can substitute for the problematic foods, such as boiled potatoes.

If you are on side with the "Treat Day" concept, your child can look at the foods offered on each day and choose which day to eat everything that the other children are eating. Then, mark "Treat Day" on the appropriate day of the menu plan.

Your son or daughter can take the menu plan, which the two of you have gone over, to camp and refer to it as needed. Your child can also use the menu plan as a calendar and mark off the days at camp so that they will know when "parents' visitor day" or the "last day at camp" is.

Step 5

It's all well and good if you and your child create an excellent meal plan but if the appropriate adults don't know about it, the plan is useless. You will need to ask the camp owner or manager which employees of the camp need to be notified of the plan. Most likely, you will learn that the camp nurse, cook and your child's counselor are the ones that need to be informed. Do not assume that one of the employees will inform the others of your plan unless you're specifically told that this is the case.

Step 6

Once everyone knows what your child is going to eat while at camp, you may need to pack a cooler of safe or substitute foods for your child. If your child is not eating the pancakes, are you allowing them to have toast and jam, provided for by the camp or do you want to pack your dairy-free pancakes in the cooler? This decision is specific to each family's situation.

Obviously, planning and communication are key components in your child's camp experience. Trust is also important; trust in your child and trust in the camp employees. You need to be prepared for your plan to fall through. However, if your child has food sensitivities or non-severe allergies; there is room for mistakes. If mistakes occur, your child may be fine or may be sent home early. That is the worst that can happen.

Holidays and special occasions

Food is how we celebrate; food is how we commemorate. Unfortunately, holidays are notorious for causing problems: different foods, different schedules, all the excitement... the balanced diet is thrown off because of a higher intake of sweets. Also, during the holidays there is more exposure to colourings and preservatives, which are common allergens or irritants.

We all know how much children love treats, particularly when they are surrounded by them. Depending on how sensitive your child is, there may not be a lot of treats that your child can have. If this is the case, save certain foods for when they are really needed. In our household, chocolate bars, made of carob, malt, honey and coconut are a big favourite. These chocolate bars can *only* be eaten on very special occasions. There are no ifs ands or buts! At school, when the class is celebrating a birthday with cake, my daughter has her chocolate bar or her own piece of cake from home if I've had the time to make it!

I'm going to start by discussing birthday parties, as they seem to take place the most frequently. You may use the ideas and philosophy from this birthday section, in dealing with all other holidays and special occasions.

Birthdays
Your child is invited to a party

Your child receives an invitation to a birthday party. What do you do? Some parents may tell their child they cannot attend "because of the food". It is certainly your prerogative to make that call. Who needs the hassles, right? I would like to show you an easy approach to allowing your child the pleasure of attending a birthday party, without your child suffering repercussions.

1. When you call to RSVP for the party (not a separate call), tell the parent that your child is very excited to attend Timmy's party and that your child will be there. Then say, for example, "Taylor has food sensitivities, so I would like to provide her own food for the party. Do you know at this point what you'll be serving? I'd like to bring her version of what the other children are eating." Insist that you bring your own food. You do not want you or your child to be a hassle to anyone. People have enough on their plates without worrying about what to feed your child.

2. The other parent will tell you what they are serving or call you once they know. There is a healthy substitute for every "regular" meal served. Decide what you are going to bring for your child so that they feel they are eating something close to what the other children are eating. In my experience, this is what is usually served at birthday parties, with a list of their healthy equivalents:

– Hotdogs or Hamburgers	– Turkey, chicken, tofu or vegetable hotdogs or hamburgers on spelt, kamut or rice buns
– Chicken fingers	– Chicken/turkey dipped in egg/yogurt, covered in spelt/kamut crumbs
– Pizza	– Spelt/kamut/rice pizza crust with rice/goat/soy cheese and vegetables and spices
– Sandwiches	– Sandwiches (turkey, chicken, egg etc) maybe cut differently than usual
– Cake	– Cake (See recipes in Appendix)
– Cupcakes	– Cupcakes (See recipes in Appendix)
– Ice cream	– Ice cream (Soy Dream, Rice Dream etc)
– Popsicles/Freezies	– Popsicles (homemade) or freezies (Cool Fruits)
– Vegetable/fruit platter	– Vegetable/fruit platter (yeah!)

Packing some plain potato chips is also a good idea, if your child is okay with them, as flavoured chips are often served. You may want to keep some "safe" pre-cut cake or cupcakes in your freezer so you can grab some when needed, as opposed to making a cake or cupcakes for every party your child is invited to. Lastly, it would be a good idea to bring one of your child's treats or something new to try at the party.

3. When your child is young, you will, most certainly, accompany your child to birthday parties. My advice to you is to not say a word about your child eating differently unless asked! When the other children are eating chips or candy, give your child their own chips or safe treat. Once the other children are being served their main course, give your child their version of the main course. You may hear this and think, what will everyone else think? Will it be obvious how different my child is being treated? Not at all. Even if it's a small group of kids, I have found that the excitement in the air and the constant chatter amongst the kids and parents creates a rather chaotic atmosphere where a lot can go unnoticed. If someone does ask you what you are doing, simply answer, "My child reacts to certain foods" or "My child has food sensitivities" very matter of factly and do not elaborate while everyone, particularly your child, is listening. If a parent wants to question you about it further, ask that you take the conversation to another room so that your child doesn't hear. Some parents are such kind souls and quick thinkers that they actually will say to your child, upon seeing his or her food, "That looks so good and what you are eating is so healthy!" Bless those souls! When this happens to us, I make sure I thank those individuals, even if I just mouth the words to them over my child's head.

4. Lastly, parents must contend with the infamous loot bag. Many parents will prepare a loot bag for your child devoid of all food; based on the conversations you had with them prior to the party. If, however, they don't have time to think about that detail, your excited child may come running over to you at the end of the party, waving a wonderful looking package in your face, pleading, "Can I eat this candy?" You have three choices of answer:

A) "Yes"–that candy may be alright for your child to consume

B) "Let's talk about it in the car, okay?" In the car, you will need to remind your child how they will feel once the candy is eaten. Also, remind them of the treats already consumed at the party and the fun that was had.

C) "Yes–on treat day" (See Chapter #6) You will usually find that if your child knows they can eat the candy at some point, your child will be happy.

You might ask, "Why not ask the parent to make your child a special loot bag or one without candy?" and avoid this whole fiasco? If you do this, you'd be forgetting the cardinal rule. The only thing that you ask of others is that your child be allowed to eat their own food. That's it. It's that simple.

Your child is having a birthday party

1. Your child may have minor food sensitivities that cause only minor reper-cussions. If this is the case, you may be able to host a birthday party the same way everyone else does and know that it's only one day of treats; you'll just be careful over the next few days.
2. Your child may just have one sensitivity, (e.g. to dairy) in which case, all of the children can be served the same foods at your child's birthday party.
3. Your child has multiple food sensitivities or allergies. That is the subject of this section.

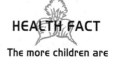

HEALTH FACT

The more children are surrounded by healthy foods, the better—for their bodies and their minds.

When you are hosting the party, my general rule of thumb is to serve "regular" foods to all the children, except yours and for your child to eat their version (See chart in last section) of those foods. You are probably shocked to hear this! You may be thinking, "my poor child". Here is the thing, if you serve everyone your child's foods, the other kids will undoubtedly say they do not like those foods, and we all know that chil-dren are not quiet about things they do not like! This results in one party causing a lot of harm to your child's overall existence. Your child likes their own food; it's what your child is accustomed to and it's healthy! You do not want your child's food marred by one event.

Okay, you are resigned to the fact that you are going to make your child's version of all the foods. Cupcakes are always a great idea to serve, because you can make your child's one way and the rest of the cupcakes the usual way. You would be surprised at how similiar you can make them look. You can also serve "make your own" ice cream sundaes and use soy, rice or even homemade ice cream for your child. Trust me when I say that the only way others will notice that your child is eating some-thing different than the rest of the children, is if you say that it's the case.

Now, the loot bags. Simply make up loot bags that have no candy inside. If you give out loot bags with candy, you are giving your child the message that candy is okay for others to eat. Occasionally, it is and what other parents do is their busi-ness. However, you need to pay attention to the message you are giving your child by putting candy in the other children's treat bags. You've already learned that having food sensitivities or allergies keeps your child healthy. The more children are surrounded by healthy foods, the better–for their bodies and their minds.

Halloween

For some, Halloween seems the hardest holiday to manage.

Every year when my children were young, a few weeks before Halloween, I would go shopping for new treats for my girls. This entailed going to a couple of health food stores as each store carries different items. I always bought treats I knew they were okay with, as well as something they hadn't had before. In later years, I added a bit more risk to the equation. I also purchased a few items that I was confident about but I ensured that there was only one new ingredient to test. For example, I bought a few treats with sugar in them. That way, my girls received new treats and if they reacted afterwards, I knew it was the sugar that was the problem. After carefully selecting the treats for my daughters, one or two nights before Halloween, I knocked on the neighbours' homes that we knew and asked them if they would give my treats to my daughters when they came to their door. Everyone was happy to help out. Most of them thought this was a great idea, realizing that my girls were being raised healthily, even on Halloween. Some neighbours were even good enough to add Halloween colouring books, fancy pencils or books to my girls' loot-bags! They knew that children have a lot of loves besides food!

Of course, as my girls became older, they wanted to go to more houses so each year, I began adding at least two houses to my list of ones that we visited. These were people that I'd seen around but did not know well. Again, when I explained to them that my girls had food sensitivities, they were happy to help out by giving my treats to the girls. The trouble was that they did not know which of the trick or treaters were my kids. So, I just made sure that I was the person taking the girls to those houses rather than my husband. They recognized me and knew to give the treats that I had delivered for my girls.

When Taylor was 4, she decided that 10 houses were not enough for her to visit. I needed a new plan, so this is what we did. After we'd gone to the 10 houses and she asked to go to more, we told her that she and her sister would need to use new trick or treat bags and that these next houses did not know about their food sensitivities. We told them that whatever treats they received would be for Dad. The girls were most excited to be able to get treats for Dad! Off they went and when they came home, they handed their bags to their father. He showed his excitement and thanked them for helping him out because dads aren't allowed to trick or treat, you know.

Some might say that knocking on doors ahead of time leaves a bit to chance—would everyone remember your child's special bag? What if someone adds something they think would be okay? In the five years that we did this, we never had a problem, but having a child with food sensitivities is different than having a child with severe food allergies. Some allergic children cannot even go near a pack-aged candy with peanuts inside. Therefore, trick or treating would not be an option for them.

You can also let your child bring home treats like everyone else and then hand them over to you. In return, you give them an identical bag back filled with treats that your child can eat.

Another idea is to let your child trade treats for trinkets or even something big that they have chosen ahead of time. One of my friends told me that the "Halloween fairy" visits her house every Halloween and removes the children's candy, replacing it with a gift. I tried this idea once my children were able to eat the candy and only experience minor symptoms, such as nightmares. Taylor was 8 and Paige was 5. They were thrilled to be able to eat candy on Halloween night and then have the Halloween or candy fairy visit the next night, leaving them toys I was sure they would adore. Don't forget that you will need to tell your child that you have made special arrangements with a candy fairy and that not all families have these arrangements!

In my mind, all siblings should be handled the same, whichever method you choose.

Halloween at school

For pre-schoolers, Halloween is easy. All you need to do is give them a cute costume, a pumpkin, and some easy craft projects and the whole occasion is a raving success.

For elementary students, Halloween can be even more fun. Never underestimate the power of stickers and other small gifts for children of this age. Halloween goody bags with orange and green play dough (for making pumpkins, witches and ghouls; of course), stickers, and little toys thrill the little ones. Be sure to tell your child that the treats others will be eating will be gone in a matter of minutes, but their special goody bag will last for weeks.

You can bake "healthy" cookies or cupcakes that your little one can bring into share with the class. Children are delighted by the way things look, almost more than the way they taste. You can add non-edible pumpkins made of orange icing to a dairy-free cake, use cookie cutters in Halloween shapes with your version of pudding inside or make chocolate dixies (See Appendix) filled with health food store candy. Halloween plates and napkins also add a special touch.

Christmas

Christmas celebrations are not as focused on treats as Halloween or Easter, but certainly food plays a large role at this time of year!

It is easy to cook turkey, squash, potatoes and other vegetables for your child's dinner, without using common allergens. Dessert can be "safe" ice cream, caramel popcorn balls, gingerbread cookies or homemade fudge, just to give you a few ideas. Using your child's "safe" ice cream, you can fill a gingerbread man cookie cutter with softened ice cream, decorate it however you choose and return it to the freezer. After at least an hour, run a knife around the edges of the mold, carefully lift it out and it is ready to be served.

Christmas stockings need only be filled with small gifts and maybe some Christmas tangerines; there is no need for them to contain sweets. If you did want to give your child some treats, there are candies like jelly beans and "worms" at the health food store that taste really good and are dairy, gluten and chemical free and made with fruit juice. Carob Santas and snowmen are also tasty treats.

The best advice I can give you for Christmas's busy season, is to prepare ahead of time! Cooking and freezing individual portions of your child's meals will come in very handy when you are invited to others' for dinner.

Easter

It can feel a little sad not to be able to fill a child's Easter basket with a chocolate bunny. Just remember, when your child is young, it only feels sad to you. Your child is happy to receive anything from the Easter bunny and it doesn't necessarily need to be food. You can fill Easter baskets with small toys from the dollar store or hide them for your child to find. The fun is in the hunt, not in the items found. Hiding pennies can even be a thrill for young children! Keep in mind that there are Easter bunnies made of maple syrup or carob if your child has a problem with chocolate, dairy or chemicals.

Travelling

Vacations require careful planning to ensure a pleasurable time. Whether your trip is long or short, travelling with food sensitivities or allergies requires pretty much the same degree of preparation. It's a lot of work.

Even with careful menu planning, the change in schedule, excitement of taking a trip and exposure to different foods can upset the balance for any child. Children or adults can become constipated just from taking a flight. Others can throw up from excitement, worry or from sheer exhaustion. If this is the case with your child, try to maintain a regular schedule for sleeping and eating. It is important that your child gets plenty of rest and avoids over-stimulation, as much as possible. If you are traveling, make certain your little one drinks plenty of filtered water. Airplanes and other air-conditioned places are dry environments.

Most children are happy with the simple food they enjoy at home and understand that the fun part of the trip will be the experience, not the treats. As parents, we want them to have it all, which means actively seeking out the places where our children can enjoy a "safe" meal.

The ideas in this next section will help you to travel with children that react to numerous foods.

Finding and contacting health food stores

You can begin this search by using the Internet and looking for health food stores in the area you will be traveling to, particularly within North America. You can also call the hotel where you will be staying and ask the concierge if they know of any health food stores within a short drive from your hotel.

Once you have the name and phone number of the closest health food store to your hotel, you may want to put together a wish list of the items you hope the store will carry so that when you call them, you remember what it is you need to ask. Health food stores are usually the safest places to ask questions pertaining to food. They are in the business of understanding food and selling health. If they do not carry the brand names you are used to, you may need to ask them a few questions about what they do carry that your child can eat. Of course, when you call across the miles, you will need to rely on luck that you will reach a helpful person that has time to remain on the line with you for a while. The best advice I can give you is to be extremely polite and even apologetic for calling. Then you might say, "My child has food sensitivities and we will be travelling to your area. I am very worried about what I will be able to feed her while I am there. Do you have time to answer some questions as to what you have in your store? Is there a better time for us to speak, because I can call back?" Whatever happens, if you end up talking to a rude employee or the store does not carry the items you require, you know you will need to bring those items yourself or do without. Some health food stores will be so helpful that they will even allow you to pre-order fresh bread and other groceries to ensure they are there when you arrive at the store. The less you have to pack the better. Whatever you purchase at your destination will always be fresher than what you could bring from home.

You will probably want to visit the store the day that you arrive at your destination or the day after, so that you do not need to worry for long about how you are going to feed your child while away. When you do visit the health food store, the employees are the best people to ask about restaurants in the area that serve health food.

Packing a cooler or thermos

Another way to prepare for a trip is to pack one of those large plastic rectangular coolers. Being able to take a cooler on your trip allows you to have control over the food your child is consuming. Coolers are especially helpful for camping or travelling by car or motor home. If you are flying within North America, you can usually check a cooler with your baggage. Be sure to call the airline that you'll be travelling with and find out for certain. I've packed "safe" cooked hamburgers, chicken nuggets, chicken drumsticks, thermoses filled with soup, pasta, lasagna, and casseroles. If your child loves hotdogs but can only eat certain brands, boil the dogs ahead of time and put the water and dogs in a thermos. They will stay hot and delicious for hours. Pack a bun and you're done. Don't forget to pack snacks, desserts and drinks, in addition to meals.

Traveling to foreign countries

I would strongly suggest emailing or calling Customs in the country to which you are traveling, in order to find out what restrictions they have on bringing in food. When we traveled to Cuba, we could not check a cooler. They also restrict what

foods can be brought into the country. They did not allow us to bring fruit, vegetables, milk or meat and all other foods had to be in their original packaging (so,
no homemade food).

When we went there, we brought the following with us:
- Cartons of rice or almond milk (they allow these milks),
- Packages of rice or spelt crackers
- Rice, kamut or spelt cakes
- Rice or granola bars
- Various dips such as hummus, tofu spread, pesto
- Loaves of bread
- Almond or other nut butter and jam
- Box of cereal
- Cans of beans or soup
- Baby food
- Snacks–plastic containers of apple sauce, nut or seed bars, fruit bars, veg-
  etable chips, "safe" suckers and chocolate bars, nuts, and cookies

Luckily, my girls can eat eggs and were able to have them for breakfast, cooked
in different ways, along with some fruit. Each lunch consisted of the foods that I
brought from home along with raw vegetables that were in the restaurants we
visited. Dinners were plain fish or poultry, rice and vegetables. I correctly assumed
that I would not find acceptable foods and I packed accordingly.

Booking Accommodations
You will need to choose accommodations that have a kitchenette or at the very
least, a fridge. A microwave would also be of benefit to those who use them.

Seeing friends
If you're travelling to visit friends or relatives, you could consider shipping some
favourite foods to their house before you arrive. This ensures you have what you
need and saves you the hassle of extra luggage.

Two rules of thumb when travelling with children with multiple food sensitivities
1. Avoid airline meals.
2. Avoid buffets.

You never know the ingredients or the freshness of what is being served and
there is unlikely anyone around that you could ask about the ingredients, not that
you would do so after reading my earlier advice on that subject!

Packing for the airplane

I suggest packing a meal for yourself, as well as your child, for the plane. This ensures that you both have healthy, fresh meals and that your child does not feel singled out, being the only person unable to have an airline meal. You can pack your child's lunch bag with a cold or hot pack. Then, pack the lunch bag in a knap-sack, along with a number of treats, books and activities for occupying your child during the flight. Assume there will be delays and pack more food than you think necessary. Lollipops (maple syrup) or homeopathic gum are a good idea for chil-dren to make taking off and landing easier on the ears.

Postponing a trip

You're all packed and ready to go and then, your child becomes sick. In fact, when you think about it, he or she didn't seem well over the past few weeks. I would suggest that before every trip, you take a long look at how healthy your child has been in the month prior to your vacation. If you decide to cancel, tell your child that you've postponed the trip, if that is the case. The idea is to not put undue emphasis on your child's health. You don't want a child to grow up thinking the world revolves around their health issues, although it would certainly seem as if our parental world does. A cheerful matter-of-fact approach is always best.

Your family's trip can be every bit as safe, exciting and memorable as other families'. Enjoy yourself!

How to make the best use of this chapter's information

1. If you read this whole chapter, you will know how to feed your child healthily, no matter where you are in the world.
2. You may choose to read just a few sections, in order to know how to feed your child differently in certain situations.

CHAPTER 9

HELP IS OUT THERE!

How Alternative Therapies Can Improve Your Child's Health

Conventional Medicine versus Complementary/ Alternative Medicine

There are four reasons we, as parents, seek outside professional health care for our children. Your child has:

- An injury
- Ongoing symptoms or a condition e.g. asthma
- Become sick recently
- Need of a checkup

Conventional medicine is the clear choice when it comes to broken bones, lacerations, organ failures and emergencies, but when it comes to immune system disorders and chronic illness, other experts are often needed. Medical doctors are not trained in nutrition or the link between food and symptoms, conditions or disease.

> "Over the past few years pediatricians have begun to see children with severe malnutrition as a result of ill-advised diets. This has caused great concern among the medical profession and led some doctors to mount what can only be described as a crusade against the whole idea of food intolerance as a commonplace illness."[1]

Doctors are afraid that parents will eliminate major food groups from their children's diets and not replace them with alternatives, thereby losing valuable nutrients. This is why they deny the existence of food sensitivities or intolerances.

Why do so many of us turn to doctors with every health question that we have? Nobody knows everything and doctors are no exception. Yet, the majority of people think doctors know all there is to know about health. We, as a society, gave them that power.

You may ask why doctors do not train themselves in the areas in which they are lacking knowledge. The physicians in Canada are so overworked and under-paid, is it any wonder that they don't spend a lot of time doing self–study? Also, the doctors that *do* become heavily involved in natural therapies risk losing their medical licenses! Dr. Josef Krop is a perfect example; you may be interested in reading about his court cases on the Internet.

HEALTH FACT

Doctors are afraid that parents will eliminate major food groups from their children's diets and not replace them with alternatives, thereby losing valuable nutrients.

There are some physicians that have achieved a nice balance between their medical advice and natural therapies, but those doctors' practices are often full. Other doctors who are fed up and frustrated with trying to get the medical establishment to take note of their findings, have written books covering all sorts of different health and nutrition topics. At least by writing these books, they give the public the chance to judge for themselves whether a given therapy is worth their while.

Dr. Rona's book *Childhood Illness and the Allergy Connection* points out that in Europe, complementary approaches are on the rise and often are integrated into conventional medical practices.

> He states that, "A recent study by the *British Medical Journal* revealed some staggering numbers:
> - In Belgium, eighty–four percent of all homeopathy and seventy-four percent of all acupuncture treatment is provided by conventional doctors.
> - The use of homeopathic remedies is growing by twenty percent each year in Great Britain and thirty percent each year in Greece and Portugal. "[2]

The trend is a positive one and gives us hope that there will be a synthesis of the medical and alternative systems in North America, to form a new system called Integrated Medicine. Both areas of health care need to know the relationship of the patient to their diet and environment if they plan to improve the health of mankind.

For the time being, the North American medical system is generally impersonal in its diagnosis and treatment of illness. Treatments are applied to all patients, more or less universally, sometimes without regard to their individuality. The system is primarily drug and surgery oriented and only treats symptoms rather than the underlying cause.

Typically, parents take their children to their family doctor first. Then, if the doctor is not able to help, they tell themselves not to worry about their children's symptoms. If the child's symptoms persist or become worse, that is often when a parent tries to see other doctors and possibly, eventually seek complementary care. In my mind, doctors should be the last resort for ongoing symptoms or health conditions–imagine how much our health care expenditures would decrease if the majority believed this! Invasive treatments and drugs can actually complicate your child's health problems further. That is not to say that a doctor shouldn't be part of your health care team.

Many parents who never considered alternative care prior to having children, have a hard time starting once children arrive. Many do not want to try treatments or remedies for their child if it's their first time experiencing a complementary practitioner! However, what do you do if your child is sick and your medial doctor doesn't have any solutions or if your child reacts to drugs? As I told you, my eldest daughter became constipated and in pain when I gave her Children's Tylenol, Triaminic or any other drugs. I needed to find a way to help ease her suffering without using drugs. This is when I learned all about natural remedies and cures.

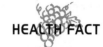

HEALTH FACT

Invasive treatments and drugs can actually complicate your child's health problems further.

Complementary or Alternative Health Care

"Alternative" and "complementary" mean the same thing. These words describe a type of care in which the patient is more actively involved in his or her own health care.

Hundreds of thousands of books have been written about the various disciplines available to you but my objective is simply to give you a quick overview of what some of the alternative professions are about and tell you, from a mother's point of view, how they *can* help your child.

Be careful who you see

It is important to know though, that not all complementary practitioners are the same, just as all family physicians differ. There are some complementary practitioners out there who are not as knowledgeable as others and, unfortunately, dealings with those practitioners get the most publicity.

Homeopaths are not regulated. There were a few homeopaths that I dealt with in order to help with Taylor's constipation. Their remedies did not work on her. After a few tries, I gave up on homeopaths. Then, when I was pregnant and overdue with my second child but not wanting to be induced, my labour coach recommended that I call a classical homeopath that she knew. She told me the homeopath could prescribe a remedy to bring on labour, if my body *and* baby were ready. Within 24 hours of taking the remedy that matched my personality and feelings at the time, I was holding my second daughter in my arms. As you can imagine, I had a whole new perspective on the powers of homeopaths. They cannot all be painted with the same brush.

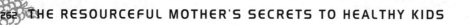

I strongly suggest that you see a practitioner who comes highly recommended to you and preferably, someone that works on a regular basis with children. If no one that you know can recommend anyone, your best bet is to call or visit a complementary clinic where there are a number of practitioners on staff who have chosen to work with one another due to each others' success rates or good reputations.

Important things to know about complementary practitioners

HEALTH FACT

I strongly suggest that you see a practitioner who comes highly recommended to you and preferably, someone that works on a regular basis with children.

Shorter amount of time in waiting room

Taking your child to numerous doctors and specialists and sitting in waiting rooms cannot be described as an uplifting experience, never mind the actual examination part. I have usually found the wait to be shorter at the offices of complementary practitioners. If there is a wait, it's often more pleasant because people trying to prevent poor health and fewer that have already contracted a sickness, often surround you.

Non-invasive

Examinations and treatments performed by complementary practitioners are usually non-invasive, which makes things particularly appealing for children.

Longer appointments because of holistic approach

You will find that your appointments with complementary practitioners will be significantly longer than at the doctors' offices because these experts examine your **whole child**, physically, mentally and emotionally by studying your child's diet, lifestyle, activity level, and environment. They recognize the link between all aspects of a human being in identifying and treating the **root cause** behind your child's symptoms. These experts then take the time to educate patients. This is why it is called a **holistic approach**. You will find that complementary practitioners help eliminate your child's symptoms but more importantly, build your child's immunity and improve their overall health.

Knowledge of sensitivities and allergies

Complementary practitioners acknowledge the role of food and chemicals in triggering chronic illness. Many use non-conventional forms of testing to determine which foods or chemicals are culprits for your child e.g. Elimination-provocation, IgG-RAST (Radio-Allergo-Sorbent-Tests), ELISA (Enzyme-Linked Immunosorbent Assay) tests, electro acupuncture, pulse testing, and others.

Interested in the root cause of illness

With the use of blood, urine, and hair tests, complementary therapists investigate and determine if your child has vitamin and mineral deficiencies, too much bad bacteria, a digestive enzyme inadequacy, absorption problems, leaky gut syndrome, candida, parasites and other conditions (See Chapter #3).

Unique and effective treatments

Complementary practitioners use treatments such as chemical and food avoidance, rotation diets, avoidance of drugs if possible, organic foods, detoxification programs, vitamins and mineral therapies, and herbal remedies. These practitioners acknowledge the fact that frequent use of antibiotics and vaccinations may have something to do with the immune system becoming impaired.

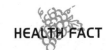

HEALTH FACT

Complementary practitioners help eliminate your child's symptoms but more importantly, build your child's immunity and improve their overall health.

> You have read a number of quotes from Dr. Zoltan Rona in this book. Dr. Rona is a medical doctor who also uses complementary medicine in his practice. He explained the difference between conventional and complementary treatment approaches by saying,
>
> "A good example of the different approaches of a conventional and complementary doctor can be found in the treatment of recurrent ear infections in children. The conventional treatment involves repetitive prescriptions for broad-spectrum antibiotics and, in the most resistive cases, the surgical implantation of plastic tubes into the middle ear to provide continuous drainage. Treatment depends entirely upon drugs and/or surgery–a simple matter of swallowing pills and/or lying anesthetized in the operation room. A natural health care practitioner, on the other hand, would advise the elimination of sugar, refined carbohydrates, milk, and other potential food allergy triggers or suppressors of the immune system. He or she may also recommend a friendly bacterial culture such as **lactobacillus acidophilus,** herbs (Echinacea, goldenseal, calendula, garlic, parsley, hypericum, and others), vitamins (A, B complex, and C), minerals (zinc, selenium), or other substances (colloidal silver, propolis). "[3]

It is also important to keep in mind that if your child is older and has a number of complications, many forms of alternative medicine could take some time in order to work. However, natural medicine is often **more effective and most definitely has fewer side effects** than prescription drugs. You may even see symptoms worsen for a short while before they get better; that can actually be a good sign. However, if your child is young and has only a few symptoms, natural treatment (usually involving dietary changes) can work extremely quickly. If you are working with classical homeopathy, an acute remedy should work really fast or it is not the right remedy! Maintaining your diary and recording the changes you see in your child while trying a complementary treatment, often proves to be extremely useful.

If your child has taken conventional medication on a long-term basis, ***a complementary practitioner should be able to prescribe a treatment that works in conjunction with your child's medication.*** This enables your child to gradually come to a point where they might not need to take as much or eventually eliminate the need for medication at all. Certainly, coming off long-term medication cold turkey is not advised.

Not approved of by the majority of mainstream health professionals

Complementary practitioners are usually opposed by medical associations, the pharmaceutical industry, licensing boards, the FDA, dieticians, insurance companies, and bureaucrats.

Imagine that you take your child to a complementary therapist and have great success. Maybe you want to share this terrific news with your doctor so that they may be able to help others. Be forewarned that most doctors will tell you that complementary therapies are not proven to be safe and effective in the same way that prescription drugs are. In actual fact, there are numerous studies that testify to the effectiveness of complementary methods. Unfortunately, these studies are small because the funding is not as great as it is with the drug companies. Even when the studies are published, they are often not read by or trusted by North American doctors. In addition, doctors have never been taught about these alternate methods, so why should they believe in them? Please do not take their rejection of your ideas or actions personally.

What should you do if everything your complementary practitioner prescribes or does for your child doesn't work? What if you or your child does not feel comfortable with the practitioner you have chosen; this could seriously hamper the success of your child's treatment. Please, try someone else! Do not give up on complementary therapies!

There are so many different complementary practitioners—how do you decide whom your child should see? Some will say that you only need to see one. That is not what my girls have taught me. Our children see a chiropractor, classical homeopath, cranial osteopath or cranial sacral therapist and a naturopath on an *as needed* basis. Don't forget, I am a nutritionist with reiki training, so we have those components, as well. I am going to tell you about these complementary practitioners, but there are many other kinds of complementary practitioners that I could mention. These are just the ones that my family visits.

You might be thinking, "There is just no way I'm taking my children to see all of those people!" and you may not have the need or even the interest. Please understand that I am not suggesting you see all of these practitioners! However, because of life circumstances, I have come to learn about the work of these practitioners and feel compelled to share our knowledge and experiences with you.

Nutritionists

Nutritionists go to school for up to two years. All they study is food and the body. It is a very intensive program yet at the end of it, they still don't know *all* there is to know about nutrition!

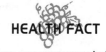

HEALTH FACT

There are numerous studies that testify to the effectiveness of complementary methods.

I believe that every parent should see a nutritionist, unless they have done a lot of research themselves on how to feed their family healthily. It is particularly important to see a nutritionist if you believe your child has an issue with food. I now know that the first person I should have taken Taylor to when she was in so much pain with constipation was a nutritionist. Unfortunately, like most people, I didn't know that we needed a nutritionist.

I thought our family was eating healthy foods. In fact, I was wrong. In addition, I learned that healthy foods for one person can be completely unhealthy for another.

The job of a nutritionist is to help you identify and eliminate any health issues that your child is experiencing by recognizing symptoms. If they believe your child needs further testing or help, nutritionists will recommend you to other complementary practitioners.

Nutritionists can help you detect food sensitivities or nutritional deficiencies and then assist you in devising a plan to change your child's diet. If they do not perform the testing themselves, they will refer you to someone who will. They also know about elimination diets and can help you implement an elimination diet, step-by-step, for your child.

If you determine the foods to which your child reacts and your findings include one of the major food groups, such as dairy and wheat, you might ask yourself, "What can I feed my child?" A nutritionist will teach you exactly what to feed your child, what the alternatives are and ensure that your child does not miss out on any important nutrients. They will even supply you with recipes and books to assist you, so that you do not need to do any of your own research if you don't want to! However, all things happen for a reason. If I had the help of a nutritionist, I wouldn't have done my own research and wouldn't be writing this book right now.

Again, in choosing a nutritionist, you will want to make an appointment with someone that has been recommended to you. One that has his or her own children would also be best, as children do have different interests, when it comes to food, than adults do. You may often find that nutritionists, who are also mothers, became nutritionists because of issues they were trying to get to the bottom of with their own children.

Why don't I recommend that you see a dietician? What is the difference between a nutritionist and a dietician? A dietician knows a lot about food and is linked with the medical field. They recommend dairy, along with other foods that have been proven to present problems for the majority of people. Dieticians also

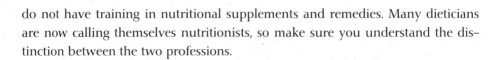

do not have training in nutritional supplements and remedies. Many dieticians are now calling themselves nutritionists, so make sure you understand the distinction between the two professions.

Naturopaths

Naturopaths are the family doctors of complementary medicine. They go to school for a minimum of 4 years, on top of their undergraduate education. Naturopathy or "natural medicine" was formally developed in the late nineteenth century, but it incorporates healing techniques that are far older. Naturopaths are knowledgeable in all areas of healing (and most have at least one area of particular expertise) such as clinical nutrition, homeopathy, acupuncture, herbal medicine, hydrotherapy, therapeutic touch, spinal and soft-tissue manipulation, physical therapies involving electric currents, ultrasound and light therapy, and lifestyle counselling. Their services are often covered under company benefit plans.

Naturopaths focus on underlying causes not on disease. Many perform hair, sweat, saliva, urine and blood testing in order to determine the areas of your child's body that are out of balance. Some have the capability to test every organ and give you an overall grading for each, so it is clear where the problems lie. Naturopaths work with diet, supplements and often, herbs and homeopathic preparations to boost children's immune systems and correct imbalances. They can determine which vitamins and minerals your child is lacking. They can even give you an indication of which supplements will work best with your child by testing the supplement for compatibility against your child.

I believe that children benefit from seeing a naturopath once a year, just like your annual doctor visit. If you have a child whose food sensitivities are not healing fast enough for your liking, through dietary changes alone, I would highly recommend that you take your child to a naturopath. A naturopath will help cleanse your child's body so that they can absorb the good nutrition you are trying to put into their body. When I was told Taylor needed cleansing, I remember thinking, "She's a child; how could she need cleansing or detoxing? I thought only adults needed to do this." I forgot about everything that she inherited from her parents that went into her genetic makeup!

HEALTH FACT

I believe that children benefit from seeing a naturopath once a year, just like your annual doctor visit.

Naturopaths often use UNDA drops for cleansing. Taylor went on one round of these drops and I notice a marked improvement in how she handled foods as a result. These '"healing drops" and others that naturopaths recommend are in alcohol-based solutions. Both my children reacted, over time, to the alcohol in these solutions (My naturopath explained this to me and commented on the degree of sensitivity in my children) so beware of that possibility. If this happens in your family, ask your naturopath for help in finding an alternative.

Manipulative healing therapies—Chiropractors

The modern-day chiropractic system and theory was founded in the United States in 1895. Today, chiropractors are better known and accepted than many of the other complementary therapists. They have only *started* to become widely accepted in caring for babies and children. When chiropractors work with children, they use a much more subtle and gentle technique than with adults because children's bones have not developed fully. When children of any age have chiropractic adjustments, all they feel is the gentle pressure of the chiropractor's hands or instrument on their vertebrae. When my girls were babies, they were often smiling or laughing throughout their five-minute treatments.

Chiropractic therapy emphasizes the connection between illness and maladjustments in the spine. It is useful in eliminating any symptom experienced in the body. Chiropractors believe that certain corrections relax the nervous system. The nervous system regulates all functions of the body. The theory behind it is that when vertebrae are even subtly out of place, a break in proper nerve impulse transmission results (i.e. subluxation). When a chiropractor realigns the vertebrae, using well-controlled and specific techniques, the nervous system is restored to a healthy state.

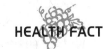

HEALTH FACT

When chiropractors work with children, they use a much more subtle and gentle technique than with adults because children's bones have not developed fully.

There are all different kinds of chiropractic care; the primary feature of all chiropractic treatment is the chiropractic adjustment. One type of adjustment is the manual adjustment where a joint is gently stretched to just beyond its normal range of motion and a "click" is heard. A child will notice that they have more movement in that area and any pain will quickly disappear. Some chiropractors use "non-force techniques", applying gentle touch along the spine, skull and pelvis. No clicking or popping sounds are heard with this technique. Other chiropractors use a hand held instrument called an Activator or Integrator that gently moves the vertebrae. Another type of chiropractor uses applied kinesiology, which helps balance opposing muscles, making adjustments more effective. "Network chiropractors" are newer to the chiropractic field. They combine a variety of chiropractic techniques depending on the subluxation particulars.

Chiropractors can turn babies around from a breech position. They help newborns, checking to make sure that no vertebrae misalignment or abnormal cranial moulding occurred while going through the birth canal. Chiropractic adjustments can even help in cases where babies have poor sucking capabilities and are not able to properly breastfeed.

Children having falls or even jumping on trampolines or into pools can end up with subluxations and need the help of a chiropractor. Any child experiencing a symptom, condition or disease can benefit from a chiropractor's care. Chiropractors can assist with colic, ear infections, eczema, chronic fatigue, headaches, muscle spasms, asthma and attention deficit disorder, just to name a few.

> "An experiment enrolled 81 children with asthma. After 2 months of chiropractic care, 90% showed a significantly improved quality of life."[4]

One time, Taylor was having troubles breathing. I had no idea why, but thought I would see if our chiropractor could help. It turns out Taylor had some subluxations in her neck and as soon as those were adjusted, she was able to breath normally again. As you know, our chiropractor was a tremendous help in eliminating Taylor's other symptoms i.e. gas, fussiness, colic and constipation. I still needed to address the root cause with food, but her symptoms were completely eliminated with each chiropractic visit.

Manipulative healing therapies—Cranial Osteopathy

One of the major sub-specialties of Osteopathic Manipulative Medicine is "Cranial Osteopathy." It was developed in the United States by William Sutherland, D.O. in the 1930's. All other cranial therapies, including "Cranio-sacral therapy", are derived from Cranial Osteopathy.

The goal of Osteopaths is to remove all restrictions to full body motion and circulation, thereby improving the functioning of the immune system. This hands-on healing therapy removes remnants of old physical and emotional traumas, restoring energy flow and balance in the body and motion to the bones. Osteopathy enhances alignment, overall well being and reduces pain. It creates faster recovery rates and keeps the nervous system working optimally.

Cranial Osteopathy and Cranial Sacral therapy are uniquely suited to treat problems related to the skull and brain, yet these therapies can heal any trauma or sickness in the body. Even an almost imperceptible alteration of the skull's natural configuration can lead to such disorders as colic, the inability of a baby to swallow, frequent spitting up or delayed development. Trauma affecting this mechanism in adults can lead to lower back problems, headaches, breathing difficulties, digestive disorders, joint pains, menstrual disorders and repetitive stress injuries. These therapies are extremely helpful in eliminating symptoms of food sensitivities or allergies, digestive challenges, migraines, spinal and joint difficulties, asthma, developmental delays and learning disorders.

HEALTH FACT

I recommend that every child see one of these experts shortly after birth because of the trauma experienced in the birth canal.

I recommend that every child see one of these experts shortly after birth because of the trauma experienced in the birth canal. Obviously, if your child's birth experience is particularly traumatizing or your child's head becomes misshapen in the process, all the more reason to see a cranial osteopath or cranial sacral therapist.

The great part about this therapy is that your child simply needs to lie on a table. Babies can even be breastfed, lying on the table, while the technique is applied to them. If you hear your child take some deep breaths or even fall asleep on the table, you know that the technique is working. This reminds me of all the babies who are not sleeping well and whose parents are past the point of exhaustion, caring for their little one. Take your child to a recommended cranial osteopath or cranial sacral therapist and see the difference in how much your child sleeps!

When Taylor was in so much pain with her constipation, a cranial osteopath helped her experience no pain until I could determine and eliminate the root cause. When Paige smashed her head on our glass coffee table and when my husband had a head concussion from playing hockey, it was one appointment with a cranial sacral therapist that helped them return to normal. When Paige had parasites from our trip to Mexico and began ripping out her hair, creating a large bald spot at her crown, it was cranial work that relieved her body of the stress it was experiencing.

Essentially, cranial osteopaths and cranial sacral therapists can help with everything that a chiropractor can. Certainly, if you are not getting the results you hoped for after seeing a recommended chiropractor a few times, then I recommend you see a cranial osteopath or cranial sacral therapist.

Healing therapies involving remedies—Homeopathy

Homeopathy is a European system based on the theory that like cures like. I have used homeopathy to help my daughters more often than any other complementary therapy. Homeopathic remedies are completely natural and safe. They also happen to be the least costly of all of the alternative disciplines.

In 400 BC Greece, Hippocrates mentioned homeopathy in his writings. By 1900, almost 25% of American physicians practiced homeopathy! Frustrated with the barbaric and ineffective treatments offered by orthodox medicine, doctors were using homeopathy as a safe, gentle and effective alternative. This diminished the use of mass produced and marketed drugs. As a result, the American Medical Association (AMA) was organized with the explicit purpose of eliminating the practice of homeopathy in the United States. It wasn't many years later that the bond between the AMA, allopathic physicians and the pharmaceutical industry was cemented. Homeopathy was not unique; it was merely the first in a long line of alternative health care methods the medical association singled out for elimination.

Almost a century later, homeopathy became a powerful force for healing individuals again. ***Homeopathy works by stimulating the body's own ability to heal itself***. There are over 3000 different homeopathic remedies (tiny white pellets, the size of a pierced earring hole, that taste good), all made from natural materials (plants, minerals and elements). Homeopathy helps the body heal itself more effectively and faster. It is particularly effective in children because their bodies are so clear and responsive. Remedies can help with any symptom, condition or disease involving the immune system. Homeopathic remedies contain no molecular structure, they are purely energy and therefore, they can be used safely, without the risk of side effects or interfering with prescription medications. This is what makes homeopathic remedies distinct from other forms of alternative medicine.

There are **acute remedies** available through homeopathy. For example, Aconite may be considered for a sudden illness or trauma such as an earache if symptoms coincide. Antibiotics may clear up an ear infection but the long-term effects of the drugs on your child's body are far reaching, as you now know. Sometimes antibiotics don't even clear up an ear infection, which means another trip to the doctor and waiting to see if the next antibiotic makes the difference. In the mean time, your child might be in pain or lose hearing. The acute homeopathic remedy that is right for your child's symptom is fast acting.

HEALTH FACT

What makes homeopathy so effective is that each remedy is chosen for the unique symptoms of each individual.

There are also **constitutional remedies**. For example, Lycopodium is based on symptoms unique to your child, taking personality into account. These remedies can eliminate imbalances in the body and mind (i.e. chronic ailments). Constitutional remedies are known for their long-term health benefits.

What makes homeopathy so effective is that each remedy is chosen for the unique symptoms of each individual. That's why two children with the same ailment or illness may receive a different remedy. When my first daughter had the chicken pox, she suffered terribly, one night in particular. The next day, I called our homeopath and asked for a remedy. After hearing all of Taylor's symptoms, the homeopath prescribed the acute remedy called Rhus Tox. Within hours of giving the remedy to Taylor, her pox scabbed over, the itchiness went away and she was on the mend. When my second daughter caught the chicken pox from Taylor, hearing her symptoms, our homeopath prescribed Sulphur. Paige experienced the same quick recovery as her big sister. I could give you countless examples of the fast acting healing power of homeopathic remedies.

Without the use of complementary therapy, children have to just suffer through the chicken pox. Some might say, "Well, what's wrong with that?" My belief is that there are enough challenges in the world that each individual is faced with, so why create unnecessary challenges? I believe our role as parents is to do whatever we can to eliminate our children's suffering.

Every member of our family of four has been on a constitutional homeopathic remedy. Taylor takes hers once a week. I took one about every three months. Everyone is different in terms of which constitutional remedy is needed and how often it is required. Taylor's remedy diminished her fears. My remedy relaxed me and helped me to see things more clearly. Paige's remedy helped her become less sensitive in general but particularly to foods.

Don't just take my word for it. Simply try giving your child a dose of the home-opathic remedy called Arnica the next time your child is in pain (e.g. bangs their head) and watch how quickly his pain is relieved. Every child can benefit from homeopathy.

> An article written for *Mothering Magazine*, described how a mother found that homeopathy healed her sons of anxiety and tics and twitches, and states, "Homeopathy's long and venerated history in the U.S. includes successful treatment of numerous epidemics of the 1800s, such as flu, cholera, typhoid and smallpox outbreaks."[5]

I felt it necessary to list some of the homeopathic remedies that I have found to make a huge difference in my children's lives. Some homeopaths may not appreciate the simplicity of this section. However, homeopathic remedies are being sold in the health aisle at the Superstore now for anyone to purchase. I think it makes sense that you know what some of these remedies do and then make use of them. Each remedy has two names i.e. Apis mellifica but I will refer to the most commonly used name of each remedy.

Acute Remedy	Ailment	Example of its use
Apis	Sting, bite or hives	Your child is stung by a bee or mosquito or is experiencing itchiness/redness/swelling/ hives from eating strawberries, cheese, shellfish or citrus foods or has reacted to penicillin.
Arnica	Pain	Your child is sore anywhere on their body.
Arsenicum	Food poisoning	Your child is throwing up/has stomach cramps/diarrhea.
Belladonna	Fever	Your child has an intense and high fever. There are other fever remedies if this one doesn't bring it down.
Chamomile	Needs calming	Your child is worked up i.e. colic/can't sleep/has a nightmare/is teething.
Pulsatilla	Dehydration	Your child has been sick and not drinking much and you want to replenish the fluid in their body quickly.
Coccolus	Nausea	Your child is having motion sickness in the car, plane, boat or train.
Euphrasia	Eye discomfort	Your child's eye/eyes are sore, red or pussing from food, pool water or infection.
Gelsenium	Flu	Your child feels sick, their limbs are sore, and they are thirstless and drowsy.
Hepar Sulph/ Spongia	Croup	Your child has a persistent barking cough.
Rhus Tox	Chicken pox	Your child has the chicken pox and/or is itchy. This is not the only remedy for the chicken pox but is the most well known.

Healing therapies involving remedies—Bach Flower

"Behind all disease lies our fears, our anxieties, our greed, our likes and dislikes," wrote English physician, Edward Bach, in the early 1930's. Today, numerous studies have confirmed Dr. Bach's theory. Dr. Bach then said, "Treat people for their emotional unhappiness, allow them to be happy, and they will become well".[6]

He began to investigate the healing potential of wildflowers, discovering that thirty-eight of them improved underlying psychological and emotional states that influence physical illness. Those thirty-eight Bach flower remedies form the basis of all flower remedies today.

These remedies are like homeopathic remedies in that they trigger the body's own healing process and move the body's healing in the direction it needs to go in order to reach homeostasis. The remedies are in the form of drops and can be placed under a child's tongue. I have not delved too much into this area but I wanted to make you aware of the fact that these remedies can do wonders in helping children and are readily available in most health food stores.

"Rescue Remedy" has been used for over 50 years and contains five of the flower remedies. It is absolutely incredible for calming a child in a crisis or acute situation. It will help your child manage physical trauma, fears, anxiety and bereavement. I encourage you to look further into its benefits and then add it to your first aid kit.

It is the relief from physical or emotional stress that these flower remedies provide that may enable a child to overcome reactions to foods.

Aromatherapy oils, extracted from plants, are similar in terms of their use and results.

Healing therapies involving touch—Massage

I believe that massage is the most widely known and accepted complementary therapy. There are many different types of massage. Infant massage is a very simple set of techniques that parents can perform on their own with their babies. I recommend that every parent attend an Infant Massage Class. Infant massage helps relax the nervous system, helping babies and children to sleep longer and deeper. Massage can relieve colic or gas, help stimulate digestion and circulation. Massage also helps to eliminate symptoms from food, remove toxins from the body, get the bowels moving, reduce pain (because it releases endorphins), and helps heal a physical injury. It also improves the immune system, overall. Do not forget that massage is also a great way to spend time with your child and bestow the powers of physical touch upon your son or daughter, when you might not be a "touchy feely" person.

Different oils are used in the massage process. Using flax oil to massage your child is a great way to help essential fatty acids be absorbed by his or her body.

Healing therapies involving touch—Reiki

Reiki, an ancient Japanese technique, is the simplest of all healing techniques. It involves the placing of hands on the body in order to channel healing energy. It allows anyone, including children, to tap into their unseen, yet infinite "life force energy" to promote healing and relaxation in the body. Life force energy is what keeps each of us alive.

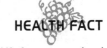

HEALTH FACT

Life force energy is what keeps each of us alive.

When I told my girlfriend about the pain Taylor was experiencing with her constipation, she suggested that I learn Reiki. After receiving the same advice from another person, I took a Level One class. Every time I put my hands on Taylor's tummy, she relaxed, which often resulted in her having a bowel movement within 24 hours of our five-minute "session"! I also noticed that she slept more soundly after the Reiki. It wasn't long before her overall well being noticeably improved.

Reflexology and therapeutic touch are other effective methods for helping children's bodies heal themselves and overcome reactions to foods.

Healing therapies involving touch—Polarity Therapy

This is an area of expertise that is not well known but is *most* responsible for my personal healing. I would be remiss if I did not extol its virtues. Polarity therapy is rooted in Indian sciences but was discovered by an Austrian born chiropractor and naturopath, Dr. Randolph Stone in the 1950s. It is based on the principal that symptoms are physical manifestations of patterns of energy. It works with the electromagnetic field and the five elements, being fire, earth, air, ether and water. This healing therapy believes that repressed emotions create an imbalance, which in turn affects digestive fire. When digestive fire is low, abnormal immune reactions (i.e. allergies) may occur. When digestive fire was put back into my body, my stomach began to growl! I had not heard that sound in years. Can you believe it? What a difference this work made to my ability to digest food. When a child continually needs to see a chiropractor, for example, polarity therapists believe that the underlying patterns of energy and thought are not being addressed. Polarity therapists address the blockages in energy or flow through hands–on healing, certain exercises and nutrition.

Holistic Allergists—Please don't skip reading this section just because you haven't heard of these people!

For those of you that want a quick fix, this may be the answer for you! Holistic allergists are trained at the Institute of Natural Health Technologies to perform Bioenergetic Intolerance Elimination (BIE). This organization does not believe that a leaky gut is the cause of allergies. It believes that the energy of food reacts with the energy of an individual's body. This new approach is based on traditional Chinese medicine. It won't replenish your child's body with good bacteria but it can take the stress off of the immune system. It can eliminate sensitivities and allergies simply, effectively and naturally. It is used on acupressure points and blends the principles of electro-acupuncture and homeopathy. Unlike the Nambudripad's Allergy Elimination Techniques, also known as NAET, this technique may have longer lasting results and is far less costly.

When Paige became allergic to dairy and began suffering from joint pain, I didn't feel it was right or healthy for her to experience such a reaction after being exposed to such small amounts of an allergen. Remember, that I believe in moderation, ("Treat Days") which means having dairy occasionally. So we tried the B.I.E. method and after the first treatment, Paige was able to eat ice cream without any repercussions. After the second treatment, she was fine with all dairy foods, with the exception of cheese. I worked on my problem with dairy and found no improvement after one treatment. I went back for a second one and learned that my issue with dairy was an emotional one. I won't get into how we tackled that one, but we did and after two treatments I am fine with small amounts of dairy, for the few times that I choose to consume the food. Others that have tried the technique, have eliminated their children's reactions to chicken, eggs, and nuts, to name a few.

The way it works is that a lightweight device transmits a low electronic frequency onto various acupressure points on the body to stimulate and clear any blockages in energy that an individual has with a specific food. At the same time that this device is being used, the substance that your child reacts to is in a glass vial lying on his or her stomach. While the blockages are clearing, the body's cells are literally being reprogrammed to recognize the samples' frequency so that the body will no longer react when exposed to a culprit food. The whole process takes about half an hour.

It takes around 1 to 4 sessions to clear the symptoms of a sensitivity and possibly, even an allergy. In each session, up to 5 problematic substances can be cleared at once. Success is dependant on the stress level, strength of the immune system, level of toxicity, and level of hydration of the individual. 80–85% of clients feel relief from their symptoms after the first appointment.

Clinical Ecology or Environmental Medicine

An organization was formed in 1965, called The Society of Clinical Ecology. A medical doctor named Dr. Theron G. Randolph was the pioneer and founder of this organization. Today, clinical ecologists are called environmental medicine specialists. Because of their work, many previously unrecognized allergy sufferers are being successfully diagnosed and treated. Much of the "new" knowledge concerning food allergies and sensitivities has been around for more than 50 years but it was not made available to the public!

There are two kinds of allergists–the traditional allergist who, in accordance with the antigen-antibody theory, links allergy to immunoglobin E or other immune-mediated conditions. If there is no measurable rise in IgE or other immunoglobin, there is no allergy. The other kind is the clinical ecologist, who uses a wider definition of allergy. They actually developed the concept of sensitivity (you'll see it differs from our use of the word), which encompasses allergies recognized by the traditional allergist *and* altered reactions to substances that cannot be explained by the antigen–antibody theory. Their primary focus in treating allergies is to eliminate or neutralize the cause of allergy.

Traditional allergists usually offer two types of treatment, allergen avoidance and immunotherapy (allergy shots), whereas clinical ecologists' treatments are much more comprehensive. For example, they will not just tell you to avoid feeding your child a given allergen; they will also help you implement a rotational diet so that your child does not develop any new food allergies. As well, they will check your child's digestive system, which may play a role in his or her allergies. They prescribe vitamins and minerals and a diet to bolster your child's immune system and help it function more effectively. They speak out about prescribing drugs other than in emergency situations.

The clinical ecologist recognizes that an allergic response can occur in any human organ, including the stomach and the brain. They use tests not performed by traditional allergists to pick up otherwise unidentified sensitivities. They do use Neutralization Therapy, which involves injecting children with the food, chemical or substance they have a problem with, an invasive process, in order to neutralize their reaction.

Environmental medicine specialists have done a huge amount of research on allergies and sensitivities and really should be commended for the number of people they have helped over the years. To keep the world informed of their research, clinical ecologists publish and contribute to The Archives of Clinical Ecology, a well-respected publication.

In Conclusion

Alternatives to traditional medicine are constantly appearing on the scene–chelation therapy, anti–candida and allergy-free diets and megavitamin therapy, and other alternatives to drugs and surgery. One would think that the medical establishment would look into these therapies, take what is valuable and leave what is not. Sadly, this is not always the case, although more and more doctors are beginning to open up to the idea of complementary health care. Those doctors are becoming aware that we, in the natural medicine world, are not going away. In fact, we are gaining in popular usage.

It is important that people begin to realize that they can learn to take care of themselves in many areas of health. Individuals can choose to make doctors their partners in the health care process, convincing them of the need for a new approach to chronic illness. For millions of people, this alternative approach to healing cannot come too soon.

Some people do not want the responsibility for taking care of themselves. They would rather have bypass surgery than cut down on red meat, dairy and sugar products or they would rather drink that extra coffee, smoke that cigarette, and let someone try to patch them up later. For these people, the symptom–suppressing approach of modern medicine is not only adequate, it is just what they want. Not everyone is like that, though. There are people willing to change in order to improve their quality of life. They just need the knowledge of how to do so. Many of us are trying to fulfill that need in our society and provide that access.

Hopefully, reading this material is only one of the steps you are taking in order to assume responsibility for maintaining your own health and that of your child.

"The doctor of the future will give no medicine but will interest his patients in the care of the human frame, in diet and in the cause and prevention of disease." Thomas Edison (1847–1931)[7]

How to make the best use of this chapter's information

1. The first priority is always to ensure your child is eating the foods that are right for his or her body. Then you will be giving your child the supplements discussed in Chapter #6. Simultaneously, you may want to be seeking alternative or complementary health care discussed in this chapter.

2. You may not feel it is important to see a nutritionist after having read this book, however, a nutritionist can provide you with a specific protocol for your child's unique health challenge(s). Also, sometimes people need to discuss ideas for improving health, as opposed to just reading about them. Besides, there is always more to learn about health.

3. If you would like your child tested, your child is sick or you are in more of a hurry to cleanse your child's body and return it to health, I would recommend seeing a naturopath. Don't forget to simultaneously improve the foods your child is eating.

4. I believe that every child can benefit from seeing a chiropractor simply from undergoing the process of being born. And then if your child has symptoms and your chiropractor is unable to address them, I suggest seeing a cranial osteopath.

5. The other sections of this chapter provide other options for helping your child remain the healthiest possible.

CHAPTER 10

THE FOOD-LOVE CONNECTION

When food is a form of nurturing

How to help your child be nurtured at mealtimes

Many of us, with our busy lifestyles, have forgotten that eating is much more than a physical process. Maybe we never even knew. The environment in which our food is grown, prepared, served and eaten affects our bodies, minds and spirits. If we eat consciously, we not only allow food to feed us, we allow food to nourish us. "Imagine if we could remember how it felt to be held in our mother's arms, close to the same familiar heartbeat we listened to in the womb, being nourished with warm milk, totally safe and supported. Not only are babies nourished by the milk they drink, they are also fed by their close contact with people. Ideally, every baby would experience this profound and total nourishment as her or his first engagement with the physical world. If you have ever nursed or fed a baby, then you know how incredible it is to watch the baby take in the nourishment of milk. The body completely relaxes and the baby falls into a deep sleep, smiling a celestial smile. All is right with the world. This the purest face of nourishment."[1]

Imagine feeding your five–year old child natural, alive, good quality foods today while holding them in your loving arms. As you visualize this scene, I know you can see how far many of us have strayed from allowing ourselves to be nourished by food. Let's try visualizing again:

"Dinner in my home begins with everyone in the kitchen. Since the time my children were very young, I've always engaged every family member in the preparation of our meals. From opening a can to washing potatoes, stirring a pot, taking out the compost, and setting the table, everyone is part of the meal. Sitting down at the table has always been a special time for our family. No matter what's going on in our lives, dinner is an opportunity to come together. We light a candle and hold hands. Either someone offers a blessing over the food, or we silently make our own individual blessings. And then we eat."[2]

There are simple ways to recreate this scene in your own home. Here are some ideas:

1. Involve the whole family in the preparation of a meal, at least some of the time. Wearing the aprons lovingly made by their grandmother seems to increase the enjoyment of my children working in the kitchen immensely! My girls thoroughly enjoy the tactile aspects of the kitchen. They cut vegetables, grind spices with a pestle and mortar, crack the pepper, stir the food while it cooks and then, set the table. My husband cleans the dishes that we use, brings and removes the food from the table. The cleaner and more orderly your kitchen, the more peaceful you will feel as you prepare the food.

2. When your family has a meal, make eating your only activity–avoid eating separately in different rooms of the house, in the car, or in front of the television. There is no need for young children to be distracted from eating with toys or playing games with their food; this interferes with your child's assimilation of food. When the main focus is food, the digestive system comes to understand this and knows just what to do.

3. Set your table attractively, with a nice tablecloth, cloth napkins, fresh flowers, and candles.

4. Encourage your family members to sit silently, relax and take a deep breath for a couple of moments before you begin eating. This allows everyone to quiet their minds and open their bodies and hearts to fully receive the food's nourishment. You see, there is another purpose for 'saying grace'. You or your child can select or write a blessing to say before each meal. You can thank the universe or God or all beings that helped provide your food, including the plants and animals, the farmers who grew it and perhaps, the person that prepared it for you.

5. Suggest to your family that they feed themselves slowly, chew well, taking the time to really tune into the smells, tastes and textures of their food and ensure you do the same!

6. This next idea is where your spouse or other adults present at the table will give you a hard time unless you have a word about it ahead of time! Teach your children to have an inner dialogue with themselves as they eat, telling themselves that this food is being transformed into life energy for their use. Encourage them to picture themselves becoming healthier and more beautiful as a result of eating the food before them. Help them create a mantra. They might say, "I am good to my body and my body is good to me."

7. Loving, positive conversation amongst family members goes a long way towards the enjoyment and digestion of a meal. If your dinner conversation starts heading in a negative direction, bring it back to the positive. When we eat, we are ingesting our thoughts and emotions, as well as our food.

8. Encourage your family members to stop eating when they notice that they are starting to feel full, yet still have some space in their tummies.

9. Take a few moments after you have all finished your meal to enjoy the warmth in your tummy and feel the satisfaction and contentment within.

10. Ensure your next meal is two to three hours away and that you maintain a regular routine with a balance between eating, activity and rest.

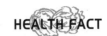

HEALTH FACT

The more often you and your family members tune into your food this way, the better your digestion will fare and the more good health and inner peace you will create for yourselves.

> *Creative Visualization* states, "Eating is really a magic ritual, an amazing process in which various forms of energy from the universe are transformed into the energy that forms our bodies. Whatever we are thinking or feeling at the time is part of the alchemy."[5]

The more often you and your family members tune into your food this way, the better your digestion will fare and the more good health and inner peace you will create for yourselves.

How to help your child be nurtured by food itself

There are names for the foods that nurture us: high life force, high vibration, vital essence, life enhancing, pranically charged, healing or natural, alive, good quality foods. I have talked about these foods throughout the book but not shared all of these other important names with you until now. The foods that energize our children's bodies and awaken their spirits to creativity and meaning are: organic, seasonal vegetables and fruit, whole grains, nuts and seeds, legumes, fish caught in the wild, organic chicken and eggs, hormone and antibiotic-free meat and dairy products, high quality olive oil, flax oil and filtered drinking water.

> *If the Buddha Came to Dinner* states, "The fundamental purpose of food is to provide us energy—energy for walking, talking, being creative, running in the park with our children, living our lives. This same energy is also used for digesting food. The more energy that's required for digestion, the less energy we have for living. We ordinarily expend a great deal of energy digesting foods that are difficult for our system—these include processed meats and foods that

are fried, refined, loaded with sugar, salt and chemicals. When people consume less of these foods and more vital essence foods that are easier to digest, they're always amazed by the increase in their vitality. Instead of all the energy they normally would have needed to just digest their food, that energy is freed up for other areas of their lives."[4]

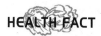

HEALTH FACT

Food harmonizes, stabilizes, and stimulates our mind, body and spirit.

Food harmonizes, stabilizes, and stimulates our mind, body and spirit. The main guideline for ascertaining if a food fuels your child in all of these ways is to contemplate the question: How does my child feel one to two hours after eating? If their energy is still strong, if they feel vibrant, focussed and emotionally balanced, then you know that particular food is good fuel for them. If your son or daughter feels lethargic, irritable, unable to focus, and craves more of that same food, then you know that that food depletes them. It is important to determine the foods that encourage the flow of life energy in your child and those that block the flow.

The mental and emotional effects of each food are actually astounding. Eating red meat can make us feel more aggressive, as opposed to eating almonds or dates, which create more loving and harmonious feelings. Even the way food is prepared impacts the food your child eats. Baking a potato for your child is so much more gentle and loving than frying a potato. Simple but amazing, isn't it?

Dr. Michael Lyon describes food as information in *Is Your Child's Brain Starving?*

He says, "Everyone knows that food is used by the body to make and to build and rebuild organs. However, it might come as a surprise that food is also an important source of information. It communicates life-giving messages to our cells.

Magnesium "communicates" to the blood vessels telling them to relax, lowering blood pressure. Bioflavonoids, plant chemicals found in fruits and vegetables, "instruct" brain cells to increase their production of neurotransmitters, improving brain function. Omega–3 fatty acids "converse" with our cells and encourage them to cool it with the inflammation!

There are thousands of examples of how natural, health–giving foods "speak" this amazing molecular language understood by our bodies. In a very real way, natural food is full of intelligence. In contrast, fast foods, junk foods, and over processed foods, can be considered unintelligent, and illiterate, because they lack important phytochemicals, fibre, vitamins and minerals. They lack the messages that the body depends upon."[5]

Ways to make your child's meals more interesting

If your food–reactive child is unable to eat the variety of foods or have as many "tasty" foods as other children, the way you display your child's food plays a large role. Believe it or not, the display and layout of a meal goes a long way towards any child's enjoyment of food. It can make your child's meal more appealing and it can give your son or daughter something to be excited about, even if it isn't the food itself. I used these techniques in particular when Taylor was only eating 19 foods. Just ensure that you don't use these ideas on a daily basis or your child will come to believe that every snack or meal should be served in an interesting way!

HEALTH FACT

Believe it or not, the display and layout of a meal goes a long way towards any child's enjoyment of food.

Here are some unique ideas to try:
- Use fancy plates, cups, utensils, straws, tablecloths, napkins, place mats and centerpieces, including candles. Lit candles can even go on non–birthday cupcakes or cake!
- Have your child's stuffed animals or dolls join them at a meal.
- Serve various foods on a platter, with or without dividers i.e. fruits and nuts or rice crackers, vegetables and dips.
- Put snacks into your child's snack or lunch bag with their favourite character on it.
- Pack soup, stews, hotdogs or drinks into a brightly coloured thermos.
- Package your child's snacks in patterned cellophane bags with ribbons for parties or special occasions.
- Picnics anywhere and everywhere are always a huge joy for children and they don't always need to be outside. (A plastic mat is very helpful if you are going to try this!)
- Eat in different places within the house. It's fun and takes the focus off the meal itself. Setting up a little table and chairs for our children with its own tablecloth made eating exciting for the girls for months.
- Make interesting shapes, animals, letters or people out of your child's food.

Ways to help your child appreciate food

There are other ways to help your child increase their appreciation of food, over and above the ideas we've discussed for mealtimes, the foods you choose and its attractive presentation.

They include:
- Planting, cultivating and eating the foods from a vegetable garden in your own backyard

- Teaching your child where food comes from by visiting farms or farmer's markets
- Discussing how meals are made, including different ingredients
- Planning meals together
- Grocery shopping together, letting your child choose some of your purchases
- Cooking and baking together
- Taking your children to real restaurants (not the restaurant chains) to discuss the menus together and eat real food

Our relationship to food mirrors our relationship to life

A happy life and a positive attitude are just as important as the food your child eats. If your child is not happy inside, he or she cannot derive nourishment and benefits from the food they eat. Do you ever notice that when you are upset or stressed, you either don't want to eat at all or you find yourself trapped in the void of emotional eating, consuming copious amounts of chocolate, chips or sugar? Children who are upset or stressed are no different. My littlest one, Paige, had troubles with a girl at school and starting eating only half her sandwich and no water at all. This was my cue to start asking questions. Lo and behold, once we got to the bottom of it, Paige started eating and drinking normally again.

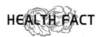

HEALTH FACT

A happy life and a positive attitude are just as important as the food your child eats.

Some children are scared to eat, have phobias, are surrounded by negativity or anger or are such picky eaters that there is no way that they are able to receive the necessary vitamins, minerals and pleasure from their food. In my practice, I have seen children fed intravenously as babies, who now subconsciously feel that they will be saved if they don't eat the right foods or enough. Do you pressure or cajole your child to eat food, creating a power struggle within your child and putting that guilt and control into your child's food? Or, do you simply need to spend more time honing your cooking skills so that your child enjoys your meals more?

When your child feels safe emotionally, he or she can allow food to provide the nourishment and love we all require. What I have learned in the decade that I have been raising and helping children heal is that it is easiest and best to address a child's physical health first. If you cannot make improvements or get to the bottom of the challenge your child is facing, then it's time to look into their emotional health. My experience has been that most of the emotional challenges children face can be overcome in time and often, using very simple methods. For example, if you decide to go full tilt and integrate every idea in this book into your lifestyle right away, you and your child's emotional well-being will suffer and it will be impossible for you or your child to flourish. Implement changes gradually, one step at a time and everyone reaps the rewards.

Our relationship to food mirrors our relationship to life. Every individual has a different way of processing life, as well as foods. The health of your child is actually more than the elimination of symptoms, conditions and disease. It is experiencing the inherent joy in life, having healthy and happy relationships and experiencing love each and every day. When your child is being nourished in these ways, in addition to the foods they are eating, watch your child's relationship to food thrive.

All parents are on a joint journey of learning and discovery with their children. We have our unique challenges to overcome but those challenges help us grow, as individuals. The goal is to be grateful for each and every one, even when you're in the midst of them.

"The body's natural inclination is for health, well-being and vitality and its natural wisdom is to perpetually strive for balance. It's a beautiful thing. All we have to learn to do is get out of the way!"[6]

How to make the best use of this chapter's information

This is the shortest chapter in the book and hopefully, because of that, you are able to read it in its entirety. If you understand the concepts in this chapter, and combine it with the information that you gleaned from the rest of the book, you will know in your heart, that you have all the information you need in order to feed your child with love and respect. For, feeding your child with love and respect is *your responsibility* as your child's parent. There is no greater accomplishment than raising a healthy and happy human being.

APPENDIX

Scrumptious Recipes

Initially, it might seem that your child does not have the variety of foods to choose from that other children have. Children eating differently from the majority certainly cannot go into any store or restaurant and eat whatever is on the shelves or the menu. However, there is a way to make children their own version of every single meal or dessert that others are eating. It simply means being creative and remaining open to alternatives such as coconut milk and flours such as spelt, kamut, amaranth, or arrowroot. Even a child who reacts to all of the common allergens can have their own versions of almost any food.

Trying new recipes

I, for one, have many interests other than cooking. Why I had two children that I need to cook for on a regular basis, is beyond me. Well, of course that is not true. I wouldn't have chosen to be a nutritionist if I didn't see why this happened to me! My children do, however, inspire me to keep finding new food ideas for them. I enjoy getting my children excited about new recipes, always letting them choose between a few options.

The recipes that we use are always simple because:
- They are easy for my girls to follow
- The food is ready faster
- My girls feel empowered after they have effortlessly followed a recipe and created a masterpiece
- We have more time to play together once we're done in the kitchen.

I find a marking system to be very helpful. I read through each of my new cookbooks as soon as I purchase them and use sticky notes to mark the recipes in the following manner:

Blue sticky notes–Recipes to try, where we usually have the ingredients on hand

Red sticky notes–Recipes to try, where we need to purchase the ingredients

Yellow sticky notes–Recipes to try, where we have the ingredients but want to test them on our children

Green sticky notes–Recipes that we've tried and love

As soon as a recipe is ready, we each try the new concoction. If my older child likes it, my younger will usually like it. If the older doesn't like it, the younger one won't either. The amount of copying that goes on still astounds me. I have tried letting the younger one taste the food first, stating her opinion before the older one even has a taste but eventually the younger one always figures out that her older sibling is not eating the food, so she stops eating it too. I wait to see if the girls like the food. If they do not like it and I do not like it either, I simply tell the girls, "This is horrible. Luckily we had fun making it though" and we laugh our heads off. No matter what, the preparation of a meal or baked good becomes a bonding experience.

Healthy Recipe Substitutions

1 cup white sugar	= ¾ cup maple syrup
	= ¾ cup molasses + ¼ tsp baking soda
	= 1 cup sucanat
	= 1 cup date sugar
	= ½ tsp stevia
	= ¾ cup brown rice syrup and a pinch of baking soda
	= ½ cup apple juice concentrate, rice or barley malt syrup
	= 2 mashed and blended bananas
Butter or margarine	= Equal amounts of sesame oil or cold-pressed, extra virgin olive oil or coconut oil (closest consistency to butter) or ghee (clarified butter)
Hydrogenated fats, lard, shortening and refined oils	= Equal amounts of cold pressed, expeller pressed and unrefined oils
1 cup cow's milk	= Equal amounts of almond, hemp, nut, soy, rice or coconut milk
1 cup sour cream	= 1 cup of sweet non-dairy milk + 1 Tbsp lemon juice or vinegar
	= 1 cup plain yogurt
	= ½ cup tofu and ½ cup yogurt, blended
Baking chocolate square	= 3 Tbsp carob powder + 2 Tbsp water heated in 1 ½ tsp oil
	= 3 Tbsp carob chips (milk-free)
Cocoa	= Powdered carob in equal amounts
Cornstarch	= Equal amounts of arrowroot flour, agar agar, or tapioca flour.
1 Tbsp. all purpose flour (thickener)	= 1 ½ tsp cornstarch
	= 1 ½ tsp arrowroot flour
	= 1 Tbsp tapioca flour
	= ½ Tbsp rice flour
	= 1 egg
1 cup white or whole wheat flour	= 1 cup spelt/kamut/amaranth flour
	= 1 1/3 cups ground rolled oats
	= 1 1/8 cups oat flour
	= 1 ¼ cups rye flour
	= 5/8 cup potato flour

	= ¾ cup potato starch
	= ¾ cup bean flour
	= 1 cup barley/millet/tapioca flour
	= 7/8 cup rice flour
	= ¾ cup corn meal/cornstarch
	= 7/8 cup buckwheat
	= Equal amounts of ground nuts or seeds
White rice	= Brown or wild rice, quinoa
Peanut butter	= Nut butters like sesame, almond, macademia, cashew, sunflower or pecan and Sunbutter
Salt	= Himalayan salt (other flavours are garlic, fine herbs), Spike, sea salt or herb seasonings
Vinegar	= Apple cider vinegar, brown rice vinegar, lemon or lime juice
1 tsp baking powder	= 1 tsp aluminium-free and corn-free baking powder
	= 1 tsp cream of tartar
	= 2 tsp arrowroot powder
1 tsp baking soda	= 1 tsp aluminium-free and corn-free baking soda
	= 1 tsp cream of tartar
	= 2 tsp arrowroot powder·
1 egg	= 1 Tbsp of ground flax seeds in 2 Tbsp water and leave to settle for a few minutes
	= ½ a mashed ripe banana
	= ¼ cup applesauce or pureed fruit
	= 1 Tbsp arrowroot powder mixed with 2 Tbsp water
	= Kingsmill Foods egg replacer
Luncheon meats	= Organic or nitrate free chicken or turkey sliced meat

Terrific Recipes for Children

The following recipes are extremely simple, healthy and yummy! If your child reacts to any of the foods listed in these recipes, remember to refer to the healthy substitution list for alternatives to flours, eggs, sweeteners or oil.

Breakfast Ideas
Flip-flapping Pancakes

1 cup	Spelt flour
¾ cup	Rice milk
1 Tbsp	Baking powder
¼ tsp	Sea salt
2	Eggs
½ cup	Blueberries, raspberries, apples, bananas (optional)
¼ cup	Olive oil
To taste	Maple syrup

- Blend wet ingredients, adding maple syrup for extra sweetness, if desired
- Add dry ingredients and blend until mixed
- Fry in pan using olive oil
- Spread pancakes with jam, agave syrup, maple syrup or carob chips

Note: Blueberries make purple pancakes and raspberries make pink pancakes.

Funky French Toast

To make batter, mix one ripe banana with 2 eggs and ¾ teaspoon cinnamon. Add some rice milk if too thick. Dip spelt bread or any alternative bread into batter and fry in cold pressed extra virgin olive oil.

Banana Mama Muffins

3	Bananas (approx 1 cup) mashed
¾ cup	Sucanat
1	Egg
1/3 cup	Olive oil
1 ½ cups	Spelt flour
1 tsp	Baking soda
1 tsp	Baking powder
½ tsp	Sea salt
½ cup	Chocolate or carob chips

- Preheat oven to 375 degrees F
- Mash bananas
- Add sucanat, egg and olive oil to bananas
- Mix the rest of dry ingredients together and add to moist ingredients
- Fold in chocolate chips
- Oil muffin tins with paper towel
- Bake in for 18–20 minutes

All Star Zucchini Muffins

3 cups	Zucchini, grated
3	Eggs, beaten
3 cups	Spelt or nut flour
1/3 cup	Coconut oil, melted
½ – 2/3 cups	Maple syrup
2 tsp	Cinnamon
1 tsp	Baking soda
½ tsp	Salt

- Preheat oven to 350 degrees F
- Mix flour, melted coconut oil, syrup and zucchini
- Add beaten eggs, cinnamon, salt and baking soda and mix well
- Bake in muffin tins, lined with papers for about 20 minutes or until done

Marvelous Muffins

1 ¼ cup	Almonds, finely ground
1 cup	Coconut, shredded
2 tsp	Baking powder
1 tsp	Almond extract
½ tsp	Cinnamon
½ tsp	Sea salt
½ cup	Fruit puree (see next recipe)
¾ cup	Maple syrup
½ tsp	Safflower oil

- Preheat oven to 350 degrees F
- In a mixing bowl, mix the dry ingredients with a whisk
- Add the wet ingredients and combine them well with the dry ingredients, using a spoon or spatula
- Allow the batter to rest for 30 minutes
- Line muffin tin with paper muffin baking cups
- Spoon the mixture into the baking cups, until they are each 2/3 full
- Bake for 25 or 30 minutes
- They can be served with jam or on their own
- Variations of this recipe can be used to make fruit bars or a cake

Fruit Puree

Fall/winter ingredients:

1 pear

1 apple

1 banana

½ cup rice milk

or

Spring/summer ingredients:

1 peach/2 apricots

1 plum

1 pear

1 banana

½ cup rice milk

- For either combination, put all ingredients in a blender and blend until smooth and the consistency of a milkshake
- Four or five pieces of fruit will yield enough puree for 2 batches of muffins, fruit bars or cake
- The puree will keep for 5 days in a tightly covered container in the fridge or you may want to treat yourself to this milkshake right away!

Oaty Granoly Bars

4 cups	Rolled oats
1 ½ cups	Assorted nuts and seeds, chopped
½ cup	Chopped fruit (dates, raisins, apricots)–optional
½ cup	Sucanat
1/3 cup	Maple syrup
½ cup	Brown rice syrup
½ cup	Coconut oil
2 tsp	Cinnamon

- Preheat oven to 325 degrees F
- Grease a cookie sheet or place parchment paper on it
- Combine oats, nuts, seeds and/or fruit in a bowl
- Melt the coconut oil in a saucepan
- Add the sweeteners, stirring until blended
- Stir the wet mixture into the dry mixture and combine thoroughly
- Press into prepared pan and bake for 20–25 minutes until browned
- Let cool completely before removing from pan and cutting into squares or bars

Nutty Banana Bread

3 cups	Nut flour (almond)
3	Eggs, beaten
¼ cup	Coconut oil, melted
½ cup	Maple syrup
1 tsp	Baking soda
2	Extra ripe bananas, mashed

- Preheat oven to 350 degrees F
- Mix all ingredients
- Pour into a greased baking pan and bake for 30–35 minutes

Treat Ideas

Crunchy Chocolate Chippers

2 1/3 cup	Spelt flour
½ tsp	Baking soda
¾ – 1 ¼ cup	Apple juice concentrate, depending on the degree of sweetness desired or simply add maple syrup (to taste)
½ cup	Olive oil
¾ cup	Dark chocolate chips or milk–free carob chips (optional)

- Preheat oven to 350 degrees F
- If you like your cookies fairly sweet, boil 1 ¼ cup apple juice concentrate down to ¾ cup in volume and allow it to cool
- For minimally sweetened cookies, use ¾ cup apple juice concentrate
- Stir together the flour and baking soda in a large bowl
- Mix the oil and apple juice concentrate and stir them into the flour mixture until they are just mixed in
- Fold in the carob or chocolate chips
- Drop the dough by heaping teaspoons onto a lightly oiled baking sheet
- Bake them for 10–14 minutes or until they begin to brown

Must Eat Carrot Cake

2	Eggs, beaten
½ cup	Olive oil
½ cup	Maple syrup
½ tsp	Cinnamon
1-1/4 cup	Carrots, grated
1-1/4 cup	Spelt flour
2 tsp	Baking powder

- Preheat oven to 350 degrees F
- Grease and flour a 9 X 13 baking pan
- In large bowl, mix ingredients in the above order
- Bake 25–30 minutes

Huggable Honey Cake

1	Egg
3 Tbsp	Olive oil
¾ cup	Honey
½ cup	Rice milk
1 ½ cup	Spelt flour
½ tsp	Baking soda

- Preheat oven to 325 degrees F
- Grease or flour a loaf pan
- In a large bowl, mix ingredients in the above order
- Bake for 45 minutes until loaf begins to pull away from sides of pan
- This recipe could also be used to make a dozen cupcakes that are ready in 20 minutes

Clap Your Hands Carob Cake

1 cup	Amaranth flour
½ cup	Arrowroot flour
¼ cup	Carob or cocoa powder
1 tsp	Baking soda
2/3 cup	Warm water
1/3 cup	Olive oil
1/3 cup	Maple syrup
1 Tbsp	Lemon juice
1 tsp	Vanilla extract

- Preheat oven to 350 degrees F
- Mix the flours, carob and baking soda in a large bowl
- Whisk together the water, oil, maple syrup, lemon juice and vanilla in a small bowl
- Pour wet ingredients into the bowl containing the dry ingredients and mix quickly
- Pour mixture into a well greased square baking pan
- Bake for 30 minutes until some cracks appear on top and the inside is moist. Do not over bake
- To make brownies, reduce the water to ¼ cup so that the batter is thick. Spread thinly in a rectangular baking pan and bake at same temperature for 20–25 minutes. Again make sure you don't over bake. Brownies should remain moist inside.

Awesome Icing

½ cup	Water
1 cup	Raw tahini
4 Tbsp	Maple syrup
3 Tbsp	Raw carob powder
1 tsp	Vanilla

- Use a blender to mix all ingredients, ensuring you put the water in first
- Spread the icing evenly over a cake or cupcakes or use a decorating bag
- Decorate with fruits, berries and nuts
- Chill

Try combining some of this icing with frozen bananas for a great tasting ice cream.

Delectable Carob Fudge

1 ¼ cups	Maple syrup or fruit concentrate
1 cup	Sesame tahini or nut butter (can use ½ cup of each)
1 ¼ cups	Carob powder
1 cup	Sesame seeds or shredded coconut
8–14 drops	Peppermint extract
2 Tbsp	Arrowroot powder
2 tsp	Vanilla extract

- Heat the nut butter and liquid sweetening on low to medium heat until hot and soft
- Remove from heat and stir in remaining ingredients
- Press the mixture into a lightly oiled 9 or 10 inch glass pie plate or similar pan
- Press extra sesame seeds or coconut on top
- Chill thoroughly in fridge
- Cut and serve
- Keeps up to 3 months refrigerated

Sticky Caramel Popcorn

4 cups	Popped popcorn
2 Tbsp	Coconut oil
1 ½ tsp	Vanilla extract
2–3 Tbsp	Maple syrup
1 Tbsp	Molasses
1 Tbsp	Cinnamon

- In a saucepan over low heat stir together coconut oil, vanilla, syrup and molasses until completely melted
- Add cinnamon
- Pour mixture over popcorn, tossing to cover kernels

So Tasty Carob Almond Spread

1 cup	Almond butter
½ cup	Carob powder
½ cup	Mashed banana
2 tsp	Vanilla

- Mix together and put in refrigerator
- You could use this spread on crackers or bread
- You could shape it into balls, roll them in cinnamon and press a walnut half on top of each ball to make a kind of candy

Golden Gingerbread Cookies

3 cups	Spelt flour
¾ tsp	Baking Soda
¼ tsp	Lemon juice
½ tsp	Ginger
¼ tsp	Nutmeg
¾ cup	Molasses
½ cup	Olive oil

- Preheat oven to 350 degrees F
- Combine the spelt flour, baking soda, lemon and spices in a large bowl
- Stir together the molasses and oil and mix them into the dry ingredients to make a stiff dough
- Roll the dough out on a floured board
- Cut the dough into gingerbread men and women and transfer them to an ungreased baking sheet using a spatula
- Bake them for 10–15 minutes

Humble Hemp Cookies

2/3 cup	Sucanat
1	Egg, beaten
½ cup	Melted coconut oil, cooled
½ cup	Spelt flour
1 tsp	Cinnamon
1 cup	Hemp seeds

- Preheat oven to 350 degrees F
- Blend the top three ingredients together
- Mix in the spelt flour
- Gradually add cinnamon and hemp to oil mixture
- Bake for 7 minutes

No-No Bake Cookies

10	Dried dates, chopped
10	Pitted prunes, chopped
½ cup	Walnuts, chopped
2 Tbsp	Apple juice
1 Tbsp	Ground cinnamon

- Mix the dates, prunes and walnuts
- Stir in the apple juice and cinnamon
- Shape into balls

Crazy Cranberry Baked Apples

4	Apples (peaches can be substituted as well)
2 Tbsp	Cranberries, dried
¼ cup	Pecans
½ tsp	Cinnamon
¼ cup	Oats

- Preheat oven to 400 degrees F
- Wash apples and chop them into large pieces
- Mix apple with remaining ingredients in a casserole dish
- Bake for a minimum of 20 minutes or until apples are soft

Meringue Kisses

2	Egg whites
1 cup	Maple syrup
1 cup	Grated coconut or chopped nuts

- Preheat oven to 250 degrees F
- Beat egg whites until stiff and dry
- Slowly add syrup and coconut or nuts
- Drop by spoonfuls into paper cupcake holders
- Bake for 1 hour

Chocolate Bottom Cups

2 cups	Dark chocolate or carob chips
2 Tbsp	Olive oil

Pudding or ice cream (rice, soy or hemp)

- Fill a cupcake tin with paper cupcake baking cups
- Melt carob chips and oil together in a pan on low heat
- Stir until blended and smooth
- Put a heaping spoonful of chocolate or carob mixture in the centre of each baking cup
- Using a small spatula, spread the chocolate or carob so it completely coats the bottom and sides of the cup
- Put the whole cupcake tin in the fridge and chill for at least 30 minutes
- When the chocolate or carob cups feel firm, carefully peel off the paper baking cups
- Fill your chocolate or carob cups with pudding or ice cream and top with a cherry or berry

Quick As A Bunny Crisp

1 can (12 oz)	Sliced peaches/apples/pears
3 Tbsp	Tapioca flour
1 Tbsp	Olive oil
1 tsp	Barley malt sweetener or 3 Tbsp raw sugar
2 Tbsp	Quick cooking oats
½ tsp	Cinnamon

Dash of nutmeg and ginger

- Preheat oven to 350 degrees F
- Pour peaches into a small baking dish
- Top with rest of ingredients, except for the oil, and mix well
- Brush top with oil
- Bake for 30 minutes

Doublicious Chocolate Pudding

1 ½ cups	Enriched rice milk or almond milk
3 Tbsp	Tapioca flour
¼ cup	Cocoa or carob powder
¼ cup	Maple syrup
¼ tsp	Vanilla extract

- Whisk all ingredients in a pot over medium heat, stirring occasionally until pudding thickens.

Healthy Rice Crispy Squares

3 cups	Puffed spelt, kamut, millet or corn
½ cup	Almond butter
¼ cup	Honey
¼ cup	Olive oil

- Melt all wet ingredients together in a pan
- Mix in the puffed grain
- Stir well until grain is coated
- Place in 6x6 inch pan and refrigerate

Drink Ideas

Healthy Coke

1 ½ Tbsp	Maple syrup
2 cups	Seltzer, club soda or sparkling water

Ice

- Pour maple syrup into a cup
- Fill the remainder of the cup with carbonated liquid of choice
- Add ice and stir
- A straw makes it even more fun!
- You can make any flavour of pop (cranberry, apple, grape) in this way

Ginger Ale

4 cups	Seltzer, club soda or sparkling water
¾ cup	Ginger root, peeled and chopped
2 Tbsp	Pure vanilla extract
1/4 tsp	Stevia powder

- Mix all ingredients together and add crushed ice if desired.

Hot Chocolate or Carob

4 cups	Rice or almond milk
1 Tbsp	Maple syrup
½ tsp	Vanilla extract
3 Tbsp	Cocoa or carob powder

- Blend ingredients until smooth. Heat if desired but do not boil.

Fruit Smoothie

¼ cup	Rice/goat/almond/hemp milk
1 tsp	Flax oil
1	Banana
A handful	Berries, peaches, mango etc.

- Mix all ingredients together in a blender. Then taste and make adjustments as needed.

Shrek Shake (Green drink)

2 cups	Rice/goat/almond/hemp milk
1 cup	Filtered water
1 tsp	Spirulina powder
½	Banana
½	Avocado
12 approx	Spinach leaves
2 inches	Cucumber
6 approx	Ice cubes

- Mix all ingredients in a blender, then taste and make adjustments
- You can substitute the green vegetables for any other green vegetables, adding more milk or banana for additional sweetness

Meal Ideas
MEAT RECIPES
Bake or poach chicken, turkey or fish.

You could add any combination of the following for more flavour: lemon, honey, mustard, olive oil, tomato or tamari sauce.

Healthy Shake n' Bake

Kamut or spelt bread crumbs or
Finely ground almonds and flour (2:1) mixture
Egg or yogurt
Chicken, Turkey or Fish
Olive oil

- Rinse and dry meat and cut into thin strips
- Crack open an egg or two into a bowl or fill a bowl with yogurt
- Coat meat in egg or yogurt
- Put bread crumbs into a bag
- Add a few pieces of meat at a time, shaking them in the bag so that they are completely coated in bread crumbs
- Put coated meat into a skillet or bake meat until cooked through

Salmon Bits

1 tsp	Sesame oil
1 tsp	Olive oil
1	Garlic clove, finely chopped
500g/1lb	Salmon fillet, boneless and skinless, cut into small pieces
1 Tbsp	Tamari
4 Tbsp	Filtered water

- Heat the oils with the garlic in a medium frying pan over medium heat until the garlic begins to turn translucent, about 2 minutes
- Add the salmon, stir, then add the remaining ingredients
- Stir until the salmon is cooked through and the liquids have evaporated by half, 4–6 minutes

Tangy Tuna Casserole

4 cans	Raincoast Trading Company tuna
4 Tbsp	Spectrum organic canola mayonnaise
4 Tbsp	Spelt breadcrumbs
1 stalk	Celery, thinly sliced
1	Red pepper, chopped
½ cup	Goat cheese, grated (optional)
To taste	Salt and Pepper

- Preheat oven to 400 degrees F
- Mix tuna and mayonnaise together until smooth
- Add vegetables
- Layer bottom of casserole dish with half of the mixture
- Sprinkle half of the breadcrumbs and cheese on top of the mixture
- Add the rest of the mixture, sprinkling the rest of the breadcrumbs and cheese on top
- Put the lid on top of the casserole and put in the oven for 15 minutes or until it is lightly browned

Chock Full O' Chicken Noodle Soup

4 cups	Chicken broth (Imagine or Pacific brand in 1 litre container)
2/3 cup	Shredded and cooked chicken breast
One	Handful of cooked rice or spelt pasta
1	Diced carrot
1	Diced green onion
1 Tbsp	Thyme, fresh (1 tsp dried)
To taste	Salt and pepper

- Cook chicken and rice or pasta separately.
- Add carrot, onion, broth and thyme to a medium pot of water and bring to a boil
- Mix all ingredients together and simmer for 10 minutes.

Satisfying Shepherd's Pie

2 tsp	Olive oil
1 cup	Ground chicken or turkey
½ cup	Carrots, thinly sliced
1 cup	Tomatoes, diced
1 ½ cup	Celery, diced
1 cup	Corn
1	Onion, chopped
1 ½ Tbsp	Thyme, fresh, chopped
½ cube	Chicken or vegetable stock cube, dissolved in water
8–10	Medium potatoes, red
¼ cup	Rice or almond milk
¼ tsp	Paprika
To taste	Pepper and garlic salt

- Chop potatoes and boil until tender
- Heat oil in non–stick fry pan, add ground poultry and stir–fry for 5 minutes or until browned
- Stir in carrots, tomato, celery, onion, tomatoes, thyme and stock
- Reduce heat, cover and cook, stirring often for 15 minutes
- Drain potatoes and place in a bowl with milk, pepper and garlic salt and mash until smooth
- Place turkey or chicken mixture into a casserole dish and arrange mashed potato over mixture
- Broil for 2 to 3 minutes or until the pie is golden brown
- Sprinkle with paprika and serve

Soy Recipe

Maple Tofu Fingers

1 block	Firm or extra firm tofu (La Soyaire)
½ cup	Tamari sauce
3 Tbsp	Maple syrup
1 Tbsp	Fresh ginger
½ cup	Spelt bread crumbs
1 tsp	Olive oil

- Preheat oven to 350 degrees F
- Mix tamari, syrup and ginger in saucepan and heat thoroughly
- Slice tofu lengthways about ¼ inch thick
- Dip each piece of tofu into sauce, coating it well
- Cover each piece of tofu in bread crumbs
- Grease baking tray with oil and place tofu on it in a single layer
- Bake for 20 to 30 minutes depending on how crispy you like it

Legume Recipes

Scrumptious Bean Spread

1 cup	Chickpeas
1 cup	Black beans
1 stalk	Celery, minced fine
1	Green onion, minced fine
2 Tbsp	Fresh squeezed lemon juice
3 tsp	Parsley, fresh, minced fine
2 tsp	Tamari (soy) sauce
¼ cup	Ground roasted sunflower or sesame seeds

- Toast the seeds by stirring in a skillet over medium heat until they smell and taste nutty. Do not over-brown.
- Grind the seeds in a blender
- Mash beans
- Mix all ingredients together
- Spread on rice cakes or crackers or pita bread

Homerun Chickpea Balls

12 oz	Cooked chickpeas
1 tsp	Curry powder
1 tsp	Mustard, prepared or dijon
1	Egg

Olive oil

- Place the chickpeas in a blender or food processor and blend until they are finely ground
- Add the remaining ingredients and blend until everything is thoroughly mixed
- Heat the oil in a medium, heavy-bottomed saucepan or wok over medium-high heat until it is hot
- Form marble-sized balls with the chickpea mixture
- Fry them in small batches until they are golden, 3–4 minutes
- Transfer to a plate lined with paper towels to drain

Yummy Burgers

2 tsp	Olive oil
3	Green onions, chopped
2 cloves	Garlic, minced
1 tsp each	Oregano and chili powder
1 cup	Red pepper, sliced
½	Tomato, chopped
1 can (19 oz)	Chickpeas, drained and rinsed
1/3 cup	Spelt or kamut bread crumbs
2 Tbsp	Fresh cilantro or parsley, chopped

Salt and pepper to taste

- In a non-stick skillet, heat 1 tsp of the oil over medium heat and cook onions, garlic, oregano, and chili powder, stirring for 2 minutes
- Add red pepper and tomato
- Cook, stirring for about 3 minutes or until pepper is tender and liquid is evaporated
- In food processor, mix pepper mixture with chickpeas and transfer to bowl
- Stir in breadcrumbs, parsley and salt and pepper to taste until well combined
- Shape into 4 burgers
- In non-stick skillet, heat remaining oil over medium heat
- Cook burgers for 4 minutes on each side or until heated through

Vege Chili

1¼ cups	Onions, chopped
1 cup each	Red and green pepper, chopped
¾ cup each	Celery and carrots, chopped
3 cloves	Garlic, minced
1 can (28 oz)	Tomatoes, undrained, cut up
1 can (19 oz)	Black beans, drained and rinsed
1 can (19 oz)	Chickpeas, drained and rinsed
1 can (12 oz)	Kernel corn
1 Tbsp	Ground cumin
1½ tsp each	Dried oregano and basil
½ tsp	Cayenne pepper (adjust to taste)

- Spray a large saucepan with non-stick spray
- Add onions, peppers, celery, carrots, and garlic
- Cook over medium heat, stirring often, until vegetables are softened (about 6 minutes)
- Add tomatoes, beans, chickpeas, corn, cumin, oregano, basil and cayenne pepper and stir well
- Bring to a boil. Reduce heat to medium-low. Cover and simmer for 20 minutes, stirring occasionally
- You can always add ground chicken to this recipe

Grain Dishes
Vege Filled Lasagne

One box	Spelt or kamut lasagne noodles (12)
12	Mushrooms, sliced
3	Peppers (red and green)
2	Garlic cloves, pressed
1½	Zucchini, sliced
1	Onion, chopped
1	Block of goat's cheese (cheddar/mozzarella), grated
½	Carrot
½	Celery
1	Large preserve jar of tomato sauce (~ 24 oz)
1 Tbsp	Olive oil

Salt and pepper to taste

- Preheat oven to 320 degrees F
- Boil lasagne noodles al dente and rinse
- Stir fry vegetables with olive oil and salt and pepper
- Pour thin layer of tomato sauce into bottom of large casserole dish
- Add a little olive oil on top of tomato sauce
- Put one layer of noodles on top of sauce
- Completely cover layer of noodles with strained vegetable stir fry
- Add a layer of goat cheese
- Add three more layers of tomato sauce, pasta, vegetables and cheese
- Cover with foil, put in oven and bake for one hour
- Remove foil and return to oven, broiling for 5–10 minutes

Yeast-free Pizza

2 cups	Spelt or rice flour
2/3 cups	Water
¼ cup	Olive oil
1 tsp	Sea salt

Pizza fixings of your choice

- Preheat oven to 400 degrees F
- Blend all ingredients together in a bowl
- Use a rolling pin and shape dough into a circle or rectangle
- Put dough on a baking tray that has been greased with olive oil
- Bake for 10 minutes
- Add tomato sauce or hummus and vegetables and/or pre-cooked meat
- Bake for another 10 minutes

Four Ingredient Mac & Cheese

1 bag/12 oz	Spelt/kamut/rice pasta
5 oz	Goat's cheese (cheddar/mozzarella)
¾ cup	Water
4½ tsp	Arrowroot flour

- Boil pasta al dente
- Blend the other three ingredients in a blender until smooth
- Pour the mixture into a saucepan and heat over medium heat until it thickens slightly and boils a little
- Pour the sauce over pasta or vegetables

Condiments

Dairy Free Sour Cream

½ cup	Cashews
⅓ cup	Boiling water
2 Tbsp	Lemon juice
1 tsp	Honey
¼ tsp	Tamari sauce

- Place nuts in a blender and grind to a fine powder
- Add the water and blend on high for 2 minutes, stopping once to scrape the bottom and sides of the container
- Add the lemon juice, honey, and tamari and blend briefly
- Chill before serving

Oh-So-Sweet Potato Hummus

1 cup	Chickpeas, cooked and drained
½ cup	Water
½ cup	Cooked sweet potato
2 Tbsp	Tahini
2 Tbsp	Olive oil
1 Tbsp	Lemon juice
1 tsp	Garlic, minced
1 tsp	Cumin
¾ tsp	Sea salt

- Blend all ingredients except for the sweet potato
- Add the sweet potato and blend until smooth
- Serve on crackers, bread or with vegetables

Infant Formulas
Coping with Food Intolerances

Goat's Milk Formula

1 quart	Goat's milk
1–2 mg	B complex (dissolve 50 mg tablet in 1 oz. Dropper bottle and use 1 dropper each day)
200 micro grams	Folic acid
1/4 tsp	Flax seed oil
1 drop	Beta carotene (5000 iu)
1 drop	Vitamin E (25 iu)

Dry Mix for Rice Formula

1 jar	ProRice or Medipro
45 caps	Calcium (aspartic acid chelate) or citramate 9 L–carnitine caps
(150 mg/cap)	(330 mg/ cap)
1 tsp	Salt (sodium/potassium chloride)

References

Chapter #1
From Reaction to Pro-Action: Recognizing and Making Sense of Common Food Reactions

1. Bateson-Koch DC ND, Carolee. *Allergies, Disease in Disguise*. Alive Books. 2002: page 30

2. Brostoff MD, Jonathon and Gamlin, Linda. *Food Allergies and Food Intolerance – The Complete Guide to their Identification and Treatment*. Crown Publishers, Inc. 2000: page 6

3. Bateson-Koch DC ND, Carolee. *Allergies, Disease in Disguise*. Alive Books. 2002: page 22

4. Randolph MD, Theron and Moss MD, Ralph. *An Alternative Approach to Allergies – The New Field of Clinical Ecology Unravels the Environmental Causes of Mental and Physical Ills*. Harper & Row Publishers. 1989: page 272

5. Randolph MD, Theron and Moss MD, Ralph. *An Alternative Approach to Allergies – The New Field of Clinical Ecology Unravels the Environmental Causes of Mental and Physical Ills*. Harper & Row Publishers. 1989: pages 26 and 27

6. Rivera MD, Rudy and Deutsch, Roger Davis. *Your Hidden Food Allergies are Making You Fat*. Prima Publishing. 2002: page xxv

7. Rivera MD, Rudy and Deutsch, Roger Davis. *Your Hidden Food Allergies are Making You Fat*. Prima Publishing. 2002: page 103

8. Rona MD, Zoltan. *Childhood Illness and The Allergy Connection*. Prima Publishing. 1996: page 18

9. Lyon MD, Michael. *Is Your Child's Brain Starving?* Mind Publishing Inc. 2002: page 61

10. Lyon MD, Michael. *Is Your Child's Brain Starving?* Mind Publishing Inc. 2002: page 153

11. Thom ND, Dick. *Coping with Food Intolerances*, Fourth Edition. Sterling Publishing Company Inc. 2002: page 17

12. Weintraub ND, Skye. *Allergies and Holistic Healing. A Comprehensive Reference for Everything on Allergies—from Nutritional Causes to Natural Treatments*. Wooland Publishing. 1997: page 57

Chapter #2
Getting to Know All About You: Understanding the Culprits in Foods and Other Substances

1. Colbin, Annemarie. *Food and Healing*. Ballantine Books, a division of Random House, Inc. and simultaneously Random House of Canada Limited. 1986: page 213

2. Reid, Daniel. *The Tao of Detox*. Simon & Schuster UK Ltd. 2006: page 251

3. Reid, Daniel. *The Tao of Detox*. Simon & Schuster UK Ltd. 2006: page 251– 252

4. Rona MD, Zoltan. *Childhood Illness and The Allergy Connection*. Prima Publishing. 1996: page 78

5. Weintraub ND, Skye *Allergies and Holistic Healing. A Comprehensive Reference for Everything on Allergies—from Nutritional Causes to Natural Treatments*. Wooland Publishing. 1997: page 165

6. Rona MD, Zoltan. *Childhood Illness and The Allergy Connection*. Prima Publishing. 1996: page 38

7. Pescatore MD, MPH, Fred. *The Allergy and Asthma Cure. A Complete 8-Step Nutritional Program* John Wiley and Sons, Inc. 2003: page 85

8. Weintraub ND, Skye. *Allergies and Holistic Healing. A Comprehensive Reference for Everything on Allergies—from Nutritional Causes to Natural Treatments*. Wooland Publishing. 1997: page 209

9. Weintraub ND, Skye *Allergies and Holistic Healing. A Comprehensive Reference for Everything on Allergies—from Nutritional Causes to Natural Treatments*. Wooland Publishing. 1997: page 181

10. Walsh MD FACA, William. *The Food Allergy Book. The Foods that Cause You Pain and Discomfort and How to Take Them Out of Your Diet*. William E. Walsh ACA Publications, Inc. 1995: page 77

11. Savill, Antoinette and Sullivan, Karen. *Allergy-free Cooking for Kids – A Guide to Childhood Food Intolerance with 80 Recipes*. Thorsons. 2003: page 8

12. Rona MD, Zoltan. *Childhood Illness and The Allergy Connection*. Prima Publishing. 1996: page 99

13. Rona MD, Zoltan. *Childhood Illness and The Allergy Connection*. Prima Publishing. 1996: page 31

14. Rona MD, Zoltan. *Childhood Illness and The Allergy Connection*. Prima Publishing. 1996: page 32

15. Savill, Antoinette and Sullivan, Karen. *Allergy-free Cooking for Kids – A Guide to Childhood Food Intolerance with 80 Recipes*. Thorsons. 2003: page 10

16. Jensen MD, Bernard. *Dr. Jensen's Guide to Better Bowel Care*. Penguin Putnam Inc. 1999: page 29

17. Fisher, Barbara Loe. *Defending Informed Consent to Vaccination in America*. Pathways to family wellness magazine. Issue 17, March 2008: page 45

18. Rona MD, Zoltan. *Childhood Illness and The Allergy Connection*. Prima Publishing. 1996: page 107

19. Fisher, Barbara Loe. *In the Wake of Vaccines*. Mothering Magazine. Issue 126, Sept–Oct 2004: page 4

Chapter #3
The Dirty Laundry List: Symptoms, Conditions and Disease Caused by Reactions to Food

1. Balch, Phyllis A. *Prescription for Dietary Wellness*. Penguin Group Inc. 2003: page xi

2. Rona MD, Zoltan. *Childhood Illness and The Allergy Connection*. Prima Publishing. 1996: page 1

3. Rona MD, Zoltan. *Childhood Illness and The Allergy Connection*. Prima Publishing. 1996: page 96

4. Rona MD, Zoltan. *Childhood Illness and The Allergy Connection*. Prima Publishing. 1996: page 112

5. Bateson-Koch DC ND, Carolee. *Allergies, Disease in Disguise*. Alive Books. 2002: page 192

6. Bateson-Koch DC ND, Carolee. *Allergies, Disease in Disguise*. Alive Books. 2002: page 193

7. Rona MD, Zoltan. *Childhood Illness and The Allergy Connection*. Prima Publishing. 1996: page 91

8. Pescatore MD MPH, Fred. *The Allergy and Asthma Cure. A Complete 8-Step Nutritional Program*. John Wiley and Sons, Inc. 2003: page 3

9. King MS MFS, Brad J. *Childhood Obesity*. Alive Magazine. September 2007: page 36

10. Shulman DC RHN, Joey. *Winning the Food Fight* John Wiley & Sons Canada Ltd. 2003: page 188

11. Walsh MD, Dr. William. *The Food Allergy Book. The Foods that Cause You Pain and Discomfort and How to Take Them Out of Your Diet*. William E. Walsh ACA Publications, Inc. 1995: page 99

12. Weintraub ND, Skye. *Allergies and Holistic Healing. A Comprehensive Reference for Everything on Allergies—from Nutritional Causes to Natural Treatments*. Wooland Publishing. 1997: page 40

13. Crook MD, William G. *Can Your Child Read…Is He Hyperactive?* Professional Books. 1975: page 44

14. Karatzas ND, Irene. *Autism*. Alive Magazine. September 2007: pages 84–85

15. Mehl-Madrona, MD PhD, Lewis. *Successful Treatments for Autism*. Mothering Magazine. January–February 2006: page 43

16. Rona MD, Zoltan. *Childhood Illness and The Allergy Connection*. Prima Publishing. 1996: page 109

17. Block DO PA, Mary Ann. *No More Ritalin*. Dr. Mary Ann Block. 1997:page 73

18. Block DO PA, Mary Ann. *No More Ritalin*. Dr. Mary Ann Block. 1997:page 74

19. Mitrea MD (Eur) ND, Lilieana Stadler. *Pathology and Nutrition*. Dr. Lileana Stadler Mitrea. 2005: page 71

20. Bateson-Koch DC ND, Carolee. *Allergies, Disease in Disguise*. Alive Books. 1994: page 63

21. Rona MD, Zoltan. *Childhood Illness and The Allergy Connection*. Prima Publishing. 1996: page 27

22. Bateson-Koch DC ND, Carolee. *Allergies, Disease in Disguise*. Alive Books. 2002: page 242

23. Georgiou CNP, Lora. *Raising Healthy Children*. Human Spirit Magazine. May/June 2004: page 18

24. Jantz PhD, Gregory L., and McMurray, Ann. *Healthy Habits. A Practical Plan to Help Your Family*. Fleming H. Revell a division of Baker Publishing Group. 2005: page 14

Chapter #4
Good Riddance: The Importance of the Elimination of Toxins

1. Jensen MD, Bernard. *Dr. Jensen's Guide to Better Bowel Care.* Penguin Putnam Inc. 1999: page 10
2. Renew Life Canada Inc. company brochure
3. Jensen MD, Bernard. *Dr. Jensen's Guide to Better Bowel Care.* Penguin Putnam Inc. 1999: page 47
4. Jensen MD, Bernard. *Dr. Jensen's Guide to Better Bowel Care.* Penguin Putnam Inc. 1999: page 46
5. Gorfinkle MD, Kenneth. *Soothing Your Child's Pain.* Contemporary Books. 1998: page 168
6. Gorfinkle MD, Kenneth. *Soothing Your Child's Pain.* Contemporary Books. 1998: page 155
7. Cain, Nancy. *Healing the Child. A Mother's Story.* Rawson Associates. 1996: page 101
8. Cain, Nancy. *Healing the Child. A Mother's Story.* Rawson Associates. 1996: page 104
9. Cain, Nancy. *Healing the Child. A Mother's Story.* Rawson Associates. 1996: page 49

Chapter #5
The Secret's Out: How to Prevent, Detect, Minimize and Eliminate Reactions to Food

1. Savill, Antoinette and Sullivan, Karen. *Allergy-free Cooking for Kids – A Guide to Childhood Food Intolerance with 80 Recipes.* Thorsons. 2003: page 10
2. Thom ND, Dick. *Coping with Food Intolerances.* Sterling Publishing Company Inc. 2002: page 16
3. Smith MD, Lendon *How to Raise a Healthy Child.* M. Evans and Company, Inc. 1996: page 66
4. Thom ND, Dick. *Coping with Food Intolerances.* Sterling Publishing Company Inc. 2002: page 17
5. Matsen ND, John. *Eating Alive. Prevention Thru Good Digestion.* Crompton Books, Ltd. 1987: page 69
6. Balch, Phyllis A. *Prescription for Dietary Wellness.* Penguin Group Inc. 2003: page 250
7. Savill, Antoinette and Sullivan, Karen. *Allergy-free Cooking for Kids – A guide to Childhood Food Intolerance with 80 Recipes.* Thorsons. 2003: page 19
8. Weintraub ND, Skye. *Allergies and Holistic Healing. A Comprehensive Reference for Everything on Allergies—from Nutritional Causes to Natural Treatments.* Wooland Publishing. 1997: page 21
9. Bateson-Koch DC ND, Carolee. *Allergies, Disease in Disguise.* Alive Books. 2002: page 60
10. Savill, Antoinette and Sullivan, Karen. *Allergy-free Cooking for Kids – A Guide to Childhood Food Intolerance with 80 Recipes.* Thorsons. 2003: page 36
11. Savill, Antoinette and Sullivan, Karen. *Allergy-free Cooking for Kids – A guide to childhood food intolerance with 80 Recipes.* Thorsons. 2003: page 36
12. Reid, Daniel. *The Tao of Detox.* Simon & Schuster UK Ltd. 2003, 2006: page 31
13. Reid, Daniel. *The Tao of Detox.* Simon & Schuster UK Ltd. 2003, 2006: page 33
14. Reid, Daniel. *The Tao of Detox.* Simon & Schuster UK Ltd. 2003, 2006: page 32
15. Reid, Daniel. *The Tao of Detox.* Simon & Schuster UK Ltd. 2003, 2006: page 32
16. Reid, Daniel. *The Tao of Detox.* Simon & Schuster UK Ltd. 2003, 2006: page 5
17. Weintraub ND, Skye. *Allergies and Holistic Healing. A Comprehensive Reference for Everything on Allergies—from Nutritional Causes to Natural Treatments.* Wooland Publishing. 1997: page 151
18. Weintraub ND, Skye. *Allergies and Holistic Healing. A Comprehensive Reference for Everything on Allergies—from Nutritional Causes to Natural Treatments.* Wooland Publishing. 1997: page 153
19. McGraw, Phil. *Family First.* Free Press A division of Simon & Schuster, Inc. 2004: page 126
20. Hewlett, Jill www.brainworksglobal.com

Chapter #6
Eat This! How to Feed Your Child

1. Bateson-Koch DC ND, Carolee. *Allergies, Disease in Disguise.* Alive Books. 1994: page 82
2. Roberts PhD, Susan, Melvin MD, Heyman, Tracy, Lisa. *Feeding Your Child for Lifelong Health.* Bantam Books. 1999: pages 8 –11
3. Lyon MD, Dr. Michael. *Is Your Child's Brain Starving?* Mind Publishing Inc. 2002: page 41

4. Olivier, Suzannah. *Healthy Foods for Happy Kids.* Simon & Schuster UK Ltd, 2004: page 28

5. McGraw, Dr. Phil. *Family First.* Free Press A division of Simon & Schuster, Inc. 2004: page 125

6. Bernard MD, Jenson and Anderson, Mark. *Empty Harvest. Understanding the Link Between our Food, our Immunity and our Planet.* Avery, a member of Penguin Putnam Inc. 1990: page 69

7. Roberts PhD, Susan, Melvin MD, Heyman, Tracy, Lisa. *Feeding Your Child for Lifelong Health.* Bantam Books. 1999: page 6

8. Twyman, James F. *Raising Psychic Children.* James F. Twyman, 2003: page 79

9. Thom ND, Dick. *Coping with Food Intolerances.* Sterling Publishing Company Inc. 2002: page 81

10. Galland MD, Leo and Buchman PhD, Dian Dincin. *SuperImmunity for Kids.* Copestone Press Inc. 1988: page 15

11. Savill, Antoinette and Sullivan, Karen. *Allergy-free Cooking for Kids – A Guide to Childhood Food Intolerance with 80 Recipes.* Thorsons. 2003: page 34

12. Liberman PhD, Shari, Xenakis MD, Alan. *Mineral Miracle. Stopping Cartilage Loss and Inflammation Naturally.* Square One Publishers. 2006: page 13

13. Weintraub ND, Skye. *Allergies and Holistic Healing. A Comprehensive Reference for Everything on Allergies–from Nutritional Causes to Natural Treatments.* Wooland Publishing. 1997: page 193

14. Haas MD, Elson. *Staying Healthy with Nutrition.* Elson M. Haas. 1992: page 257

15. Rona MD, Zoltan. *Childhood Illness and The Allergy Connection.* Prima Publishing. 1996: page 72

16. Thom ND, Dick. *Coping with Food Intolerances.* Sterling Publishing Company Inc. 2002: page 74

Chapter 7
Let's Talk About It! Recommendations for Effectively Communicating About Feeding Your Child Differently

1. McConville, Brigid and Sharma MD, Rajendra. *Your Child: Allergies.* Element Books Limited. 1999: page 29

2. McConville, Brigid and Sharma MD, Rajendra. *Your Child: Allergies.* Element Books Limited. 1999: page 26

3. Briggs, Dorothy Corkille. *Your Child's Self-Esteem.* Doubleday Inc. 1970: page 3

4. Jantz PhD, Gregory L., and McMurray, Ann. *Healthy Habits. A Practical Plan to Help Your Family.* Fleming H. Revell a division of Baker Publishing Group. 2005: page 12

5. Eldridge John and Stasi. *Captivating.* Thomas Nelson. 2005: page 207

6. Eldridge John and Stasi. *Captivating.* Thomas Nelson. 2005: page 207

7. Vesanto MS RD, Melina, Stepaniak MSEd, Jo and Aronson MS RD, Dina. *Food Allergy Survival Guide – Surviving and Thriving with Food Allergies and Sensitivities.* Healthy Living Publications. 2004: page 122

8. Thomas, Angela. *Tender Mercy for A Mother's Soul.* Tyndale House Publishers, Inc. 2001: page 105

9. Martin, Lisa. *Briefcase Moms.* Cornerview Press. 2005: page 40

10. Thomas, Angela. *Tender Mercy for A Mother's Soul.* Tyndale House Publishers, Inc. 2001: page 180

11. Martin, Lisa. *Briefcase Moms.* Cornerview Press. 2005: page 116

Chapter 8
Outside the Safety Zone: How to Feed Your Child in the Big Wide World
Not applicable

Chapter 9
Help is Out There! How Alternative Therapies Can Improve Your Child's Health

1. Brostoff MD, Jonathon and Gamlin, Linda. *Food Allergies and Food Intolerance – The Complete Guide to their Identification and Treatment*. Crown Publishers, Inc. 2000: page 138

2. Rona MD, Zoltan. *Childhood Illness and The Allergy Connection*. Prima Publishing. 1996: page xvi

3. Rona MD, Zoltan. *Childhood Illness and The Allergy Connection*. Prima Publishing. 1996: page xii

4. Newman BSCH, DC, CACCP, Kristine. *Research…Kids & Chiropractic, Naturally!!* Park Avenue Chiropractic Path to Wellness Newsletter. Last quarter 2008: page 5

5. Lansky, Ann. *To Your Health*. Mothering Magazine. January–February 2006: page 52

6. The Burton Goldberg Group. *Alternative Medicine. The Definitive Guide*. Future Medicine Publishing, Inc. 1995: page 232

7. Krop MD FAAEM, Jozef J. *Healing The Planet. One Patient at a Time*. KOS Publishing Inc. 2002: page xvi

Chapter 10
The Food–Love Connection–When Food is a Form of Nurturing

1. Schatz, Hale Sofia. *If the Buddha Came to Dinner - How to Nourish Your Body to Awaken Your Spirit*. Hyperion. 2004: page 20

2. Schatz, Hale Sofia. *If the Buddha Came to Dinner - How to Nourish Your Body to Awaken Your Spirit*. Hyperion. 2004: page 65

3. Gawain, Shakti. *Creative Visualization*. Bantam Books, Inc. 1978: page 111

4. Schatz, Hale Sofia. *If the Buddha Came to Dinner - How to Nourish Your Body to Awaken Your Spirit*. Hyperion. 2004: page 87

5. Lyon MD, Dr. Michael and Laurell PhD, Dr. Christine. *Is Your Child's Brain Starving?* Mind Publishing Inc. 2002: page 62

6. Schatz, Hale Sofia. *If the Buddha Came to Dinner - How to Nourish Your Body to Awaken Your Spirit*. Hyperion. 2004: page 172

Bibliography

Ansorge, Rick, Metcalf, Eric. *Allergy Free Naturally. 1,000 Nondrug Solutions for More Than 50 Allergy-Related Problems.* New York. Grand Central Publishing, 2001.

Balch CNC, Phyllis. *Prescription for Nutritional Healing Third Edition.* New York. Avery, 2000.

Balch CNC, Phyllis. *Prescription for Dietary Wellness Second Edition.* New York. Avery, 2003.

Bachman MD, Judy. *Keys to Dealing with Childhood Allergies.* New York. Barron's Educational Series, Inc, 1992.

Barber, Marianne. *The Parent's Guide to Food Allergies.* Canada. Fitzhenry and Whiteside Ltd, 2001.

Bateson-Koch DC ND, Carolee. *Allergies, Disease in Disguise.* British Columbia. Alive Books, 1994.

Bateson-Koch DC ND, Carolee. *Allergies, Disease in Disguise.* British Columbia. Alive Books, 2002.

Benson MD, Herbert, Stark, Marg. *Timeless Healing. The Power and Biology of Belief.* New York. Fireside, 1996.

Block DO PA, Mary Ann. *No More Ritalin.* New York. Kensington Publishing Corp, 1997.

Briggs, Dorothy Corkille. *Your Child's Self-Esteem.* New York. Doubleday: A division of Bantam Doubleday Dell Publishing Group, Inc, 1970.

Brostoff MD, Jonathon, Gamlin, Linda. *Food Allergies and Food Intolerance – The Complete Guide to Their Identification and Treatment.* New York. Crown Publishers, Inc, 2000.

Cain, Nancy. *Healing the Child. A Mother's Story.* New York. Rawson Associates, 1996.

Colbin, Annemarie. *Food and Healing.* New York. Ballantine Books: a division of Random House, Inc. / Random House of Canada (Toronto) Limited, 1986.

Crook MD, William. *Can Your Child Read? Is He Hyperactive?* Tennessee. Professional Books, 1975.

Crook MD, William. *The Yeast Connection.* New York. Random House Inc / Random House of Canada (Toronto) Limited, 1986.

Eldridge John and Staci. *Captivating.* Nashville. Thomas Nelson, 2005.

Galland MD, Leo, Buchman PhD, Dian Dincin. *Superimmunity for Kids.* New York. Copestone Press Inc, 1988.

Gawain, Shakti. *Creative Visualization.* New York. Bantam Books, Inc, 1978.

Gorfinkle MD, Kenneth. *Soothing Your Child's Pain.* Chicago. Contemporary Books, 1998.

Haas MD, Elson. *Staying Healthy With Nutrition.* California. Elson M. Haas, 1992.

Haynes, Antony, Savill, Antoinette. *The Food Intolerance Bible.* London. HarperThorsons, 2005.

Jantz PhD, Gregory L., McMurray, Ann. *Healthy Habits. A Practical Plan to Help Your Family.* Michigan. Fleming H. Revell a division of Baker Publishing Group, 2005.

Jensen MD, Bernard. *Dr. Jensen's Guide to Better Bowel Care.* New York. Penguin Putnam Inc, 1999.

Jenson, Bernard, Anderson, Mark. *Empty Harvest. Understanding the Link Between our Food, our Immunity and our Planet.* New York. Avery: a member of Penguin Putnam Inc, 1990.

Krop MD FAAEM, Jozef J. *Healing The Planet. One Patient at a Time.* Alton, Ontario. KOS Publishing Inc, 2002.

Liberman PhD, Shari, Xenakis MD ScD, Alan. *Mineral Miracle. Stopping Cartilage Loss and Inflammation Naturally.* New York. Square One Publishers, 2006.

Lyon MD, Michael, Laurell PhD, Christine. *Is Your Child's Brain Starving?* Canada. Mind Publishing Inc, 2002.

Martin, Lisa. *Briefcase Moms.* Vancouver. Cornerview Press, 2005.

Matsen ND, John. *Eating Alive. Prevention Thru Good Digestion.* Vancouver. Crompton Books, Ltd, 1987.

McConville, Brigid, Sharma MD, Rajendra. *Your Child: Allergies.* Dorset. Element Books Limited, 1999.

McGraw, Phil. *Family First.* New York. Free Press A division of Simon & Schuster, Inc, 2004.

McNichol, Jane. *The Great Big Food Experiment.* Toronto. Stoddart Publishing Co. Limited, 1990.

Mendelsohn MD, Robert. *How to Raise a Healthy Child... in Spite of Your Doctor.* New York. The Ballantine Publishing Group, 1984.

Mitrea MD (Eur) ND DNM, Lilieana Stadler. *Pathology and Nutrition First Edition Revised.* Canada. Lilieana Stadler Mitrea, 2005.

Nault, Kelly. *When You're About to Go Off the Deep End, Don't Take Your Kids with You.* West Vancouver. Stepping Stones for Life Ltd, 2004.

Null, Gary, Feldman MD, Martin. *Good Food, Good Mood – A Nutritional Guide to an Allergy-Free Happier, Healthier Life.* New York. St. Martin's Press, 1988.

Olivier, Suzannah. *Healthy Foods for Happy Kids.* England. Simon & Schuster UK Ltd, 2004.

Pescatore MD MPH, Fred. *The Allergy and Asthma Cure. A Complete 8-Step Nutritional Program.* New Jersey. John Wiley and Sons, Inc, 2003.

Petty RHN, Lisa. *Living Beauty.* Ontario. Fitzhenry and Whiteside Limited, 2006.

Rapp MD, Doris, *Is This Your Child?* New York. William Morrow and Company, Inc, 1991.

Reid, Daniel. *The Tao of Detox.* England. Simon & Schuster UK Ltd, 2006.

Rivera MD, Rudy, Deutch, Roger. *Your Hidden Food Allergies Are Making You Fat – How to Lose Weight and Gain Years of Vitality.* Roseville, California. Prima Publishing, 2002.

Roberts PhD, Susan, Heyman MD, Melvin B. Tracy, Lisa. *Feeding Your Child for Lifelong Health.* New York. Bantam Books, 1999.

Rona MD, Zoltan. *Childhood Illness and the Allergy Connection. A Nutritional Approach to Overcoming and Preventing Childhood Illness.* California. Prima Publishing, 1996.

Savill, Antoinette and Sullivan, Karen. *Allergy-free Cooking For Kids. A Guide to Childhood Food Intolerance with 80 Recipes.* Great Britain. Thorsons, 2003.

Schatz, Hale Sofia. *If the Buddha Came to Dinner - How to Nourish Your Body to Awaken Your Spirit.* New York. Hyperion, 2004.

Scott–Moncrieff MB ChB MFHom, Christina. *Overcoming Allergies.* London, England. Collins and Brown Limited, 2002.

Shulman DC RHN, Joey. *Winning the Food Fight.* Etobicoke. John Wiley & Sons Canada Ltd, 2003.

Smith MD, Lendon. *How to Raise a Healthy Child.* New York. M. Evans and Company, Inc, 1996.

The Burton Goldberg Group. Comp. *Alternative Medicine. The Definitive Guide.* Washington, Future Medicine Publishing, Inc, 1995.

Theron MD, Randolph, Moss MD, Ralph. *An Alternative Approach to Allergies – The New Field of Clinical Ecology Unravels the Environmental Causes of Mental and Physical Ills.* New York. Harper & Row Publishers, 1989.

Thom ND, Dick. *Coping with Food Intolerances Fourth Edition.* New York. Sterling Publishing Company Inc, 2002.

Thomas, Angela. *Tender Mercy for A Mother's Soul.* Illinois. Tyndale House Publishers, Inc, 2001.

Twyman, James F. *Raising Psychic Children*. Scotland. James F. Twyman, 2003.

Vesanto MS RD, Melina, Stepaniak MSEd, Jo, Aronson MS RD, Dina. *Food Allergy Survival Guide – Surviving and Thriving with Food Allergies and Sensitivities*. Summertown, Tennessee. Healthy Living Publications, 2004.

Walsh MD FACA, William. *The Food Allergy Book. The Foods that Cause You Pain and Discomfort and How to Take Them Out of Your Diet*. St. Paul, Minnesota. William E. Walsh ACA Publications, Inc, 1995.

Weintraub ND, Skye. *Allergies and Holistic Healing. A Comprehensive Reference for Everything on Allergies— from Nutritional Causes to Natural Treatments*. Utah. Wooland Publishing, 1997.

Magazines and Newsletters

Mothering Magazine, no. 126, Sept/Oct 2004.

Mothering Magazine, Special Autism Edition, Jan/Feb 2006.

Pathways to Family Wellness, Issue 17, March 2008.

Human Spirit Magazine, May/June 2004.

Newman BSCH, DC, CACCP, Kristine. *Park Avenue Chiropractic Path to Wellness Newsletter*, last quarter of 2008.

Alive Magazine, Sept 2007.

Kamp, Jurriaan. "Feed Your Brain." *Ode Magazine*, Sept 2007.

Index

This index states the *main* page numbers in which each term is discussed in the book. You will find that some of the terms are discussed *throughout* the book.

About the Author

Meredith Deasley is passionate about making a difference in the lives of children and their parents. She recognizes that the general state of our children's health is the worst it has ever been. Meredith strongly believes that the North American diet is the single most contributing factor to the pervasive poor health we are experiencing today.

After obtaining a bachelor's degree in Sociology from the University of Western Ontario and working in the corporate world for ten years, Meredith began raising two daughters with extreme food sensitivities. Her journey led her to become who she is today – *The Resourceful Mother*. Meredith is a Registered Holistic Nutritionist and Nutritional Consulting Practitioner (R.N.C.P.), specializing in pediatric nutrition since 1999. She teaches pediatric nutrition at the Canadian School of Natural Nutrition. She also conducts numerous seminars for parents and counsels them on an individual basis, teaching them how to nourish the bodies and souls of their children.

Meredith lives in Aurora with her husband, Craig and their two children, Taylor and Paige. Meredith would love to receive your feedback and/or assist you with your parenting journey. You can reach her at *www.theresourcefulmother.com*.